Essentials of Nursing Leadership & Management

SECOND EDITION

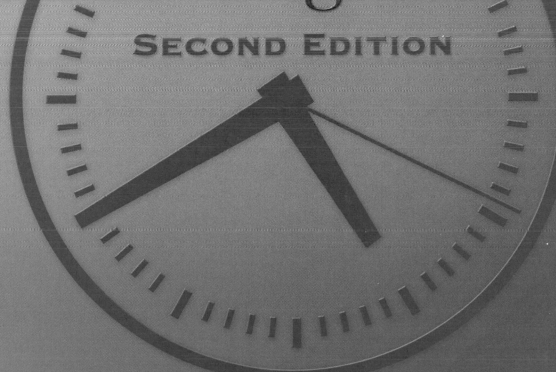

Essentials of Nursing Leadership & Management

SECOND EDITION

Patricia Kelly

Professor Emeritus
Purdue University Calumet
Hammond, Indiana

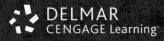

DELMAR
CENGAGE Learning

Australia • Brazil • Japan • Korea • Mexico • Singapore • Spain • United Kingdom • United States

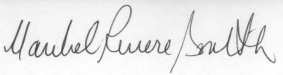

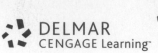

**Essentials of Nursing Leadership &
Management, Second Edition**
Patricia Kelly

Vice President, Career and Professional
Editorial: Dave Garza

Director of Learning Solutions: Matthew
Kane

Executive Editor: Stephen Helba

Managing Editor: Marah Bellegarde

Senior Product Manager: Elisabeth Williams

Editorial Assistant: Samantha Miller

Vice President, Career and Professional
Marketing: Jennifer Ann Baker

Marketing Director: Wendy Mapstone

Senior Marketing Manager: Michele
McTighe

Marketing Coordinator: Scott Chrysler

Production Director: Carolyn Miller

Production Manager: Andrew Crouth

Content Project Manager: Andrea Majot

Senior Art Director: Jack Pendleton

Library of Congress Control Number: 2008943298

ISBN-13: 978-14354-53562

ISBN-10: 14354-53565

Delmar
5 Maxwell Drive
Clifton Park, NY 12065-2919
USA

Cengage Learning products are represented in Canada by
Nelson Education, Ltd.

For your lifelong learning solutions, visit **delmar.cengage.com**

Visit our corporate website at **cengage.com**

Notice to the Reader
Publisher does not warrant or guarantee any of the products described herein or perform any independent analysis in connection with any of the product information contained herein. Publisher does not assume, and expressly disclaims, any obligation to obtain and include information other than that provided to it by the
manufacturer. The reader is expressly warned to consider and adopt all safety precautions that might be indicated by the activities described herein and to avoid
all potential hazards. By following the instructions contained herein, the reader willingly assumes all risks in connection with such instructions. The publisher
makes no representations or warranties of any kind, including but not limited to, the warranties of fitness for particular purpose or merchantability, nor are any
such representations implied with respect to the material set forth herein, and the publisher takes no responsibility with respect to such material. The publisher
shall not be liable for any special, consequential, or exemplary damages resulting, in whole or part, from the readers' use of, or reliance upon, this material.

Printed in Canada
1 2 3 4 5 XX 11 10 09

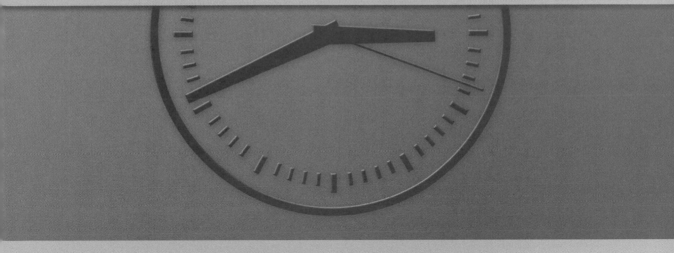

CONTENTS

CONTRIBUTORS

Rinda Alexander, PhD, RN, CS
Professor Emeritus, Nursing
Purdue University Calumet
Hammond, Indiana
and
Professor of Nursing
University of Florida
College of Nursing
Gainesville, Florida
and
Nursing Consultant
Health Care and Administration
Schererville, Indiana

Margaret M. Anderson, EdD, RN, CNAA
Professor of Nursing and Chair
Department of Nursing and Health Professions
Northern Kentucky University
Highland Heights, Kentucky

Ida M. Androwich, PhD, RN, BC, FAAN
Professor and Director, Health Systems Management
Niehoff School of Nursing
Loyola University Chicago
Maywood, Illinois

Crisamar Javellana-Anunciado, MSN, APRN, BC
Inpatient Diabetes Nurse Practitioner
Sharp Chula Vista Medical Center
Chula Vista, California

Anne Bernat, RN, MSN, CNAA
Vice President of Patient Care Services (Retired)
Arlington, Virginia

Nancy Braaten, RN, MS
Adult Health Clinical Nurse Specialist
Clinical Analyst, Nursing Information Systems
Northeast Health Acute Care Division
Troy, New York

Sister Kathleen Cain, OSF, JD
Attorney
Franciscan Legal Services
Baton Rouge, Louisiana

Martha Desmond, RN, MS, Post Masters Certificate in Nursing Education
Clinical Nurse Specialist in Critical Care
Northeast Health Acute Care Division
Troy, New York
and
Adjunct Faculty
Excelsior College
Albany, New York

Joan Dorman, RN, MS, CEN
Clinical Assistant Professor
Purdue University Calumet
Hammond, Indiana

Mary L. Fisher, PhD, RN, CNAA, BC
Professor and Department Chair
Environments for Health
Indiana University School of Nursing
Indianapolis, Indiana

Corinne Haviley, RN, MS
Director of Medicine Nursing
Northwestern Memorial Hospital
Chicago, Illinois

Paul Heidenthal, MS
Consultant
Austin, Texas

Karen Houston, RN, MS
Director of Quality and Continuum of Care
Albany Medical Center
Albany, New York

Ronda G. Hughes, PhD, MHS, RN
Senior Health Scientist Administrator
Senior Advisor on End-of-Life Care
Center for Primary Care, Prevention, and Clinical
Partnerships
Agency for Healthcare Research and Quality
Rockville, Maryland

Mary Anne Jadlos, MS, APRN, BC, CWOCN
Coordinator, Wound, Skin and Ostomy Nursing
Service
Northeast Health Acute Care Division
Samaritan Hospital
Troy, New York
and
Albany Memorial Hospital
Albany, New York

Josette Jones, RN, PhD, BC
Assistant Professor
School of Nursing
School of Informatics
Indianapolis, Indiana

Stephen Jones, MS, RN-C, PNP, ET
Pediatric Clinical Nurse Specialist/Nurse Practitioner
The Children's Hospital at Albany Medical Center
Albany, New York
and
Founder and Principal
Pediatric Concepts
Averill Park, New York

Patricia Kelly, RN, MSN
Professor Emeritus
Purdue University Calumet
Hammond, Indiana
and
Faculty
Review Courses
Houston, Texas

Glenda B. Kelman, PhD, APRN, BC
Associate Professor and Chair
Nursing Department
The Sage Colleges
Troy, New York
and
Acute Care Nurse Practitioner
Wound, Skin, and Ostomy Nursing Service
Northeast Health Acute Care Division
Samaritan Hospital
Troy, New York
and
Albany Memorial Hospital
Albany, New York

Mary Elaine Koren, RN, DNSc
Assistant Professor
School of Nursing
Northern Illinois University
DeKalb, Illinois

Lyn LaBarre, MS, RN
Patient Care Service Director
Critical Care, Specialty and Emergency Services
Albany Medical Center
Albany, New York

Linda Searle Leach, PhD, RN, CNAA
Assistant Professor
UCLA School of Nursing
Los Angeles, California
Nurse Scientist
Kaiser Permanente
Southern California Nursing Research Program
Pasadena, California

Camille B. Little, RN, MS
Instructional Assistant Professor (Retired)
Mennonite College of Nursing
Illinois State University
Normal, Illinois

Sharon Little-Stoetzel, RN, MS
Associate Professor of Nursing
Graceland University
Independence, Missouri

Dr. Miki Magnino-Rabig, PhD, RN
Assistant Professor
University of St. Francis
Joliet, Illinois

Patsy Maloney, RN, BC, EdD, MSN, MA, CNAA
Associate Professor/Director, Continuing Nursing
Education
Pacific Lutheran University
Tacoma, Washington

Richard J. Maloney, BS, MA, MAHRM, EdD
Principal
Policy Governance Associates
Tacoma, Washington

Maureen T. Marthaler, RN, MS
Associate Professor
Purdue University Calumet
Hammond, Indiana

Judith W. Martin, RN, JD
Attorney
Franciscan Legal Services
Baton Rouge, Louisiana

**Edna Harder Mattson, RN, BN, BA(CRS), MDE,
CTSN, CAE**
President
Canadian Nursing Tutorial Services
Winnipeg, Manitoba, Canada

Mary McLaughlin, RN, MBA
Assistant Director for Case Management
and Social Work
Albany Medical Center
Albany, New York

Terry W. Miller, PhD, RN
Dean and Professor
School of Nursing
Pacific Lutheran University
Tacoma, Washington
and
Professor Emeritus
San Jose State University
San Jose, California

Leslie H. Nicoll, PhD, MBA, RN, BC, LLC
Principal and Owner, Maine Desk
Portland, Maine

Laura J. Nosek, PhD, RN
Doctor of Nursing Practice Faculty
The Bolton School of Nursing
Case Western Reserve University
Cleveland, Ohio
and
Adjunct Associate Professor of Nursing
Marcella Niehoff School of Nursing
Loyola University Chicago
Chicago, Illinois
and
Course Facilitator
Excelsior College
Albany, New York

Amy Androwich O'Malley, MSN, RN
Education and Program Manager
Medela, Inc.
McHenry, Illinois

Kristine E. Pfendt, RN, MSN
Assistant Professor of Nursing
Northern Kentucky University
Highland Heights, Kentucky

Karin Polifko-Harris, PhD, RN, CNAA
Principal/Owner
KPH Consulting
Naples, Florida

Robyn Pozza-Dollar, JD
Attorney
Cambridge, Massachusetts

Chad S. Priest, RN, BSN, JD
Attorney
Baker and Daniels, LLP
Adjunct Lecturer
Indiana University School of Nursing
Indianapolis, Indiana

Jenny Radsma, RN, PhD
Associate Professor
Division of Nursing
University of Maine at Fort Kent
Fort Kent, Maine

Jacklyn L. Ruthman, PhD, RN
Associate Professor
Bradley University
Peoria, Illinois

Patricia M. Schoon, MPH, RN
Associate Professor
Department of Nursing
Coordinator
Center of Excellence for Women
and Health
College of St. Catherine
St. Paul, Minnesota

Kathleen F. Sellers, PhD, RN
Associate Professor
School of Nursing and Health Systems
SUNY Institute of Technology
Utica, New York

Susan Abaffy Shah, RN, MS, Post Masters Certificate in Nursing Education
Adult Health Clinical Nurse Specialist
Northeast Health Acute Care Division
Albany, New York

Maria R. Shirey, MS, MBA, RN, CNAA, BC, FACHE
Principal
Shirey and Associates
Evansville, Indiana
and
Adjunct Associate Professor
University of Southern Indiana
College of Nursing and Health Professions
Evansville, Indiana

Janice Tazbir, RN, MS, CCRN
Associate Professor of Nursing
Purdue University Calumet
School of Nursing
Hammond, Indiana

Karen Luther Wikoff, RN, PhD
Assistant Professor
California State University, Stanislaus
Turlock, California

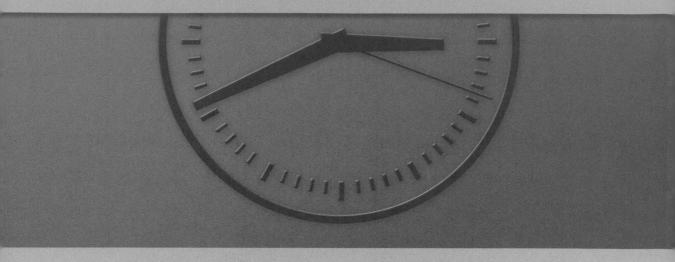

REVIEWERS

Deborah Brabham, BS, MSN
Instructional Program Manager
Florida Community College at Jacksonville
Jacksonville, Florida

Doreen DeAngelis, RN, MS
Instructor of Nursing
The Pennsylvania State University
Penn State Fayette
Uniontown, Pennsylvania

Pam Stockel, RN, MSN, FNP, PhD
Assistant Professor
School of Nursing
University of Northern Colorado
Greeley, Colorado

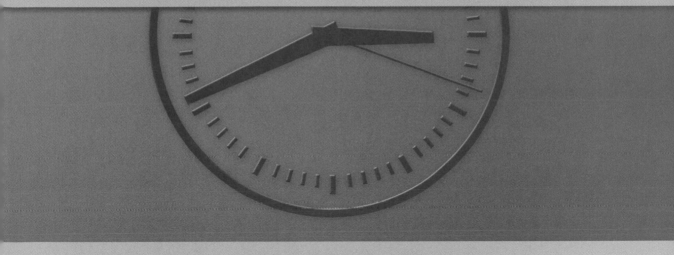

PREFACE

Nurses play a crucial role in protecting patient safety and providing quality health care. A National Academy of Sciences, Institute of Medicine (IOM) report found that "how we are cared for by nurses affects our health, and sometimes can be a matter of life and death . . . nurses are indispensable to our safety" (Institute of Medicine, 2004).

Another IOM report, *Health Professions Education: A Bridge to Quality* (2003), noted that nurses and other health professionals are currently not prepared to provide the highest quality and safest care possible. This IOM report concluded that education for the health professions is in need of a major overhaul and recommended that all programs that educate and train health professionals should adopt five core competencies. These core competencies are the ability to (1) provide patient-centered care, (2) work in interdisciplinary teams, (3) employ evidence-based practice, (4) apply quality improvement, and (5) utilize informatics (IOM, 2003).

The American Association of Critical Care Nurses convened a task force to develop standards for establishing and sustaining health work environments (2001). The Standards are skilled communication, true collaboration, effective decision making, appropriate staffing, meaningful recognition, and authentic leadership. The Standards guide the nursing leader and manager of the future.

Essentials of Nursing Leadership & Management, second edition, is designed to help beginning nurse leaders and managers develop the knowledge and skills to lead and manage nursing care delivery for patients. The text addresses the topics mentioned in the IOM Reports and prepares the beginning nurse leader and manager to move into modern day health care. The contributors to this edition include educators, nursing faculty, nursing educators, nursing consultants, clinical nurse specialists, lawyers, nurse practitioners, wound and ostomy care nurses, and nurse entrepreneurs. These contributors are from various areas of the U.S and Canada, thus allowing them to offer a broad view of nursing leadership and management. Contributors are from California, Florida, Illinois, Indiana, Kentucky, Louisiana, Maine, Maryland, Massachusetts, Minnesota, Missouri, New York, Ohio, Texas, Virginia, Washington, and Manitoba, Canada.

Each chapter of *Essentials of Nursing Leadership & Management,* second edition, discusses the latest theories relevant to its specific topic. Various points of view are presented through case studies and interviews with staff nurses, nurse practitioners, nursing administrators, nursing risk managers, nursing faculty, doctors, and patients.

ORGANIZATION

Essentials of Nursing Leadership & Management, second edition, consists of eighteen chapters arranged in a conceptual framework (see inside cover of book). The conceptual framework provides beginning nurses with an overview of the nurse's leadership and management responsibilities to the patient to the health care team, to the health care organization, and to self. The book consists of five units.

- **Unit I** introduces nursing leadership and management and then discusses the health care environment; nursing today; and decision making, critical thinking, and technology.
- **Unit II** discusses leadership and management of the interdisciplinary team, including health care communication; change, innovation, and conflict management; and power and politics.
- **Unit III** discusses leadership and management of patient-centered care, including delegation of patient care; effective staffing; budgeting for patient care; planning care; and time management and setting patient care priorities.
- **Unit IV** discusses quality improvement of patient outcomes, including quality improvement and evidence-based patient care; legal aspects of health care; ethical aspects of health care; and culture, generational differences, and spirituality.
- **Unit V** discusses leadership and management of self and the future, including NCLEX-RN preparation and your first job; and career planning and achieving balance.

Discussion of timely topics such as nurse-sensitive outcomes, evidence-based practice, the Joint Commission's National Patient Safety goals, information technology, HIPAA, magnet hospitals, interdisciplinary teamwork, quality and performance improvement, and population based care is included throughout the chapters. The real world of nursing is also embraced by presenting a variety of different views.

The second edition of *Essentials of Nursing Leadership & Management* builds on the strengths of the first edition, embraces user feedback, and accounts for the ever-changing health care landscape. Important changes include the following:

- A new conceptual framework encourages reader understanding and development of key concepts of nursing leadership and management.
- An expanded chapter on NCLEX-RN preparation and your first job, includes issues of professionalism and career planning.
- A new chapter on the health care environment (chapter 2) sets the tone for the text.
- A new section on innovation is included in the chapter on change and conflict management.
- All chapters have been revised and strengthened. Included is new information on evidence-based care, interdisciplinary teamwork, quality improvement, generational differences, balancing personal and professional needs, delegation, ethics, legal aspects, culture and spirituality, decision making, critical thinking, and technology.
- Legal charts on nursing malpractice are included to enhance learning.
- Enhanced content is offered on patient safety, health care communications, power and politics, nursing staffing, budgeting, planning patient care, time management and setting priorities, nurse-sensitive outcomes, and nursing today.
- Stronger exercises, Case Studies, Review Questions, and Activities are included for development of key concepts by the entry-level nurse.

FEATURES

Several standard chapter features are utilized throughout the text, which provide the reader with a consistent format for learning and an assortment of resources for understanding and applying the knowledge presented. Features include the following:

- Health care or nursing quote related to chapter content

- Photo that sets the scene for the chapter
- Objectives that state the chapter's learning goals
- Opening scenario, a mini entry-level nursing case study that relates to the chapter, with two to three critical thinking questions
- Key Concepts, a listing of the primary understandings the reader is to take from the chapter
- Glossary listing of important new terms presented in the chapters
- Review Questions, several NCLEX style questions at the end of chapter content
- Review Activities to apply chapter content to entry-level nursing situations
- Exploring the Web computer activities
- References
- Suggested Readings

Special elements are sprinkled throughout the chapters to enhance learning and encourage critical thinking and application:

- Evidence from the Literature with synopsis of key findings from nursing and health care literature
- Real World Interviews with nursing leaders and managers, including bedside nursing staff, clinicians, administrators, risk managers, faculty, nursing and medical practitioners, patients, nursing assistive personnel (NAP), and lawyers
- Critical Thinking exercises regarding an ethical, legal, cultural, spiritual, delegation, or quality improvement nursing or health care topics
- Case Studies to provide the entry-level nurse with a clinical nursing leadership/management situation calling for critical thinking to solve an open-ended problem
- Exploring the Web exercises, which guide the reader to the Internet and give Internet addresses for the latest information related to the chapter content
- Review activities, which encourage students to think critically about how to apply chapter content to the workplace and other "real world" situations. These activities provide reinforcement of key leadership and management skills. Exercises are numbered in each chapter to facilitate using them as assignments or activities.
- A case study that provides a "real world" illustration of the chapter's topic
- Tables and figures, which appear throughout the text and provide convenient capsules of information for the student's reference

ONLINE COMPANION (OLC)

A new online companion accompanies *Essentials of Nursing Leadership & Management*, second edition. Each chapter includes a discussion of the opening chapter scenario. Suggested responses are also included by chapter to all Case Studies, Review Questions, Critical Thinking exercises, and Review Activities.

The instructor side of the OLC assists faculty in planning and developing their programs and classes for the most efficient use of time and resources. Three components include:

- Lecture slides in PowerPoint® presentations for each chapter to enhance classroom discussions.
- A test bank of several hundred questions, in NCLEX-RN format, with answers, rationales, and cognitive level.
- A transition guide to facilitate switching lecture notes from the first to the second edition of the text.

REFERENCES

American Association of Critical Care Nurses. (AACN). (2001). *Standards for establishing and sustaining healthy work environments.* Available at www.aacn.org/WD/HWE/Docs/ExecSum.pdf.

Institute of Medicine. (IOM). (2003). *Health Professions Education. A Bridge to Quality.* Washington, DC. The National Academies Press.

Institute of Medicine (IOM) Committee on the Work Environment for Nurses and Patient Safety. (2004). *Keeping patients safe; Transforming the work environment of nurses.* Washington, DC: The National Academies Press.

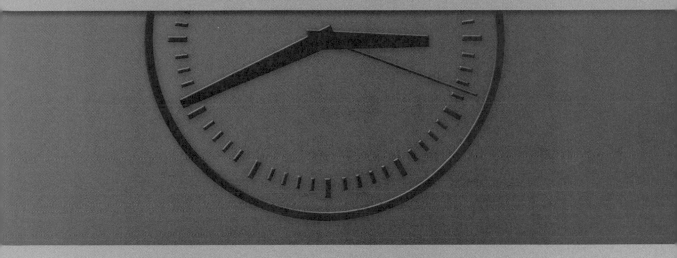

ACKNOWLEDGMENTS

A book such as this requires great effort and the coordination of many people with various areas of expertise. I would like to thank all of the contributors for their time and effort in sharing their knowledge gained through years of experience in both the clinical and academic setting. All of the contributing authors worked within tight time frames to share their expertise. I especially thank Jo Reidy, Mercy Health Care, Chicago, Illinois; Corinne Haviley, Northwestern Hospital, Chicago, Illinois; and Dawn Moeller, Advocate Good Shepherd Health Care, Barrington, Illinois, for their help in arranging some of the photographs for the text. Thanks also to Jane Woodruff for her computer support.

I thank the reviewers for their time spent critically reviewing the manuscript and providing the valuable comments that have enhanced this text. Special thanks go to my Dad and Mom, Ed and Jean Kelly; my sisters, Tessie Dybel and Kathy Milch; my Aunt Pat and Uncle Bill Kelly (who convinced me to start writing); my Aunt Verna and Uncle Archie Payne; my nieces, Natalie Dybel Bevil, Melissa Milch Arredondo, and Stacey Milch; my nephew, John Milch; my grand nephew, Brock Bevil; my grand niece, Reese Bevil; and my dear friends, Patricia Wojcik, Florence Lebryk, Lee McGuan, and Dolores Wynen, who have supported me throughout the writing of this book and much of my life. Special thanks to my wonderful nursing friends, Zenaida Corpuz, Dr. Mary Elaine Koren, Dr. Barbara Mudloff, Dr. Patricia Padjen, Jane McKeon, Kerrie Ellingsen, and especially to Gerri Kane, Janice Klepitch, Sylvia Komyatte, and Julie Martini, as well as Anna Fizer, Judy Ilijanich, Trudy Keilman, Judy Rau, Lillian Rau, and Mary Kay Moredich, who have supported me throughout the writing of this book and during our forty-seven years together as nurses. Special thanks to my faculty mentors, Dr. Imogene King, Dr. Joyce Ellis, and Nancy Weber.

I would like to acknowledge and sincerely thank the team at Delmar Cengage Learning who worked to make this book a reality. Beth Williams, Senior Product Manager, is a great person who worked tirelessly and shared her knowledge, guidance, humor, and attention to help keep me motivated and on track throughout the project.

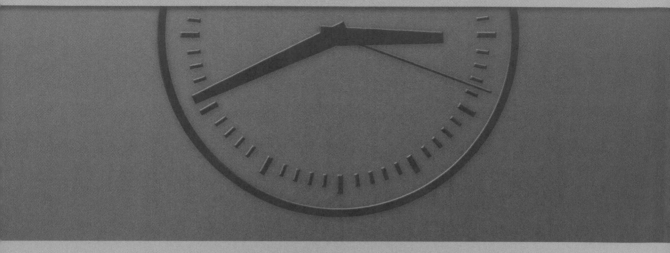

ABOUT THE AUTHOR

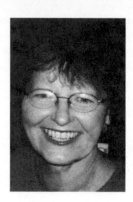

Patricia Kelly earned a Diploma in Nursing from St. Margaret Hospital School of Nursing, Hammond, Indiana; a Baccalaureate in Nursing from DePaul University in Chicago, Illinois; and a Master's Degree in Nursing from Loyola University in Chicago, Illinois. Pat is Professor Emeritus, Purdue University Calumet, Hammond, Indiana. She has worked as a staff nurse, school nurse, and nurse educator. Pat has traveled extensively in the United States, Canada, and Puerto Rico, teaching conferences for the Joint Commission, Resource Applications, Pediatric Concepts, and Kaplan, Inc. She currently teaches nationwide NCLEX-RN review courses and works part-time as an emergency room staff nurse in Chicago, Illinois.

Pat was Director of Quality Improvement at the University of Chicago Hospitals and Clinics. She has taught at Wesley-Passavant School of Nursing, Chicago State University, and Purdue University Calumet, Hammond, Indiana. She has taught Fundamentals of Nursing, Adult Nursing, Nursing Leadership and Management, Nursing Issues, Nursing Trends, Quality Improvement, and Legal Aspects of Nursing. Pat is a member of Sigma Theta Tau, the American Nurses Association, and the Emergency Nurses Association. She is listed in *Who's Who in American Nursing, 2000 Notable American Women,* and the *International Who's Who of Professional and Business Women.*

Pat has served on the Board of Directors of Tri City Mental Health Center, St. Anthony's Home, and the Quality Connection. She is the author of *Nursing Leadership & Management*, 2nd edition, Delmar Cengage Learning (2008), *Nursing Leadership & Management*, Delmar Cengage Learning (2003), *Essentials of Nursing Leadership & Management*, Delmar Cengage Learning (2004), *Delegation of Nursing Care*, 2nd edition, Delmar Cengage Learning (2010), *Delegation of Nursing Care*, Delmar Cengage Learning (2005). Pat contributed a chapter on "Preparing the Undergraduate Student and Faculty to Use Quality Improvement in Practice" to *Improving Quality*, second edition, by Claire Gavin Meisenheimer. Pat also contributed a chapter on obstructive lung disease to *Medical Surgical Nursing*, by Rick Daniels. Pat has also written several articles, including "Chest X-Ray Interpretation" and many articles on quality improvement. She has served as a National Disaster Volunteer for the American Red Cross and as a volunteer at several church food pantries in Austin, Texas, and Chicago, Illinois. She has also gone on health care relief trips to Nicaragua. Throughout most of her career, she has taught nursing at the university level. Pat has been licensed and has worked in many states during her career, including Indiana, Illinois, Wisconsin, Oklahoma, New York, and Pennsylvania. Pat may be contacted at patkh1@aol.com.

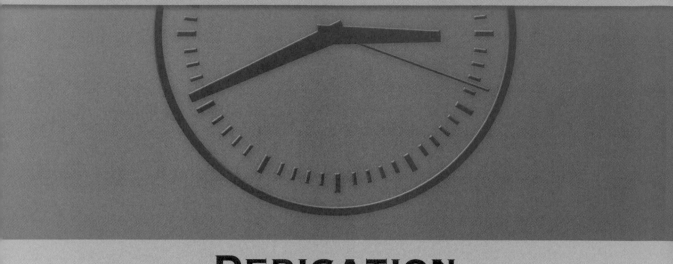

DEDICATION

This book is dedicated to my loving Dad and Mom, Ed and Jean Kelly; to my super sisters, Tessie Dybel and Kathy Milch; to my dear aunts and uncles, Aunt Verna and Uncle Archie Payne and Aunt Pat and Uncle Bill Kelly; to my nieces, Natalie Dybel Bevil, Melissa Milch Arredondo, and Stacey Milch; to my nephew, John Milch; and to my grand nephew, Brock Bevil and grand niece, Reese Bevil.

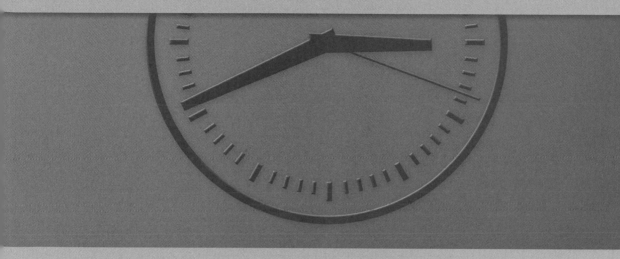

How to Use This Book

Quote

A nursing or health care theorist quote gives a professional's perspective regarding the topic at hand; read this quote as you begin each new chapter and see whether your opinion matches or differs, or whether you are in need of further information.

Objectives

These goals indicate to you the performance-based, measurable objectives that are targeted for mastery upon completion of the chapter.

OBJECTIVES

Upon completion of this chapter, the reader should be able to:

1. Identify theories of leadership.
2. Differentiate between leaders and managers.
3. Discuss management.
4. Discuss Benner's Model of Novice to Expert.
5. Discuss motivation theories.

You are a new nurse on a 30-bed medical unit that uses primary nursing as the care delivery model. There are 40 employees who work full and part time on this unit with vacancies for 8 additional full-time staff. The current schedule does not accommodate any 12-hour shifts. There are five long-term staff members who are threatening to leave if they are forced to work 12-hour shifts. You have heard there are several new graduates who will come to work on the unit only if there are 12-hour shifts.

How can the needs of both groups of staff be accommodated?

What effect will the 12-hour shifts have on the care delivery model?

Opening Scenario

This mini case study with related critical thinking questions should be read prior to delving into the chapter; it sets the tone for the material to come and helps you identify your knowledge base and perspective.

CASE STUDY 11-1

A patient developed a rash from a new medication, unbeknownst to the medication nurse, who never asked about any signs of problems. The treatment nurse noticed the rash during a routine dressing change, but never thought to inquire about any new dietary or medication changes. It was not until the time of discharge when the patient read the drug information sheet advising that any skin changes be reported that the patient asked the discharge planning nurse if the week-old rash was significant.

What could have been done differently?

Was anyone at fault? Who?

Why is good communication especially important in a situation in which there is a division of labor by function?

What types of problems could you expect if staff members focused on their own tasks and failed to communicate with each other about the patient's physical, emotional, psychosocial, educational, and discharge needs?

Case Study

These short cases with related questions present a beginning clinical nursing management situation calling for judgment, decision making, or analysis in solving an open-ended problem. Familiarize yourself with the types of situations and settings you will later encounter in practice, and challenge yourself to devise solutions that will result in the best outcomes for all parties, within the boundaries of legal and ethical nursing practice.

Evidence from the Literature

Study these key findings from nursing and health care research, theory, and literature, and ask yourself how they will influence your practice. Do you see ways in which your nursing could be affected by these literature findings and research results? Do you agree with the conclusions drawn by the author?

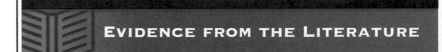

EVIDENCE FROM THE LITERATURE

Citation: Sirota, T. (2008). Nurse/Physician Relationships: Survey Report. July, 28–31.

Discussion: More than half of respondents (57%) to this survey of nurses say they're generally satisfied with their professional relations with physicians; a significant minority, 43%, reports dissatisfaction. Although relationships have improved some since an earlier survey in 1991, respondents' comments indicate that they perceive several factors to be at play here:

- male physicians' perceptions of traditional gender and cultural roles
- physicians' arrogance and feelings of superiority
- nurses' feelings of inferiority
- hospital culture or policy reinforcing a subordinate role for nurses

Important ways to improve nurse/physician overall collaboration identified in the article includes workplace empowerment for nurses, nurse/physician rounds, team meetings, collaborative educational programs, and collaborative membership on hospital committees.

The article states that the bottom line is that nurses aren't expendable. In the current nursing shortage, the climate is ripe for nurses to speak up as a group and let facility administrators know that they need to pay attention to nurses' legitimate concerns about nurse/physician collaboration, and then correct deficiencies.

Perhaps most important, improving relationships between nurses and physicians will benefit both professional groups by improving job satisfaction and productivity, and will benefit patients by enhancing their overall safety, welfare, and clinical progress. This can be accomplished by promoting greater nurse/physician professional respect, improving communication and collaboration, educating physicians about nursing roles and skills, and addressing physician misconduct (Rosenstein, 2002).

Implications for Nursing: Nursing and medical practitioner communication has improved since the 1991 survey. Good communication by all members of the health care team affects patient safety and must be facilitated by nursing, medical, and hospital team members to build an environment for patient safety.

Critical Thinking

Ethical, cultural, spiritual, legal, delegatory, and performance improvement considerations are highlighted in these boxes. Before beginning a new chapter, page through and read the Critical Thinking sections and jot down your comments or reactions; then see whether your perspective changes after you complete the chapter.

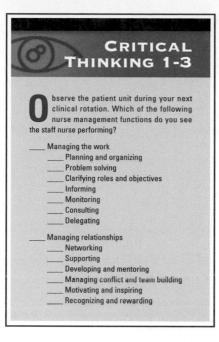

CRITICAL THINKING 1-3

Observe the patient unit during your next clinical rotation. Which of the following nurse management functions do you see the staff nurse performing?

____ Managing the work
____ Planning and organizing
____ Problem solving
____ Clarifying roles and objectives
____ Informing
____ Monitoring
____ Consulting
____ Delegating

____ Managing relationships
____ Networking
____ Supporting
____ Developing and mentoring
____ Managing conflict and team building
____ Motivating and inspiring
____ Recognizing and rewarding

REAL WORLD INTERVIEW

It was a Monday. The Emergency Department was very busy as usual. A new patient, a 69-year-old African-American female, was admitted by ambulance following a motor vehicle accident. I went to assess this patient and noted that blood was dripping from a small laceration on her forehead. She was awake, alert, and oriented. She had no pain or nausea. She told me that she was feeling fine, but I noticed that her lips and mouth were pale. I told the charge nurse that I believed that the patient's hemoglobin level was below 5, and I asked her to please tell the physician to come to the room soon to assess the patient. As I believed this patient was not stable, I immediately took the lead and inserted a large-bore intravenous heplock in her vein and collected blood samples for a CBC, BMP, PT, PTT, INR, and type and cross match, just in case. I started a liter of 0.9% normal saline intravenous fluid and connected the patient to the cardiac monitor as well as to the blood pressure, pulse, and pulse oximeter monitors. The patient now began to complain of nausea. At this point, the doctor had not come to see the patient yet. I went and told the doctor to please come to the patient's room and assess her now. I told him that the patient was bleeding and that I believed that her hemoglobin would be reported as below 5. He then came to the room and assessed the patient. He removed the head laceration dressing, which was now soaked in blood. He noted a 1-inch laceration on her forehead that was still bleeding. He sutured the wound and finally ordered the CBC. I asked him if he was sure he only wanted the CBC. He said yes. When the CBC results came back, the patient's hemoglobin was 3.8. I felt good about my assessment and intervention with this patient. The physician then ordered a type and cross match for 4 units of blood and a CT of the head. After the patient received two units of blood, she was transferred to the ICU.

Nirmala Joseph, RN
Staff Nurse
Houston, Texas

Real World Interviews

Real World Interviews with nurses, doctors, staff, patients, and family members are included. As you read these, ask yourself whether you have ever considered the point of view being represented on the given topic. How would knowing another person's perspective affect the care you deliver?

KEY CONCEPTS

- Nurses are leaders and make a difference to health care organizations through their contributions of expert knowledge and leadership. Leadership development is a necessary component of preparation as a health care provider.

- Leadership is a process of influence in which the leader influences others toward goal achievement. Leadership can be formal or informal.

- Leadership and management are different.

- Leadership styles are described as autocratic, democratic, and laissez-faire and have been studied by examining job-centered or task-oriented approaches as well as employee-centered or relationship-oriented approaches.

Key Concepts

This bulleted list serves as a review and study tool for you as you complete each chapter.

Key Terms

Study this list prior to reading the chapter, and then again as you complete a chapter to test your true understanding of the terms and concepts covered. Make a study list of terms you need to focus on to thoroughly appreciate the material in the chapter.

KEY TERMS

autocratic leadership
consideration
contingency theory
democratic leadership
emotional intelligence
employee-centered leadership
formal leadership
Hawthorne effect
informal leader
initiating structure
job-centered leaders

REVIEW QUESTIONS

1. Why is leadership important for nurses if they are not in a management position?
   A. It is not really important for nurses.
   B. Leadership is important at all levels in an organization because nurses have expert knowledge and are interacting with and influencing others.
   C. Nurse leaders leave their jobs sooner for other positions.
   D. Nurses who lead are less satisfied in their jobs.

Review Questions

These questions will challenge your comprehension of objectives and concepts presented in the chapter and will allow you to demonstrate content mastery, build critical thinking skills, and achieve integration of the concepts. Multiple choice, and other types of NCLEX-RN questions are included.

Review Activities

These thought-provoking activities at the close of a chapter invite you to approach a problem or scenario critically and apply the knowledge you have gained.

REVIEW ACTIVITIES

1. Take the opportunity to learn about yourself by reflecting on five predominant factors identified as being influential in a nurse's leadership development: self-confidence, innate leader qualities/tendencies, progression of experiences and success, influence of significant others, and personal life factors. Consider what reinforces your confidence in yourself. What innate qualities or traits do you have that contribute to your development as a nurse leader? Consider what professional experiences, mentors, and personal experiences or events can help you develop your leadership ability. How can you obtain these experiences?

EXPLORING THE WEB

Search the Web, checking the following sites.

- Emerging Leader:
  www.emergingleader.com
- Leadership Directories: Who's who in the leadership of the United States:
  www.leadershipdirectories.com
  Search for nursing leaders.
- Health Leadership Associates:
  www.healthleadership.com
- LeaderValues:
  www.leader-values.com
- Don Clark's Big Dog Leadership:
  www.nwlink.com/~Donclark

Exploring the Web

Internet activities encourage you to use your computer and reasoning skills to search the Web for additional information on quality and nursing leadership and management.

References

Evidence-based research, theory, and general literature, as well as nursing, medical, and health care sources, are included in these lists; refer to them as you read the chapter and verify your research.

REFERENCES

American Nurses Association. (ANA). (2003). Nursing Social Policy Statement. Available at nursingworld. org/Books/pdescr.cfm?cnum=7#9781558102149.

American Nurses Association. (ANA). (2008). What is Nursing? Silver Spring, MD.

Budd, K., Warino, L., & Patton, M. (2004). *Traditional & nontraditional collective bargaining strategies to improve the patient care environment.* Online Journal of Issues in Nursing, (9). Retrieved from www .nursingworld.org/ojin/topic23/tpc23_5.htm (2/25/07).

SUGGESTED READINGS

Joint Commission. (2005). The SBARR technique: Improves communication, enhances patient safety. *Joint Commission's Perspectives on Patient Safety, 5*(2), 1–2.

Leonard, M., Graham, S., & Bonacum, D. (2004). The human factor: The critical importance of effective teamwork and communication in providing safe care. *Quality and Safety in Health Care 2004, 13,* 85–90.

Murray, T., & Kleinpell, R. (2006). Implementing a rapid response team: Factors influencing success. *Critical Care Nursing Clinics of North America, 18*(4), 493–501.

Smith, M. K. (2005). Bruce W. Tuckman—forming, storming, norming and performing in groups. *Encyclopedia of Informal Education.* Retrieved April 23, 2006, from www.infed.org/thinkers/tuckman.htm.

Williamson, S. (2006). Training the team: Talk is cheap—but vital in keeping patients safe. *Inside: Duke University Medical Center & Health System Newsletter, 15*(5).

Suggested Readings

These entries invite you to pursue additional topics, articles, and information in related resources.

Photos, Tables, and Figures

These items illustrate key concepts.

TABLE 6-3	STRATEGIES FOR CHANGE	
Strategy	**Description**	**Example**
Power-coercive approach	Used when resistance is expected but change acceptance is not important to the power group. Uses power, control, authority, and threat of job loss to gain compliance with change—"Do it or get out."	Student must achieve a passing grade in a class project to complete the course requirements satisfactorily.
Normative-reeducative approach	Uses the individual's need to have satisfactory relationships in the workplace as a method of inducing support for change. Focuses on the relationship needs of workers and stresses "going along with the majority."	A new RN who is working eight-hour shifts is encouraged by the other unit staff to embrace a new unit plan for twelve-hour staffing.
Rational-empirical approach	Uses knowledge to encourage change. Once workers understand the merits of change for the organization or understand the meaning of the change to them as individuals and the organization as a whole, they will change. Stresses training and communication. Used when little resistance is anticipated.	Staff are educated regarding the scientific merits of a needed change.

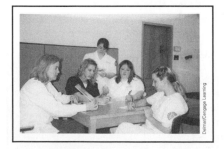

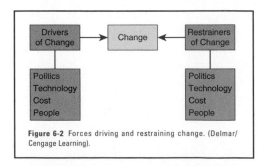

Figure 6-2 Forces driving and restraining change. (Delmar/Cengage Learning).

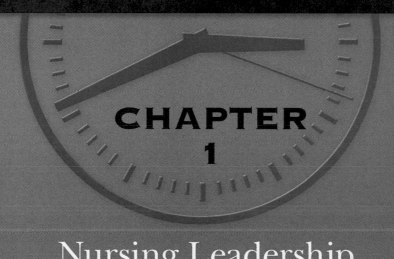

CHAPTER 1

Nursing Leadership, Management, and Motivation

Leadership is the essence of professionalism and should be considered an essential component of all nurse and other professional roles.

(Joyce Clifford, PhD, RN, FAAN)

OBJECTIVES

Upon completion of this chapter, the reader should be able to:

1. Identify theories of leadership.
2. Differentiate between leaders and managers.
3. Discuss management.
4. Discuss Benner's Model of Novice to Expert.
5. Discuss motivation theories.

Ed Harley was admitted to the cardiac observation unit. He had been diagnosed previously with heart disease and had experienced episodes of ventricular arrhythmias. That evening, while Mr. Harley was talking to his wife on the phone, and as Maria, a new RN, was walking to his bedside, he suddenly stopped talking and went into cardiac arrest. Maria reacted immediately and started cardiopulmonary resuscitation (CPR). Mr. Harley recovered and a normal sinus rhythm appeared on the monitor before anyone else could respond to the code. Mr. Harley was then transferred to the coronary care unit (CCU).

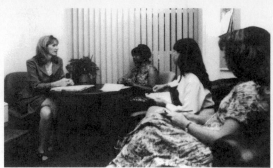

Delmar/Cengage Learning

Maria's leadership and quick action saved this patient's life and prevented the nurse-sensitive outcome of cardiac arrest. In nursing, patient assessment and nursing intervention are part of a nurse's ordinary work. Yet, it is quite extraordinary work.

What leadership characteristics did Maria demonstrate in preventing a nurse-sensitive outcome of cardiac arrest and death?

Why is Maria considered a leader, even though she is not in a formal leadership position?

Why is leadership important at all levels throughout a health care organization?

Professionals use their expertise and specialized knowledge to perform leadership and management roles. Many people think leaders and managers are only top corporate executives and administrators, political representatives, military generals, or those who lead and manage organizations. This is because these leaders and managers are highly visible and hold high-profile positions. We need leaders and managers though at all levels of an organization. Leadership and management are basic competencies needed by all health professionals. Leadership and management development is a necessary part of the preparation of health care providers.

Nurses make a critical difference every day in leading and managing the care of their patients and patients' families. Nurses often believe those accomplishments are ordinary work, yet those accomplishments often prevent the occurrence of nursing-sensitive patient outcomes. **Nursing-sensitive patient outcomes** are measures that reflect the outcome of nursing actions to rescue patients from death due to such complications as pneumonia, shock, cardiac arrest, urinary tract infection, gastrointestinal bleeding, sepsis, and deep vein thrombosis. Nurses make a critical difference whether they are working with an individual patient or managing a patient care unit or an entire nursing department. Nurses manage and lead patient care and by doing so provide caring expertise that is extraordinary. This chapter discusses leadership, management, and organizational management perspectives. Theories of motivation are also discussed.

LEADERSHIP AND MANAGEMENT

Leadership and management are different. Leadership influences or inspires the actions and goals of others. One does not have to be in a position of authority to demonstrate leadership. Not all leaders are managers. Bennis and Nanus (1985) popularized the phrase, "leaders are people who do the right thing; managers are people who do things right." Both roles are crucial, but different. Bennis stated that he often observes people in top positions doing the wrong things well. It is important to avoid thinking that leadership is important and management is insignificant. People need to be managed, as well as inspired and led. Leadership is part of management, not a substitute for it. We need both.

LEADERSHIP

Leadership is commonly defined as a process of interaction in which the leader influences others toward goal achievement (Yukl, 1998). Influence is an instrumental part of leadership. Leaders influence others, often by inspiring, enlivening, and engaging others to participate. The process of leadership involves the leader and the follower in interaction. This implies that leadership is a reciprocal relationship. Leadership can occur between the leader and another individual; between the leader and a group; or between a leader and an organization, a community, or a society. Defining leadership as a process helps us to better understand leadership than does the traditional view of a leader being in a position of authority, exerting command, control, and power over subordinates. What this means for nurses as professionals is that they function as leaders when they influence others toward goal achievement. Nurses are leaders. There are many more leaders in organizations than there are leaders who are in positions of authority in those organizations. Each person has the potential to serve as a leader.

Today's nurse must know how to lead. Leading is one of four managerial functions, along with planning, organizing and staffing, and controlling. Whereas management is more formal and relies on tools such as planning, budgeting, and controlling, leading involves having a vision and goals for what the organization can become, and then getting the cooperation and teamwork from others to achieve those goals (DuBrin, 2000).

Leadership ability grows in the beginning nurse who may demonstrate leadership in working with other staff; for example, the new nurse speaks up about the need for improvement in an element of care delivery. Leadership ability often grows as the nurse becomes more confident and experienced in working with others.

Leadership can be **formal leadership**, as when a person is in a position of authority or in a sanctioned, assigned role within an organization that connotes influence, such as a clinical nurse specialist (Northouse, 2001). An **informal leader** is an individual who demonstrates leadership outside the scope of a formal leadership role, such as a member of a group rather than the head or leader of the group. Staff nurses demonstrate informal leadership when they advocate for patient needs or when they take action to improve health care. Nurses also demonstrate informal leadership when they speak up to improve quality of care.

LEADERS AND FOLLOWERS

Leaders and followers are both necessary roles. Leaders need followers in order to lead. Followers need leaders in order to follow. Nurses are alternately leaders and followers when they work with other health care team members to achieve patient care goals, participate in meetings, and so forth. The most valuable followers are skilled, self-directed employees who participate actively in setting the group's direction and invest time and energy in the work of the group, thinking critically and advocating for new ideas (Grossman & Valiga, 2008). Good followers communicate and work well with others, being supportive, yet thoughtful, in their approach to new ideas.

Kotter (1990a) describes the differences between leadership and management in the following way: Leadership is about creating change, and management is about controlling complexity in an effort to bring order and consistency. He says that leadership involves establishing a direction, aligning people through empowerment, and motivating and inspiring them toward producing useful change and achieving the vision, whereas management is defined as planning and budgeting, organizing and staffing, problem solving and controlling complexity to produce predictability and order (Kotter, 1990b).

Nurses are leaders. Nurses function as leaders when they influence others toward goal achievement. RNs in staff nurse positions lead nursing practice by setting a direction, aligning people,

CRITICAL THINKING 1-1

Look for opportunities to gather data about quality clinical performance. What quality measures can you monitor in the following areas?

■ *Clinical Care:* Number of patients who are triaged within five minutes of arrival in the Emergency Department.

■ *Utilization:* Number of patients who achieve quality outcomes under normal staffing ratios.

■ *Financial:* Number of patients who meet patient care standards, budget, and so on.

■ *Quality:* Number of patients who state they are pleased with their nursing care, receive good pain management, and so on.

and motivating and inspiring others toward a vision. Nurses lead other nurses and their community to achieve a collective vision of quality health care. See Table 1-1 for examples of nurses carrying out leadership role activities.

LEADERSHIP CHARACTERISTICS

According to Bennis and Nanus (1985), effective leaders share three fundamental qualities. The first quality is a guiding vision. Leaders focus on a professional and purposeful vision that provides direction toward the preferred future. The second quality is passion. Passion expressed by the leader involves the ability to inspire and align people toward the promises of life. The third quality is integrity based on knowledge of self, honesty, and maturity that is developed through experience and growth. McCall (1998) describes how self-awareness—knowing our strengths and weaknesses—can allow us to use feedback and learn from our mistakes. Daring and curiosity are also basic ingredients of leadership from which leaders draw on to take risks, learning from what

works as much as from what does not (Bennis & Nanus, 1985).

In their landmark work, *AACN Standards for Establishing Healthy Work Environments: A Journey to Excellence,* the American Association of Critical-Care Nurses cites authentic leadership as one of the key standards and assert that authentic leadership requires skill in the core competencies of self-knowledge, strategic vision, risk-taking and creativity, interpersonal and communication effectiveness, and inspiration (AACN, 2004).

Certain characteristics are commonly attributed to leaders. These traits are considered desirable and seem to contribute to the perception of being a leader. They include intelligence, self-confidence, determination, integrity, and sociability (Stodgill, 1948, 1974). Research among 46 hospitals designated as magnet hospitals for their success in attracting and retaining registered nurses emphasized the value of leaders who are visionary and enthusiastic, are supportive and knowledgeable, have high standards and expectations, value education and professional development, demonstrate power and status in the organization, are visible and responsive, communicate openly, and are active in professional associations (McClure & Hinshaw, 2002; Scott et al., 1999; Kramer, 1990; McClure, Poulin, Sovie, & Wandelt, 1983; Kramer & Schmalenberg, 2005). Research findings from studies on nurses revealed that caring, respectability, trustworthiness, and flexibility were the leader characteristics most valued. In one study, nurse leaders identified managing the dream, mastering change, designing organization structure, learning, and taking initiative as leadership characteristics (Murphy & DeBack, 1991). Research by Kirkpatrick and Locke (1991) concluded that leaders are different from nonleaders across six traits: drive, the desire to lead, honesty and integrity, self-confidence, cognitive ability, and knowledge of the business. Although no set of traits is definitive and reliable in determining who is a leader or who is effective as a leader, many people still rely on personality traits to describe and define leadership characteristics.

TABLE 1-1	EXAMPLES OF NURSE LEADERSHIP ROLE ACTIVITIES		
Leadership is about creating change through:	**RN in a Staff Nurse Position**	**RNs Leading Other RNs**	**RNs Leading Communities/ Society**
Establishing direction and expressing a vision.	The RN read a current nursing journal on reducing ventilator-associated pneumonia (Pruitt & Jacobs, 2006). She uses this information to reduce the pneumonia rate among hospitalized patients on her unit.	The American Association of Critical-Care Nurses (AACN) adopts the strategic initiative that identified the need for a healthy work environment; that is, work and patient care environments must be safe, healthy, humane, and respectful of the rights, responsibilities, needs, and contributions of patients, their families, nurses, and all health professionals (AACN, 2004).	Nurses take action toward the goal of a health care system that is available to all.
Aligning people through empowerment.	The RN shared the article on reducing ventilator-related pneumonia with colleagues. Together they identify the infection rate among patients in their unit, and implement the best-practice interventions called the "ventilator bundle," which includes elevating the patient's head of the bed 30 degrees, sedation breaks, waking and weaning the patient, and prevention of deep vein thrombosis.	AACN provides testimony to the Institute of Medicine (IOM) Committee on Work Environment for Nurses and Patient Safety (AACN, 2003). "Ensuring patient safety and quality outcomes requires nurse leaders to prioritize strategic initiatives to cultivate a work environment of health." (Heath, Johanson, & Blake, 2004, p. 525)	The American Nurses Association (ANA) forms the American Nurses Credentialing Center to recognize excellence in the quality of professional nursing practice through the Magnet Recognition Program.

(continues)

TABLE 1-1	EXAMPLES OF NURSE LEADERSHIP ROLE ACTIVITIES (CONTINUED)		
Leadership is about creating change through:	**RN in a Staff Nurse Position**	**RNs Leading Other RNs**	**RNs Leading Communities/ Society**
Motivating and inspiring people.	The RN volunteers to help develop a pilot project that introduces the "ventilator bundle" to others who meet regularly to guide this project.	AACN establishes the following standards for establishing and sustaining healthy work environments: ■ Skilled Communication ■ True Collaboration ■ Effective Decision Making ■ Appropriate Staffing ■ Meaningful Recognition ■ Authentic Leadership See www.aacn.org, click on, Healthy Work Environments.	Research findings show that higher numbers of RN staff are associated with lower mortality (Aiken, 2002). Nurses in magnet hospitals report better quality of care than nurses in nonmagnet hospitals (Kramer & Schmalenberg, 2005; McClure & Hinshaw, 2002; Upenieks, 2003).
Producing useful change and achieving the vision.	Based on the results of the ventilator bundle project, the RN helps to change the unit's policies and procedures in order to permanently adopt this change in practice and improve health care outcomes for patients.	AACN publishes a call to action for nurses and all health professionals and organizations to participate in creating healthy work environments (AACN, 2004).	Nurses in magnet hospitals are leaders in attracting and retaining quality nurses and leaders and advancing nursing and health care in their communities.

Source: Compiled with information from Kotter, J. (1990a). *A force for change: How leadership differs from management.* Glencoe, IL: Free Press.

LEADERSHIP THEORIES

The major leadership theories can be classified according to the following approaches: behavioral, contingency, and contemporary.

BEHAVIORAL APPROACH Leadership studies from the 1930s by Kurt Lewin and colleagues at Iowa State University conveyed information about three leadership styles that are still widely

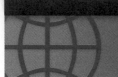

REAL WORLD INTERVIEW

It was a Monday. The Emergency Department was very busy as usual. A new patient, a 69-year-old African-American female, was admitted by ambulance following a motor vehicle accident. I went to assess this patient and noted that blood was dripping from a small laceration on her forehead. She was awake, alert, and oriented. She had no pain or nausea. She told me that she was feeling fine, but I noticed that her lips and mouth were pale. I told the charge nurse that I believed that the patient's hemoglobin level was below 5, and I asked her to please tell the physician to come to the room soon to assess the patient. As I believed this patient was not stable, I immediately took the lead and inserted a large-bore intravenous heplock in her vein and collected blood samples for a CBC, BMP, PT, PTT, INR, and type and cross match, just in case. I started a liter of 0.9% normal saline intravenous fluid and connected the patient to the cardiac monitor as well as to the blood pressure, pulse, and pulse oximeter monitors. The patient now began to complain of nausea. At this point, the doctor had not come to see the patient yet. I went and told the doctor to please come to the patient's room and assess her now. I told him that the patient was bleeding and that I believed that her hemoglobin would be reported as below 5. He then came to the room and assessed the patient. He removed the head laceration dressing, which was now soaked in blood. He noted a 1-inch laceration on her forehead that was still bleeding. He sutured the wound and finally ordered the CBC. I asked him if he was sure he only wanted the CBC. He said yes. When the CBC results came back, the patient's hemoglobin was 3.8. I felt good about my assessment and intervention with this patient. The physician then ordered a type and cross match for 4 units of blood and a CT of the head. After the patient received two units of blood, she was transferred to the ICU.

Nirmala Joseph, RN
Staff Nurse
Houston, Texas

recognized today. The three styles are autocratic, democratic, and laissez-faire leadership (Lewin, 1939; Lewin & Lippitt, 1938; Lewin, Lippitt, & White, 1939).

Autocratic, Democratic, and Laissez-faire Leadership. **Autocratic leadership** involves centralized decision making, with the leader making decisions and using power to command and control others. The *autocratic* style is used by the leader in situations in which (1) the task or outcome is relatively simple (such as telling the nursing assistive personnel (NAP) to take a temperature); (2) most team members would agree with the decision and provide consensus; and (3) a decision has to be made promptly.

Democratic leadership is participatory, with authority often delegated to others. To be influential,

the democratic leader uses expert power and the power base afforded by having close, personal relationships. In the *democratic* style, the leader will ask the opinions of the entire team, but the final decision usually lies with the leader, or there may be mutual decision making by both team members and the leader, with everyone having an equal vote. This process encourages everyone to fully accept the team's conclusion. This style allows all to have the opportunity to provide input and differing perspectives into the decision.

The third style, **laissez-faire leadership**, is passive and permissive, and the leader defers decision making. Lewin (1939) contrasted these styles and concluded that autocratic leaders were associated with high-performing groups, but that close supervision of the group was necessary and feelings of hostility were often present toward the autocratic leader. Democratic leaders engendered positive feelings in their groups; group and performance was strong whether or not the democratic leader was present. Low productivity and feelings of frustration in the group were associated with laissez-faire leaders.

Employee-Centered and Job-Centered Leaders.

Behavioral leadership studies from the University of Michigan and Ohio State University led to the identification of two basic leader behaviors: job-centered and employee-centered behaviors. Effective leadership was described as having a focus on the human needs of subordinates and was called **employee-centered leadership** (Moorhead & Griffin, 2001). **Job-centered leaders** were seen as less effective because of their focus on schedules, costs, and efficiency, resulting in a lack of attention to developing work groups and high-performance goals (Moorhead & Griffin, 2001).

The researchers at Ohio State focused their efforts on two dimensions of leader behavior: initiating structure and consideration. **Initiating structure** involves an emphasis on the work to be done, a focus on the task and production. Leaders who focus on initiating structure are concerned with how work is organized and on the achievement of goals. Leader behavior includes planning, directing others, and establishing deadlines and details of how work is to be done. For example, a nurse demonstrating the leader behavior of initiating structure could be a nurse who, at the beginning of a shift, makes out a patient assignment delegating care to the NAP.

The dimension of **consideration** involves activities that focus on the employee and emphasize relating and getting along with people. Leader behavior focuses on the well-being of others. The leader is involved in creating a relationship that fosters communication and trust as a basis for respecting other people and their potential contribution. A staff nurse demonstrating consideration behavior will take the time to talk with coworkers, be empathetic, and show an interest in them as people.

The leader behaviors of initiating structure and consideration define leadership style. The different styles nurses use include:

- Low initiating structure, low consideration
- High initiating structure, low consideration
- High initiating structure, high consideration
- Low initiating structure, high consideration

The Ohio State University studies associate the high initiating structure–high consideration leader behaviors with better performance and satisfaction outcomes than the other styles. Nurses who use high initiating structure and high consideration leader behaviors will initiate and develop clear, well-structured assignments and work considerately with their staff to achieve quality outcomes. This leadership style is considered effective, although it may not be appropriate in every situation.

Another model based on two dimensions is the managerial grid developed by Blake and Mouton (1985). Five styles identify the extent of structure, called *concern for production*, and consideration, called *concern for people*, demonstrated by the leader. Concern for both people and production can be low, moderate, or high (Figure 1-1).

The five leader styles are:

1. Impoverished leader for low production concern and low people concern;
2. Authority compliance leader for high production concern and low people concern;
3. Country club leader for high people concern and low production concern;

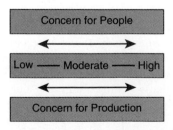

Figure 1-1 Key leadership dimensions. (*Source:* Compiled with information from Blake, Mouton, & McCanse Leadership Grid from Lussier, R. N. & Achua, C. F. [2000]. *Leadership: Theory, Application, Skill Development.* Cincinnatti, OH: South-Western College Publishing).

CASE STUDY 1-1

Among the individuals commonly identified as leaders (Table 1-2), can you identify a set of leadership traits, such as knowledge, self-confidence, determination, integrity, sociability, cognitive ability, caring, honesty, trustworthiness, flexiblity, desire to lead, and drive, that they all possess?

TABLE 1-2 LEADERS AMONG US: PAST AND PRESENT

Mother Teresa	Martin Luther King
Imogene King	John F. Kennedy
Hildegard Peplau	Sister Callista Roy
Rosa Parks	Franklin Delano Roosevelt
John Adams	Dorothea Orem
Barack Obama	Florence Nightingale
Pope Benedict	Peter Buerhaus
John McCain	Hillary Clinton
Clara Barton	Virginia Henderson
Ida Androwich	Martha Rogers
Linda Aiken	Sister Rosemary Donley
Winston Churchill	Zenaida Corpuz

Now divide your class into groups. Have each group identify someone from this list whom they see as a leader. Describe the leader's traits and then have the groups share with the class who the leaders are and their traits. Do the leaders demonstrate any traits such as drive, desire to lead, honesty and integrity, self confidence, cognitive ability, or knowledge of their business? When you work on the clinical unit, do you see any staff nurses displaying these leadership traits? How can you develop these traits in yourself?

4. Middle-of-the-road leader for moderate concern in both dimensions; and

5. Team leader for high production concern and high people concern.

CONTINGENCY APPROACHES Another approach to leadership is **contingency theory**. Contingency theory acknowledges that other factors in the environment influence outcomes as much as leadership style and that leader effectiveness is contingent upon something other than the leader's behavior. The premise is that different leader behavior patterns will be effective in different situations. Contingency approaches include Fielder's contingency theory, the situational theory of Hersey and Blanchard, path-goal theory, and the idea of substitutes for leadership.

Fielder's Contingency Theory. Fielder (1967) is credited with the development of the contingency model of leadership effectiveness. Fielder's theory of leadership effectiveness views the pattern of leader behavior as dependent upon the interaction of the personality of the leader and the needs of the situation. The needs of the situation or how favorable the situation is toward the leader influences leader-member relationships, the degree of task structure, and the leader's position of power (Fielder, 1967).

Leader-member relations are the feelings and attitudes of followers regarding acceptance, trust, and credibility of the leader. Good leader-member relations exist when followers respect, trust, and have confidence in the leader. Poor leader-member relations reflect distrust, a lack of confidence and respect, and dissatisfaction with the leader by the followers.

Task structure refers to the degree to which work is defined, with specific procedures, explicit directions, and goals. High task structure involves routine, predictable, clearly defined work tasks. Low task structure involves work that is not routine, predictable, or clearly defined, such as creative, artistic, or qualitative research activities.

Position power is the degree of formal authority and influence associated with the leader. High position power is favorable for the leader and low position power is unfavorable. When all of these dimensions—leader-member relations, task structure, and position power—are high, the situation is favorable to the leader. When they are low, the situation is not favorable to the leader. In both of these circumstances, Fielder showed that a task-directed leader, concerned with task accomplishment, was effective. When the range of favorableness is intermediate or moderate in a situation, a human relations leader, concerned about people, was most effective. These situations need a leader with interpersonal and relationship skills to foster group achievement. Fielder's contingency theory is an approach that matches the organizational situation to the most favorable leadership style for that situation.

Situational Theory.   Hersey and Blanchard's situational leadership theory (2000) addresses follower readiness as a factor in determining leadership style and considers *task behavior* and *relationship behavior.*

High task behavior and low relationship behavior is called a *telling leadership* style. A high task, high relationship style is called a *selling leadership* style. A low task and high relationship style is called a *participating leadership* style. A low task and low relationship style is called a *delegating leadership* style.

Follower readiness, called maturity, is assessed in order to select one of the four leadership styles for a situation. For example, *telling leaders* define the roles and tasks of the follower and supervise them closely. Decisions are made by the leader and announced, so communication is largely one-way. *Selling leaders* still define the roles and tasks, but seek ideas and suggestions from the followers. Decisions remain the leader's prerogative but communication is much more two-way. *Participating leaders* pass day to day decisions, such as task allocation, to the followers. The leader facilitates and takes part in decisions but control is shared with the followers. *Delegating leaders* are still involved in decisions and problem-solving but control is with the follower. The follower decides when and how the leader will be involved.

An additional aspect of this model is the idea that the leader not only changes leadership style according to followers' needs, but also develops followers over time to increase their level of maturity (Lussier & Achua, 2000).

Path-Goal Theory.   In this leadership approach, the leader works to motivate followers and influence goal accomplishment. The seminal author on path-goal theory is Robert House (1971). By using the appropriate style of leadership for the situation (that is *directive, supportive, participative,* or *achievement-oriented*), the leader makes the path toward the goal easier for the follower. The *directive* style of leadership provides structure through direction and authority, with the leader focusing on the task and getting the job done. The *supportive* style of leadership is relationship oriented, with the leader providing encouragement, interest, and attention. *Participative* leadership means that the leader focuses on involving followers in the decision-making process. The *achievement-oriented* style provides high structure and direction, as well as high support through consideration behavior.

In Path-Goal Theory, the leadership style is matched to the situational characteristics of the followers, such as the desire for authority, the extent to which the control of goal achievement is internal or external, and the ability of the follower to be involved. The leadership style is also matched to the situational factors in the environment, including the routine nature or complexity of the task, the power associated with the leader's position, and the work group relationship. This alignment of leadership style with the needs of followers is motivating and believed to enhance performance and satisfaction. The path-goal theory is based on expectancy theory, which holds that people are motivated when they believe they are able to carry out the work, they think their contribution will lead to the expected outcome, and they believe that the rewards for their efforts are valued and meaningful (Northouse, 2001).

Substitutes for Leadership. **Substitutes for leadership** are variables that may influence followers to the same extent as the leader's behavior. Kerr and Jermier (1978) investigated situational variables and identified some of these variables as substitutes that eliminate the need for leader behavior, and other variables as neutralizers that nullify the effects of the leader's behavior.

Some of these variables include follower characteristics, such as the presence of structured routine tasks, the amount of feedback provided by the task, and the presence of intrinsic satisfaction in the work; and organizational characteristics, such as the presence of a cohesive group, a formal organization, a rigid adherence to rules, and low position power. For example, an individual's experience substitutes for task-direction leader behavior (Kerr & Jermier, 1978). This theory suggests that nurses and other professionals with a great deal of experience do not need direction and supervision to perform their work. Their knowledge serves as a leadership substitute. Another substitute for leader behavior is intrinsic satisfaction that emerges from just doing the work. Intrinsic satisfaction occurs frequently among nurses when they provide care to patients and families. Intrinsic satisfaction substitutes for the support and encouragement of relationship-oriented leader behavior.

CONTEMPORARY APPROACHES Contemporary approaches to leadership address the leadership functions necessary to develop learning organizations and lead the process of transforming change. These approaches include charismatic leadership, transformational leadership theory, knowledge workers, emotional intelligence, and Wheatley's New Science of Leadership.

Charismatic Theory. A charismatic leader has an inspirational quality that promotes an emotional connection in followers. House (1971) developed a theory of charismatic leadership that described how charismatic leaders behave, as well as distinguishing characteristics and situations in which such leaders would be effective. Charismatic leaders display self-confidence and strength in their convictions, and communicate high expectations and confidence in others. These leaders have been described as emerging during a crisis, communicating vision, and using personal power and unconventional strategies (Conger & Kanungo, 1987). One consequence of this type of leadership is a belief in the charismatic leader that is so strong it takes on an almost supernatural sense and the leader is worshipped as if superhuman. Examples of charismatic leaders include Florence Nightingale, Winston Churchill, and Martin Luther King. Charisma seems to be a special and valuable quality that some people have and other people do not.

Transformational Leadership Theory. Burns (1978) defined transformational leadership as a process in which "leaders and followers raise one another to higher levels of motivation and morality" (p. 21). Transformational leadership theory is based on the idea of empowering others to engage in pursuing a collective purpose by working together to achieve a vision of a preferred future. This kind of leadership can influence both the leader and the follower to a higher level of conduct and achievement that transforms them both (Burns, 1978). Burns maintained that there are two types of leaders: the traditional manager concerned with day-to-day operations, called the **transactional leader**, and the leader who is committed to a vision that empowers others, called the **transformational leader**.

Transformational leaders motivate others by behaving in accordance with values, providing a vision that reflects mutual values, and empowering others to contribute. Bennis and Nanus (1985)

CRITICAL THINKING 1-2

As the nurse enters the room of a new post-operative patient with a radical larynge-ctomy, the patient begins to hemorrhage from his neck incision. The nurse applies direct pressure with one hand and calls for assistance. Help arrives and the patient is taken to surgery with the nurse still maintaining pressure on the hemorrhaging site. The patient lives and goes home a few days later.

How does good leadership on a patient care unit ensure positive nurse-sensitive patient outcomes in an emergency?

How can you develop your transformational leadership skills, such as belief in self as a change agent, belief in people, and being a lifelong learner to improve your ability to care for a group of patients and empower others to do so?

describe this type of leader as a leader who "commits people to action, who converts followers into leaders, and who converts leaders into agents of change" (p. 3). According to research by Tichy and Devanna (1986), effective transformational leaders identify themselves as change agents; are courageous; believe in people; are value-driven; are lifelong learners; have the ability to deal with complexity, ambiguity, and uncertainty; and are visionaries. Yet transformational leadership may be demonstrated by anyone in an organization regardless of position (Burns, 1978). The interaction that occurs between individuals can be transformational and motivate both to a higher level of performance (Bass, 1985).

Transformational leadership at the organizational level is about innovation and change. The transformational leader uses vision which is based on shared values to align people and inspire growth and advancement. It is both the inspiration and the empowerment aspects of transformational leadership that lead to commitment beyond self-interest, commitment to a vision, and commitment to action that creates change. Transformational leadership theory suggests that the relationship between the leader and the follower inspires and empowers an individual toward commitment to goals.

Nurse researchers have described nurse executives according to transformational leadership theory and have used this theory to measure leadership behavior among nurse executives and nurse managers (Leach, 2005; Dunham-Taylor, 2000; Wolf, Boland, & Aukerman, 1994; McDaniel & Wolf, 1992; Young, 1992). Additionally, transformational leadership theory has been the basis for nursing administration curriculum and for investigation of relationships such as between a nurse's commitment to an organization and productivity in a hospital setting (Leach, 2005; McNeese-Smith, 1997; Searle, 1996). Cassidy and Koroll (1998) explored the ethical aspects of transformational leadership, and Barker (1990) comprehensively discussed nursing in terms of transformational leadership theory.

Most recently, the Institute of Medicine identified transformational leadership theory as a precursor to any change initiative and stated that transformational leadership can be a crucial approach toward achieving work environments that optimize patient safety (IOM, 2003).

Knowledge Workers. The organizations that nurses are a part of are changing. They reflect the advance and the promise of the technology that enables us to perform our work. Peter Drucker (1994) identifies the organization of the future as a knowledge organization composed of knowledge workers. **Knowledge workers** are those who bring specialized, expert knowledge to an organization. They are valued for what they know. The knowledge organization will share, provide, and grow the information necessary to work efficiently and effectively. Drucker says that knowledge organizations, in which the knowledge worker is at the front lines with the expertise and the information to act, will be the dominant organizational type (Drucker, 1994; Helgesen, 1995). In organizations such as these, the ideas of leadership at the top and leadership equated with the power of a position are obsolete notions. Workers with the expertise and information to act are the organization's leaders. They provide the service, interact with the customer, represent the organization, and accomplish its goals. Leadership is needed at all levels within such an organization, not just at the top and not just with certain positions in the organization. Every nurse has knowledge and serves as a leader.

In the information age, it is the development of new knowledge and innovation and its meaningful interpretation and application that becomes the source for transactions with patients and staff. Nursing's transition to the information age is occurring within the context of rapidly advancing technology and nanotechnology and is influenced by three key trends. These trends have been termed *mobility, virtuality,* and *user-driven practices* (Porter O'Grady, 2001).

Mobility refers to the ability to change skill sets as well as having the work dispersed among a variety of work locations, rather than work occurring at fixed sites (Bennis, Spreitzer, & Cummings, 2001). Nurses are working in many new settings today and are constantly adding to their knowledge as new technologies emerge.

Virtuality means working through virtual means using digital networks, where the worker may be far from the patient but present in a digital reality. Nurses are working in outpatient settings today where they carry a computer and are in instant communication with other practitioners and patients.

User-driven practices mean that the individual, at a time when digital mediums have given us more access to information and therefore more choices, acts more independently and is increasingly accountable for those choices and actions. Nurses are constantly assessing patients using traditional assessment methods as well as newer digital methods, for example, computerized vital sign monitors, and taking action to safeguard their patients and improve their care using these assessments.

Using Knowledge.   Nurses can develop their leadership and management skills with continuing education and by increasing their knowledge and expertise in caring for a group of patients. Knowledgeable nursing leadership and management on a nursing unit fosters good patient care by providing a supportive environment for nurses to deliver care. A supportive leadership and management environment provides a clear chain of command, clear job descriptions, patient care standards, good staffing ratios, good Internet and library resources, continuing education support, and so on.

Emotional Intelligence.   **Emotional intelligence** is a component of leadership and refers to the capacity for recognizing your own feelings and those of others, for motivating yourself, and for managing emotions well in yourself and in your relationships. It describes abilities distinct from, but complementary, to academic intelligence. Many people who are "book smart" but lack emotional intelligence end up working for people who have lower IQs but excel in emotional intelligence skills (Goleman, 1998).

Emotional intelligence includes these five basic emotional and social competencies:

- Self-awareness: Knowing what you are feeling in the moment, and using those preferences to guide your decision making; having a realistic assessment of your own abilities and a well-grounded sense of self-confidence
- Self-regulation: Handling your emotions so that they facilitate rather than interfere with the task at hand, being conscientious and delaying gratification to pursue goals, and recovering well from emotional distress
- Motivation: Using your deepest preferences to move and guide you toward your goals, to help you take initiative and strive to improve, and to persevere in the face of setbacks and frustrations
- Empathy: Sensing what people are feeling, being able to take their perspective, and cultivating rapport and attunement with a broad diversity of people

■ Social skills: Handling emotions in relationships well and accurately reading social situations and networks; interacting smoothly; using these skills to persuade and lead, and negotiate and settle disputes, for cooperation and teamwork (Goleman, 1998).

Wheatley's New Science of Leadership. Margaret Wheatley, in *Leadership and the New Science* (1999), says, "There is a simpler way to lead organizations, one that requires less effort and produces less stress than the current practices." She presents us with a new view of leadership, one encompassing connectedness and self-organizing systems that follow a natural order of both chaos and uncertainty. This differs from a view that sees leadership as following a linear order in a hierarchy. Wheatley says that the leader's function is to guide an organization using vision, to make choices based on mutual values, and to engage in the culture to provide meaning and coherence. This type of leadership fosters growth within each of us as individuals and as members of a group. The notion of connection within a self-organizing system optimizes autonomy at all levels because the relationships between the individual and the whole are strong.

Wheatley (2005) discusses how people learn best when they are engaged in relationships with others and can exchange knowledge and expertise through informal, self-organized communities. Wheatley refers to these as "communities of practice" and encourages us to develop new leaders using such communities. Her notion of a community of practice represents several elements nurses are familiar with, that is, forming informal groups, using a group process of organizing, using principles of learning, and sharing information. What is unique in her description of these communities of practice is that they form via self-organization. They come together naturally. What makes these communities different from informal groups is Wheatley's characterization of a community built from relationships and participation in a way that connects nurses and allows the creation of meaning from information or the exchange of knowledge. In work done for the Center for Creative Leadership, communities of practice are described as being different from the ideas or experiences we have had with other groups, teams, and collective forming because communities of practice emerge from shared activity, shared knowledge, and ways of knowing that create meaning and thus facilitate a culture of engagement, participation, and relationships (Drath & Palus, 1994). Wheatley directs nurses to name these communities of practice that connect and bring people together, support these connections, nourish the community, and illuminate their work. These exciting notions hold great promise for health professionals as we learn how to collaborate within and across disciplines and countries to advance health care practices.

MANAGEMENT

Management is defined as a process of planning, organizing and staffing, leading, and controlling actions to achieve goals. Planning involves setting goals and identifying ways to meet them. Organizing and staffing is the process of ensuring that the necessary human and physical resources are available to achieve the planning goals. Organizing also involves assigning work to the right person or group and specifying who has the authority to accomplish certain tasks. Leading is influencing others to achieve the organization's goals and involves energizing, directing, and persuading others to achieve those goals. Finally, controlling is comparing actual performance to a standard and revising the original plan as needed to achieve the goals (DuBrin, 2000).

Descriptive research (Mintzberg, 1973; McCall, Morrison, & Hanman, 1978; Hales, 1986) about what managers do has expanded our understanding of management. Managers often seem to work at a hectic pace and sustain that effort through long hours, frequently working without breaks. Yukl (1998) says that this reflects a preference by people in management positions for continuously seeking information and being constantly engaged in interactions with others who need information, help, guidance, or approval. The typical manager is always on the go. Research by

McCall, Morrison, and Hanman (1978) showed that the daily activities of managers are diverse and fast paced with regular interruptions. Priority activities are integrated among inconsequential ones. In the scope of one morning, a nurse manager may engage in serious decisions about a critically ill patient, a staff or patient complaint, a shortage of nurse staffing, and so forth. A nurse manager's work is driven by problems that emerge in random order and that have a range of importance and urgency. These circumstances create an image of the nurse manager as a "firefighter" involved in immediate and operational concerns. A significant proportion of a manager's time is spent in interaction with others, and more of the work is concerned with handling information than in making decisions (McCall et al., 1978). Nurse managers constantly interact with other members of a health care team. This team can include nurses, various health care practitioners, unit staff, and staff from other departments who share information and assure that quality patient outcomes are achieved.

MANAGEMENT ROLES

A frequently referenced taxonomy of managerial roles is from an in-depth, month-long study of five chief executives by Henry Mintzberg. A taxonomy is a system that groups or classifies principles. Mintzberg's observations led to the identification of three categories of managerial roles: (1) information processing roles, (2) interpersonal roles, and (3) decision-making roles (Mintzberg, 1973). A role includes behaviors, expectations, and recurrent activities within a pattern that is part of the organization's structure (Katz & Kahn, 1978).

The information processing roles identified by Mintzberg (1973) are those of monitor, disseminator, and spokesperson. These roles are used to manage people's information needs. The interpersonal roles consist of figurehead, leader, and liaison, and each of these is used to manage relationships with people. The decision roles are entrepreneur, disturbance handler, allocator of resources, and negotiator. Nurse managers take on these roles when they manage care.

THE MANAGEMENT PROCESS

In the early 1900s, an emphasis on management as a discipline emerged with a focus on the science of management and a view that management is an art of accomplishing things through people (Follet, 1924). Henri Fayol described the functions of planning, organizing, coordinating, and controlling as the **management process** (Fayol, 1916/1949). His work has become a classic in the way that we define the process of managing. Gulick and Urwick (1937) defined the management process according to seven principles. Their principles form the acronym POSDCORB, which stands for planning, organizing, staffing, directing, coordinating (CO), reporting, and budgeting (Gulick & Urwick, 1937; Henry, 1992).

More recently, Yukl (1998) and colleagues (Kim & Yukl, 1995; Yukl, Wall, & Lepsinger, 1990) described 13 managerial role functions for managing the work and for managing relationships. The role functions for managing the work are planning and organizing, problem solving, clarifying roles and objectives, informing, monitoring, consulting, and delegating. The role functions for managing relationships are networking, supporting, developing and mentoring, managing conflict and team building, motivating and inspiring, and recognizing and rewarding.

The amount of time a nurse manager spends in each of these role functions varies by the level of the nurse manager's position in an organization. The staff nurse manager may spend a large part of time both giving care and monitoring a few others as they deliver care, as well as monitoring the outcomes of care given. The next highest percentage of this nurse's time is spent in planning care, with other responsibilities such as coordinating, evaluating, negotiating, and serving as a multispecialist and generalist taking less than 10% each of this nurse's time.

In contrast, the middle-level nurse manager, such as the nurse manager of critical-care nursing, may spend less time in direct care and more time in each of the other functions, particularly planning, monitoring, and coordinating. At the highest level of the organization, usually described as the nurse executive level, planning and being a

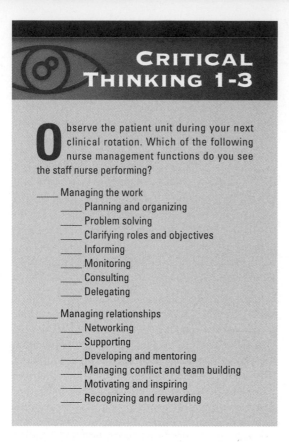

CRITICAL THINKING 1-3

Observe the patient unit during your next clinical rotation. Which of the following nurse management functions do you see the staff nurse performing?

_____ Managing the work
  _____ Planning and organizing
  _____ Problem solving
  _____ Clarifying roles and objectives
  _____ Informing
  _____ Monitoring
  _____ Consulting
  _____ Delegating

_____ Managing relationships
  _____ Networking
  _____ Supporting
  _____ Developing and mentoring
  _____ Managing conflict and team building
  _____ Motivating and inspiring
  _____ Recognizing and rewarding

generalist are a greatly expanded role function, whereas direct patient care monitoring is not as primary a role function as it is in the other two levels. Nurses in executive-level roles in health care organizations often have the title of chief nurse executive or vice president of patient care services.

MANAGER RESOURCES

Nurse managers use four types of resources to accomplish their purpose (DuBrin, 2000). Nurse managers use human resources, such as the right staff on the health care team, to complete various assignments. They use financial resources wisely to help achieve organizational goals. Nurse managers also use physical resources such as patient care equipment to complete their work. Finally, nurse managers use information resources to stay up-to-date in delivering care to their patients.

ORGANIZATIONAL MANAGEMENT PERSPECTIVES

Much of our current understanding of organizational management is based on classical perspectives that were identified in the 1800s during the industrial age as factories developed. Since then many other perspectives have emerged (Shortell & Kaluzny, 2006). See Table 1-3.

MOTIVATION

The human relations perspective in organizational management grew from the conclusion that workers were motivated and their output was greater when the worker was treated humanistically. Motivation is not explicitly demonstrated by people but, rather, is interpreted from their behavior. **Motivation** is whatever influences our choices and creates direction, intensity, and persistence in our behavior (Hughes, Ginnett, & Curphy, 1999; Kanfer, 1990). Motivation is a process that occurs internally to influence and direct our behavior in order to satisfy needs (Lussier, 1999). Motivation theories are not management theories per se; however, they are frequently considered along with management theories (Figure 1-2, Table 1-4, and Figure 1-3).

Motivation theories are useful because they help explain why people act the way they do and how a manager can relate to individuals as people and workers. When you are interested in creating change, influencing others, and managing patient care outcomes, it is helpful to understand the motivations that are reflected in a person's behavior. Motivation is a critical part of leadership because we need to understand each other in order to lead effectively. See Table 1-5 for common motivation problems and potential solutions.

FEEDBACK

Because of their professional socialization and strong achievement needs, nurses are usually motivated to deliver high-quality, excellent care to their patients. However, in order for them to know how well they are doing in this regard, they need

TABLE 1-3	**MAJOR ORGANIZATIONAL MANAGEMENT PERSPECTIVES**
Perspective	**Key Contributions**
Scientific Management Gulick & Urwick (1937) Mooney (1947) Taylor (1947)	Focuses on goals and productivity; organization is a machine to be run efficiently to increase production
	Select the right person to do job; give them proper tools, training, and equipment to work efficiently
	Uses time and motion studies to make the work efficient
Bureaucratic Weber (1964)	Focuses on hierarchical superior-subordinate communication transmitted from top to bottom via a clear chain of command
	Uses rational, impersonal management; activities are distributed among personnel
	Uses merit and skill as basis for promotion/reward
	Uses rules and regulations, focuses on exacting work processes and technical competence
	Limits personal freedom
	Emphasizes career service, salaried managers
Human Relations Argyris (1964) Barnard (1938) Likert (1967) McGregor (1960) Roethlisberger & Dickson (1939)	Focuses on empowerment of the individual worker as the source of control, motivation, and productivity in meeting organization's goals
	Hawthorne's studies at Western Electric plant in Chicago led to the belief that human relations between workers and managers and among workers were main determinants of efficiency
	The Hawthorne effect refers to the phenomena of how being observed or studied results in a change in behavior
	Emphasizes that participatory decision making increases worker autonomy and provides training to improve work
Contingency Burns & Stalker (1961) Lawrence & Lorsch (1967) Perrow (1967) Rundall, et al. (1998) Thompson (1967)	Highlights that organizational structure depends on the environment, task, technology, and the contingencies facing each unit
	Uses flexible approach; emphasizes that there is no one best way to manage work. It encourages managers to study individuals and the situation before adapting efforts and deciding on a course of action to meet the requirements of the situation
Resource Dependence Hickson, Hinings, Lee, Schneck & Pennings (1971) March & Olsen (1976) Pfeffer & Salancik (1978) Strasser (1983) Williamson (1981)	Emphasizes the need to secure necessary resources and provides reliable and valid data on patient care processes and outcomes

(continues)

TABLE 1-3	MAJOR ORGANIZATIONAL MANAGEMENT PERSPECTIVES (CONTINUED)

Perspective	Key Contributions
Strategic Management Andrews (1971) Ansoff (1965) Ouchi (1980) Porter (1980, 1985) Schendel & Hofer (1979) Shortell & Zajac (1990) Luke (2004)	Emphasizes fit or alignment between the organization's strategy, external environment, and internal structure and capabilities Links quality improvement efforts to core strategies and capabilities of the organization to meet organizational needs
Population Ecology Aldrich (1979) Delacroix & Carroll (1983) Hannan & Freeman (1985, 1989) Kimberly & Zajac (1985)	States that external environmental pressures are primary determinant of success. There is little managers and staff can do if action is not tolerable to external environment Highlights powerful role played by the external environment. Quality improvement efforts alone may not be sufficient if the organization is not well positioned for success in the environment
Institutional Alexander & Amburgey (1987) Meyer & Scott (1983) Scott (1987, 1995) Selznik (1966) Fligstein (1990) Powell & DiMaggio (1991) Scott, Ruef, et al. (2000)	States that external norms, rules, and requirements cause organizations to conform in order to receive legitimacy; organizations in a similar institutional environment come to resemble each other Emphasizes that quality improvement efforts must take into account regulatory and accreditation pressures from local, state, and federal agencies and accrediting agencies, such as the Joint Commission (JC), as well as taking into account public expectations
Social Network Uzzi (1997, 1999) Gulati (1995) Nohria & Berkley (1992) Ahuja (2000) Burt (1992)	States that all behavior is social in nature, and that successful organizations will develop and use social networks to their advantage
Complex Adaptive Systems Plsek (2001) Kauffman (1995) Anderson & McDaniel (2000) Begun, Zimmerman, & Dooley (2003) Berwick (1998)	Emphasizes that an organization is a system of interrelated unpredictable elements and if a manager adjusts one part of a system, then other parts will be affected automatically; emphasizes that the organization is an open system that constantly interacts with its environment Encourages staff to look at their activities on one unit as part of a larger picture that may affect other units. Emphasizes importance of innovation and rapid information sharing to improve performance

Source: Compiled with information from Shortell, S. M., & Kaluzny, A. D. (2006). *Health Care Management* (5th ed.). Clifton Park, NY: Delmar Cengage Learning.

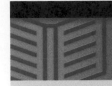

EVIDENCE FROM THE LITERATURE

Citation: Gordon, S. (2006). What do nurses really do? *Topics in Advanced Practice Nursing, 6*(1). Retrieved February 2, 2006 from www.medscape.com/viewarticle/520714.

Discussion: In this article by Suzanne Gordon, a journalist and author who writes about nursing, nurses are called upon to do a better job of accurately describing what nurses do and how they use expert knowledge acquired through scientific and technical mastery. She says, "What do nurses do? They save lives, prevent complications, prevent suffering, and save money." Her message to nurses is that there is a reason that the public has such little understanding of nursing and the importance of our work. The reason is twofold: traditional stereotypes about nursing cloud the reality of nursing as it is currently practiced, and nurses have been patterned to describe their contribution to health care in self-sacrificing and anonymous ways.

Implications for Practice: Nurses need to be clear about why it is important for the public to know what and how nurses contribute to health care. This article is an important vehicle from which nurses can begin to examine their own words and ways of discussing what nurses do and reflect upon the historical, religious, and societal practices that interfere with a clear, accurate, and realistic image of modern nursing. What nurses often think of as their ordinary work is really quite extraordinary. Nurses use scientific knowledge, expert judgment, and complex skills to make critical decisions that affect patient outcomes. Nurses need to be able to articulate how they do their work and the difference it makes.

high-quality information systems that provide feedback on a frequent basis. Such a system allows health care professionals to know not only how well they are doing, but also to enhance their confidence that they are doing things right (Kongstvedt, 2002).

Feedback can be a powerful tool to assist managers in motivating behavior; however, there are several factors that should be considered to maximize feedback effectiveness. First, for feedback to have value, nurses must truly see that their behavior needs to change. Second, feedback needs to be frequent, timely, and given at precise time intervals to sustain new behaviors. Third, feedback must be usable, consistent, correct, and of sufficient diversity. It should contain various important patient care, staffing, utilization, financial, and quality-related measures. Otherwise, behavior problems can intensify as rewards flow to improvements based on flawed feedback data (Charns & Smith Tewksbury, 1993). Last, managers should not portray the feedback as "good" or "bad." Professional nurses are knowledge workers and

know when they have missed the goal (Shortell & Kaluzny, 2006).

BENNER'S MODEL OF NOVICE TO EXPERT

Benner's (1984) model of novice to expert provides a framework that can facilitate professional development of nursing leadership and management by building on the skill sets and experience of each practitioner. Benner's model acknowledges that there are tasks, competencies, and outcomes that practitioners can be expected to have acquired based on five levels of experience. Note that the ten year rule states that it takes a decade of heavy labor to master any field (Ross, 2006).

Benner's model of novice to expert is based on the Dreyfus and Dreyfus (1980) model of skill acquisition applied to nursing. There are five stages of Benner's model: novice, advanced beginner, competent, proficient, and expert. See Table 1-6.

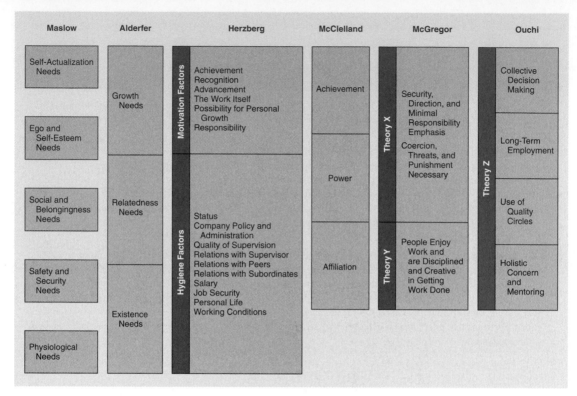

Figure 1-2 Selected theories of motivation. (*Source:* Compiled with this information from Shortell, S. M., & Kaluzny, A. D. [2006]. *Health Care Management* [5th ed.]. Clifton Park, NY: Delmar Cengage Learning; and Leadership and Management by L. S. Leach, from Kelly, P. L. [2008]. *Nursing Leadership & Management* [2nd ed.]. Clifton Park, NY: Delmar Cengage Learning).

TABLE 1-4	SELECTED MOTIVATION THEORIES

Main Contributors	Key Aspects
Abraham Maslow (1970) Hierarchy of Needs Theory	Motivation occurs when needs are not met. Certain needs have to be satisfied first, beginning with physiological needs, then safety and security, then social needs, followed by self-esteem needs and then self-actualization needs. Needs at one level must be satisfied before one is motivated by needs at the next higher level. See Figure 1-3.
Frederick Herzberg (1968) Two-Factor Theory	Hygiene maintenance factors include adequate salary, quality supervision, job security, safe and tolerable working conditions and relationships with others. When these factors are absent, people are dissatisfied; when they are present, job dissatisfaction can be avoided. However, these factors alone will not motivate people and lead to job satisfaction.

(continues)

TABLE 1-4	SELECTED MOTIVATION THEORIES (CONTINUED)
	Motivation factors include satisfying and meaningful work, development and advancement opportunities, responsibility, and recognition. When these factors are present, people are motivated and satisfied with the job. When they are absent, people have a neutral attitude about the job and the organization.
Douglas McGregor (1960) Theory X	Theory X: Leaders must direct and control, as motivation results from reward and punishment. Employees prefer security, direction, and minimal responsibility, and need coercion and threats to get the job done.
Theory Y	Theory Y: Leaders must remove work obstacles, as workers have self-control and self-discipline; the workers' reward is their involvement in work and their opportunity to be creative.
William Ouchi (1981) Theory Z	Theory Z: Collective decision making, long-term employment, mentoring, holistic concern, and use of quality circles to manage service and quality are encouraged; this is a humanistic style of motivation based on Japanese organizations.

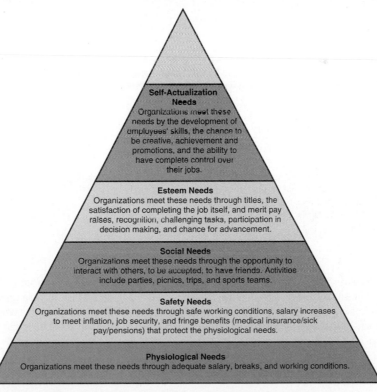

Figure 1-3 How organizations motivate with hierarchy of needs theory. (*Source:* From Lussier, R. N., & Achua, C. F. [2000]. *Leadership: Theory, Application, Skill Development* [p. 81]. Cincinnati, OH: South-Western College Publishing).

TABLE 1-5	COMMON EMPLOYEE MOTIVATION PROBLEMS AND POTENTIAL SOLUTIONS

Motivational Problems

1. Inadequate performance definition, such as lack of goals, inadequate job descriptions, inadequate performance standards, inadequate performance assessment

2. Impediments to performance, such as bureaucratic or environmental obstacles, inadequate support or resources, poor employee-job matching, inadequate job information

3. Inadequate performance-reward linkages, such as inappropriate or inadequate job rewards, poor timing of rewards, low probability of receiving rewards, inequity in distribution of rewards

Potential Solutions

– Well-defined job descriptions

– Well-defined performance standards

– Goal setting

– Feedback on performance

– Enhanced hygiene factors, such as safe and clean environment, good salary and fringe benefits, job security, good staffing, time off job, good equipment

– Pay for performance

– Increased employee involvement and participation, professional development opportunities, job autonomy, modified work schedule, recognition, praise or awards, opportunity to display skills or talents, opportunity to mentor or train others, promotions in rank or position, improved information concerning organization or department

Source: Compiled with information from Shortell, S. M., & Kaluzny, A. D. (2006). *Health Care Management* (5th ed.). Clifton Park, NY: Delmar Cengage Learning.

TABLE 1-6	BENNER'S MODEL OF NOVICE TO EXPERT

Novice

Novice nurses have no experience with situations in which they are expected to perform. They see nursing as a series of tasks with specific rules. The novice tends to rigidly follow these rules to complete tasks rather than using their judgment to apply the rules with discretion. Novice nurses work on handling pieces of the situation rather than focusing on handling the whole situation in the best way to meet patient needs.

(continues)

TABLE 1-6	BENNER'S MODEL OF NOVICE TO EXPERT (CONTINUED)

Advanced Beginner

Advanced beginner nurses have a little more experience and they demonstrate marginally acceptable performance. They may have coped with enough real situations to note, or to have pointed out to them by a mentor, the important components of a situation. These important components require prior experience in actual situations for recognition. The advanced beginner nurse uses principles based on their experience to guide their actions. They still need help setting priorities.

Competent

Competent nurses have been on the job in the same or similar situation for two or three years. Competence develops when the nurse begins to see his or her actions as part of long-range goals or plans. The conscious deliberate planning and critical thinking that is characteristic of this skill level helps the competent nurse achieve efficiency and organization. The competent nurse lacks the speed and flexibility of the proficient nurse but the competent nurse does have a feeling of mastery and the ability to prioritize and manage the many aspects of clinical nursing.

Proficient

Proficient nurses have a deep understanding of situations as a whole rather than seeing things as a series of tasks. The proficient nurse has learned from experience what typical events to expect in a given situation and how they need to modify their plans in response to these events. The proficient nurse can recognize when an expected situation does not materialize. This recognition improves the proficient nurse's decision making. Decision making becomes less labored because the proficient nurse quickly sees what is most important in a situation.

Expert

Expert nurses intuitively know what is going on with their patients. The expert nurse no longer relies on rules or guidelines. The expert nurse, with an enormous background of experience, has an intuitive grasp of each situation and zeroes in on the problem without wasteful consideration of a large range of unfruitful, alternative diagnoses and solutions. The expert nurse's performance is flexible and highly proficient. The expert uses their analytic ability in those situations where they have had no previous experience. If they get a wrong grasp of the situation and then find that events and behaviors are not occurring as expected, they can change course quickly. The expert nurse can also visualize what is possible in the future.

Source: Compiled with information from Benner, P. (1984). *From Novice to Expert.* Menlo Park, CA: Addison Wesley.

KEY CONCEPTS

- Nurses are leaders and make a difference to health care organizations through their contributions of expert knowledge and leadership. Leadership development is a necessary component of preparation as a health care provider.

- Leadership is a process of influence in which the leader influences others toward goal achievement. Leadership can be formal or informal.

- Leadership and management are different.

- Leadership styles are described as autocratic, democratic, and laissez-faire and have been studied by examining job-centered or task-oriented approaches as well as employee-centered or relationship-oriented approaches.

- Blake and Mouton's leadership model has five styles to address high or low people concerns and high or low production concerns.

- Contingency theories of leadership acknowledge that other factors in the environment in addition to the leader's behavior affect the leader's effectiveness.

- Substitutes for leadership are variables that eliminate the need for leadership or nullify the effect of the leader's behavior.

- Charismatic leadership theory describes leader behavior that displays self-confidence, passion, and communication of high expectations and confidence in others. This type of leader often emerges in a crisis with a vision, has an appeal based on personal power, and often uses unconventional strategies and emotional connections to succeed.

- Transformational leadership theory identifies two types of leaders, i.e., the transformational leader and the transactional leader.

- Nursing leadership in the future will be needed at all levels within an organization, not just at the top. Knowledge workers, with specialized knowledge and expertise are both leaders and followers in knowledge organizations.

- Organizations are self-organizing systems in which, initially, what looks like chaos and uncertainty is indeed part of a larger coherence and natural order.

- Future directions for nursing knowledge workers in organizations will continue to be influenced by technology and by the notions of mobility, virtuality, and user-driven practices.

- Management is a process used to achieve organizational goals. It involves the management functions of planning, organizing and staffing, leading, and controlling actions to achieve goals.

- Management roles are classified as the information processing role, the interpersonal role, and the decision-making role.

- Managers use human, financial, physical, and information resources to achieve goals.

- Motivation is whatever influences our choices and creates direction, intensity, and persistence in our behavior.

- Benner's model of novice to expert identifies five stages of nursing experience. The ten year rule states that it takes a decade of heavy labor to master any field.

KEY TERMS

autocratic leadership

consideration

contingency theory

democratic leadership

emotional intelligence

employee-centered leadership

formal leadership

Hawthorne effect

informal leader

initiating structure

job-centered leaders

knowledge workers

laissez-faire leadership

leadership

management

motivation

novice to expert model

nursing-sensitive patient outcomes

role

transactional leader

transformational leader

REVIEW QUESTIONS

1. Why is leadership important for nurses if they are not in a management position?
   A. It is not really important for nurses.
   B. Leadership is important at all levels in an organization because nurses have expert knowledge and are interacting with and influencing others.
   C. Nurse leaders leave their jobs sooner for other positions.
   D. Nurses who lead are less satisfied in their jobs.

2. Leadership is defined as
   A. being in a leadership position with authority to exert control and power over subordinates.
   B. a process of interaction in which the leader influences others toward goal achievement.
   C. managing complexity.
   D. being self-confident and democratic.

3. Management as a process that is used today by nurses in health care organizations is best described as
   A. scientific management.
   B. decision making.
   C. commanding and controlling others using hierarchical authority.
   D. planning, organizing, staffing, leading, and controlling actions to achieve goals.

4. Motivation is whatever influences our choices. What motivation factors did Herzberg say would lead to job satisfaction?
   A. Being offered a substantial bonus when being hired
   B. Realizing that no one ever gets fired from the organization and that job security is high
   C. Having good relationships with colleagues and supervisors
   D. Being offered opportunities for achievement and advancement

REVIEW ACTIVITIES

1. Take the opportunity to learn about yourself by reflecting on five predominant factors identified as being influential in a nurse's leadership development: self-confidence, innate leader qualities/tendencies, progression of experiences and success, influence of significant others, and personal life factors. Consider what reinforces your confidence in yourself. What innate qualities or traits do you have that contribute to your development as a nurse leader? Consider what professional experiences, mentors, and personal experiences or events can help you develop your leadership ability. How can you obtain these experiences?

2. Describe the type of manager you want to be as a staff nurse in a health care organization. Identify specific behaviors you plan to use to manage a patient's care. How will you plan, organize and staff, lead, and control patient care? In what way can transformational leadership theory help you develop your role?

3. Rate each of these 12 job factors that contribute to job satisfaction by placing a number from 1 to 5 on the line before each factor.

Very important		Somewhat important		Not important
5	4	3	2	1

_____ 1. An interesting job I enjoy doing

_____ 2. A good manager who treats people fairly

_____ 3. Getting praise and other recognition and appreciation for the work I do

_____ 4. A satisfying personal life at the job

_____ 5. The opportunity for advancement

_____ 6. A prestigious or status job

_____ 7. Job responsibility that gives me freedom to do things my way

_____ 8. Good working conditions (safe environment, nice office, cafeteria)

_____ 9. The opportunity to learn new things

_____ 10. Sensible company rules, regulations, procedures, and policies

_____ 11. A job I can do well and succeed at

_____ 12. Job security and benefits

Write the number from 1 to 5 that you selected for each factor in the appropriate column below. Total each column below for a score between 6 and 30 points. The closer to 30 your score is in each column below, the more important the factor (motivating or maintenance) is to you.

Motivating factors		Maintenance factors	
1. _____		2. _____	
3. _____		4. _____	
5. _____		6. _____	
7. _____		8. _____	
9. _____		10. _____	
11. _____		12. _____	
Totals _____		_____	

From _Leadership: Theory, Application, Skill Development_ (pp. 15–16), by R. N. Lussier and C. F. Achua, 2000, Cincinnati, OH: South-Western College Publishing.

4. How does nursing leadership & management ensure quality patient care in an emergency?

5. What leadership projects are nurses in your work setting involved in? How is information about patient quality being used to improve nursing practice? What sources of evidence from nursing science are you exploring through reading journals, attending educational conferences, using the Internet, and participating in professional nursing associations?

EXPLORING THE WEB

Search the Web, checking the following sites.

- Emerging Leader:
  www.emergingleader.com
- Leadership Directories: Who's who in the leadership of the United States:
  www.leadershipdirectories.com
  Search for nursing leaders.
- Health Leadership Associates:
  www.healthleadership.com
- LeaderValues:
  www.leader-values.com
- Don Clark's Big Dog Leadership:
  www.nwlink.com/~Donclark
- American Association of Critical-Care Nurses' Standards for Establishing and Sustaining Healthy Work Environments:
  www.aacn.org
  Click *Healthy Work Environments* under clinical practice.

- American Organization of Nurse Executives Competencies:
  www.aone.org
  Click *Resources*, and then click *AONE Nurse Exec Competencies*.
- Analyze My Career:
  analyzemycareer.com
- American Nurses Association Magnet Status Hospitals:
  www.nursingworld.org
  Search for ANCC.
- Classic management functions:
  www.1000ventures.com
  Review your character and personality, and click on other areas of interest.
- Nursing leaders:
  www.google.com
  Search for nursing leader profiles.

REFERENCES

Ahuja. G. (2000). Collaboration networks, structural holes, and innovation: A longitudinal study. *Administrative Science Quarterly, 45*(3), 425–455.

Aiken, L. H., Clarke, S. P., Sloane, D. M., Sochalski, J., & Silber, J. H. (2002). Hospital nurse staffing, patient mortality, nurse burnout, and job dissatisfaction. *Journal of American Medical Association, 288*(16), 1987–1993.

Aldrich, H. (1979). *Organizations and environments.* Englewood Cliffs, NJ: Princeton Hills.

Alexander, J. A., & Amburgey, T. L. (1987). The dynamics of change in the American hospital industry: Transformation or selection? *Medical Care Review, 44,* 279–321.

American Association of Critical Care Nurses (AACN). (2003). Written testimony to the IOM Committee on work environment of nurses and patient safety. Retrieved February 15, 2007, from www.aacn.org.

American Association of Critical Care Nurses (AACN). (2004). AACN standards for establishing and sustaining healthy work environments: A journey to excellence. Retrieved February 15, 2007, from www.aacn.org/aacn/hwe.nsf/vwdoc/HWEHomePage.

Anderson, R. & McDaniel, R. (2000). Managing health care organizations: Where professionalism meets complexity science. *Health Care Management Review 25*(1), 83–92.

Andrews, K. R. (1971). *The concept of corporate strategy.* Homewood, IL: Dow Jones-Irwin.

Ansoff, H. I. (1965). *Corporate strategy: An analytic approach to business policy for growth and expansion.* New York: McGraw-Hill.

Argyris, C. (1964). *Integrating the individual and the organization.* Hoboken, NJ: Wiley.

Barker, A. (1990). *Transformational nursing leadership: A vision for the future*. Baltimore: Williams & Wilkins.

Barnard, C. (1938). *The functions of the executive*. Boston: Harvard University Press.

Bass, B. (1985). *Leadership and performance beyond expectations*. New York: Free Press.

Begun, J. W., Zimmerman, B., & Dooley, K. J. (2003). Health care organizations as complex adaptive systems. In S. Mick & M. Wyttenbach (Eds.), *Advances in Health Care Organization Theory*, (pp. 253–288). San Francisco: Jossey-Bass.

Benner, P. (1984). *From novice to expert*. Menlo Park, CA: Addison Wesley.

Bennis, W., & Nanus, B. (1985). *Leaders: The strategies for taking charge*. New York: Harper & Row.

Bennis, W., Spreitzer, G.M. & Cummings, T.G. (2001). *The future of leadership*. San Francisco: Jossey-Bass.

Berwick, D. M. (1998). Develop and testing changes in delivery of care. *Annals of Internal Medicine*, *128*(8), 651–656.

Blake, R. R., & Mouton, J. S. (1985). The managerial grid III. Houston, TX: Gulf.

Burns, J. M. (1978). *Leadership*. New York: Harper & Row.

Burns, T., & Stalker, G. M. (1961). *The management of innovation*. London: Tavistock.

Burt, R. S. (1992). *Structural holes: The social structure of competition*. Cambridge, MA: Harvard University Press.

Cassidy, V., & Koroll, C. (1998). Ethical aspects of transformational leadership. In E. Hein (Ed.), *Contemporary leadership behavior*.

Charns, M., & Smith Tewksbury, L. (1993). *Collaborative management in health care*, San Francisco: Jossey-Bass.

Conger, J., & Kanungo, R. (1987). Toward a behavioral theory of charismatic leadership in organizational settings. *Academy of Management Review, 12*, 637–647.

Delacroix, J., & Carroll. G. R. (1983). Organizational foundings: An ecological study of newspaper industries of Argentina and Ireland. *Administrative Sciences Quarterly, 28*, 274–291.

Drath, W. H., & Palus, C. J. (1994). Making common sense: Leadership as meaning-making in a community of practice. Retrieved 2004 from www.ebookmall.com.

Dreyfus, S. E., & Dreyfus, H. L. (1980). *A five stage model of the mental activities involved in direct skill acquisition*. Unpublished report supported by the Air Force Office of Scientific Research USAF (Contract F49620-79-C-0063). University of California at Berkeley.

Drucker, P. F. (1994). *The post-capitalist society*. New York: Harper & Row.

DuBrin, A. J. (2000). *The Active Manager*. Cincinnati, OH: South-Western College Publishing.

Dunham-Taylor, J. (2000). Nurse executive transformational leadership found in participative organizations. *Journal of Nursing Administration, 30*(5), 241–250.

Fayol, H. (1916/1949). (C. Storrs, Trans.). General and industrial management. London: Pitman.

Fielder, F. (1967). *A theory of leadership effectiveness*. New York: McGraw-Hill.

Fligstein. N. (1990). *The transformation of corporate control*. Cambridge, MA: Harvard University Press.

Follet, M. (1924). Creative experience. London: Longmans, Green.

Goleman, D. (1998). Working with emotional intelligence. New York: Bantam Books.

Gordon, S. (2006). What do nurses really do? *Topics in Advanced Practice Nursing, 6*(1). Retrieved February 2, 2006, from www.medscape.com/viewarticle/520714.

Grossman, S., & Valiga, T. M. (2008) *The New Leadership Challenge: Creating the future of Nursing*. Philadelphia: F.A. Davis.

Gulati, R. (1995). Does familiarity breed trust? The implications of repeated ties for contractual choice in alliances. *Academy of Management Journal, 38*, 85–112.

Gulick, L., & Urwick, L. (Eds.). (1937). *Papers on the science of administration*. New York: Institute of Public Administration.

Hales, C. P. (1986). What managers do: A critical review of the evidence. *Journal of Management Studies, 23*, 88–115.

Hannan, M. T., & Freeman, J. H. (1985, Apr.). Structural inertia and organizational change. *American Sociological Review, 49*, 149–164.

Hannan, M. T., & Freeman, J. H. (1989). *Organizational ecology.* Cambridge, MA: Harvard University Press.

Heath, J., Johanson, W., & Blake, N. (2004). Healthy work environments: A validation of the literature. *Journal of Nursing Administration, 34*(11), 524–530.

Helgesen, S. (1995). The web of inclusion: A new architecture for building organizations. New York: Doubleday Currency.

Henry, N. (1992). Public administration and public affairs (5th ed.). Englewood Cliffs, NJ: Prentice Hall.

Hersey, P., & Blanchard, K. (2000). *Management of organizational behavior* (8th ed.). Englewood Cliffs, NJ: Prentice Hall.

Herzberg, F. (1968, January/February*). One more time: How do you motivate employees?* Harvard Business Review, 53–62.

Hickson, D. J., Hinings, C. R., Lee, C. A., Schneck, R. E., & Pennings, J. M. (1971). A strategic contingencies theory of intraorganizational power. *Administrative Science Quarterly, 16,* 216–229.

House, R. H. (1971). A path-goal theory of leader effectiveness. *Administrative Science Quarterly, 16,* 321–338.

Hughes, R. L., Ginnett, R. C., & Curphy, G. J. (1999). *Leadership: Enhancing the lessons of experience* (3rd ed.). San Francisco: Irwin McGraw-Hill.

Institute of Medicine (IOM) (2003). *Health professions education: A bridge to quality.* Washington, DC: The National Academies Press.

Kanfer, R. (1990). Motivation theory in industrial and organizational psychology. In M. D. Dunnette & L. M. Hough (Eds.), *Handbook of industrial and organizational psychology: Vol. 1* (pp. 53–68). Palo Alto, CA: Consulting Psychologists Press.

Katz, D., & Kahn, R. L. (1978). *The social psychology of organizations* (2nd ed.). New York: John Wiley.

Kauffman, S. A. (1995). *At home in the universe.* Oxford, England: Oxford University Press.

Kelly, P. (2008). Nursing leadership (2nd ed.). Clifton Park, NY: Delmar Cengage Learning.

Kerr, S., & Jermier, J. (1978). Substitutes for leadership: Their meaning and measurement. *Organizational Behavior and Human Performance, 22,* 374–403.

Kim, H., & Yukl, G. (1995). Relationships of self-reported and subordinate-reported leadership behaviors to managerial effectiveness and advancement. *Leadership Quarterly, 6,* 361–377.

Kimberly, J. R., & Zajac, E. J. (1985). Strategic adaptation in health care organizations: Implications for theory and research. *Medical Care Review, 42,* 267–302.

Kirkpatrick, S. A., & Locke, E. A. (1991). Leadership: Do traits matter? *The Executive, 5,* 48–60.

Kongstvedt, P.R. (2002). *Managed care: What it is and how it works.* Gaithersburg, MD: Aspen Publishers.

Kotter, J. (1990a). *A force for change: How leadership differs from management.* Glencoe, IL: Free Press.

Kotter, J. (1990b). What leaders really do. *Harvard Business Review, 68,* 104.

Kramer, M. (1990). The magnet hospitals: Excellence revisited. *Journal of Nursing Administration, 20*(9), 35–44.

Kramer, M., & Schmalenberg, C. E. (2005, July–Sep.). Best quality patient care: A historical perspective on Magnet hospitals. *Nursing Administration Quarterly, 29*(3), 275–287.

Lawrence, P., & Lorsch, J. (1967). *Organization and environment.* Cambridge, MA: Harvard University Press.

Leach, L. S. (2005). Nurse executive leadership and organizational commitment among nurses. *Journal of Nursing Administration, 35*(5), 228–238.

Lewin, K. (1939). Field theory and experiment in social psychology: Concepts and methods. *Journal of Sociology, 44,* 868–896.

Lewin, K., & Lippitt, R. (1938). An experimental approach to the study of autocracy and democracy: A preliminary note. *Sociometry, 1,* 292–300.

Lewin, K., Lippitt, R., & White, R. (1939). Patterns of aggressive behavior in experimentally created social climates. *Journal of Social Psychology, 10,* 271–299.

Likert, E. (1967). *The human organization.* New York: McGraw-Hill.

Luke, R. (2004). *Health care strategy.* Chicago, IL: HAP/AUPHA.

Lussier, R. N. (1999). *Human relations in organizations: Applications and skill building* (4th ed.). San Francisco: Irwin McGraw-Hill.

Lussier, R. N., & Achua, C. F. (2000). *Leadership: Theory, application, skill development.* Cincinnati, OH: South-Western College Publishing.

March, J. G., & Olsen, J. P. (1976). *Ambiguity and choice in organizations.* Bergen. Norway: Univeristetsforlaget.

Maslow, A. (1970). *Motivation and personality* (2nd ed.). New York: Harper & Row.

McCall, M. W., Jr. (1998). *High flyers: Developing the next generation of leaders.* Boston: Harvard Business School Press.

McCall, M. W., Jr., Morrison, A. M., & Hanman, R. L. (1978). *Studies of managerial work: Results and methods* (Tech. Rep.). Greensboro, NC: Center for Creative Leadership.

McClure, M., & Hinshaw, A. (Eds.) (2002). *Magnet hospitals revisited.* Washington, DC: American Nurses Publishing.

McClure, M., Poulin, M., Sovie, M., & Wandelt, M. (1983). *Magnet hospitals: Attraction and retention of professional nurses.* Kansas City, MO: American Nurses Association.

McDaniel, C., & Wolf, G. (1992). Transformational leadership in nursing service. *Journal of Nursing Administration, 12*(4), 204–207.

McGregor, D. (1960). *The human side of enterprise.* New York: McGraw-Hill.

McNeese-Smith, D. (1997). The influences of manager behavior on nurses' job satisfaction, productivity, and commitment. *Journal of Nursing Administration, 27*(9), 47–55.

Meyer, J. W. & Scott, W. R. (1983). *Organizational environments: Ritual and rationality.* Beverly Hills, CA: Sage.

Mintzberg, H. (1973). *The nature of managerial work.* New York: Harper & Row.

Mooney, J. D. (1947). *Principles of organization.* New York: Harper & Row.

Moorhead, G., & Griffin, R. W. (2001). *Organizational behavior: Managing people in organizations* (6th ed.). Boston: Houghton Mifflin.

Murphy, M., & DeBack, V. (1991). Today's nursing leaders: Creating the vision. *Nursing Administration Quarterly, 16*(1), 71–80.

Nohria, N., & Berkley, J. D. (1992). The virtual organization: Bureaucracy, technology and the imposition of control. In C. Heckseher & A. Donnellon (Eds.). *The post bureaucratic organization: New perspectives on organizational change* (pp. 32–47). Thousand Oaks, CA: Sage Publications.

Northouse, P. (2001). *Leadership: Theory and practice* (2nd ed.). Thousand Oaks, CA: Sage.

Ouchi, W. G. (1980). Markets, bureaucracies, and clans. *Administrative Science Quarterly, 24,* 129–141.

Ouchi, W. G. (1981). *Theory Z: How American business can meet the Japanese challenge.* Reading, MA: Addison-Wesley.

Perrow, C. (1967). A framework for the comparative analysis of organizations. *American Sociological Review, 32,* 194–208.

Pfeffer, J., & Salancik, G. R. (1978). *The external control of organizations.* New York: Harper & Row.

Plsek, P. (2001). Redesigning health care with insights from the science of complex adaptive systems. In *Crossing the quality chasm: A new health system for the 21st century* (pp. 309–322), Washington DC: National Academy Press.

Porter O'Grady, T. (2001). Profound change: 21st century nursing. *Nursing Outlook, 41*(1), 182–186.

Porter, M. E. (1985). *Competitive advantage: Creating and sustaining superior performance.* New York: Free Press.

Porter. M. E. (1980). *Competitive strategy: Techniques for analyzing industries and competitors.* New York: Free Press.

Powell, W. W., & DiMaggio. P. J. (Eds.). (1991). *The new institutionalism in organizational analysis.* Chicago: University of Chicago Press.

Pruitt, B., & Jacobs, M. (2006). *Best practice interventions: Learn how you can prevent ventilator-associated pneumonia.* Nursing, 36(2), 36-42.

Roethlisberger, J. F., & Dickson, W. J. (1939). *Management and the worker.* Cambridge, MA: Harvard University Press.

Ross, P. E. (August, 2006). The expert mind, *The Scientific American, 8,* 64–71.

Rundall,T., Starkweather, D., & Norrish, B. (1998). *After restructuring: Empowerment strategies at work in America's hospitals.* San Francisco: Jossey-Bass, Inc.

Schendel. D. E., & Hofer, C. W. (1979). *Strategic management: A new view of business policy and planning.* Boston: Little, Brown.

Scott, J. G., Sochalski, J., & Aiken, L. (1999). Review of magnet hospital research: Findings and implications for professional nursing practice. *Journal of Nursing Administration, 29*(1), 9–19.

Scott, W. R. (1987). The adolescence of institutional theory: Problems and potential for organizational analysis. *Administrative Science Quarterly, 32,* 493–512.

Scott, W. R. (1995). *Institutions and organizations.* Thousand Oaks. CA: Sage Publications.

Scott, W. R., Ruef, M., et al. (2000). *Institutional change and healthcare organizations: From professional dominance to managed care.* Chicago, IL: Chicago University Press.

Searle, L. (1996, Jan.). 21st century leadership for nurse administrators. *Aspen's advisor for nurse executives, 11*(4), 1, 4–6.

Selznick, P. (1966). *TVA and the grass roots.* New York: Harper & Row.

Shortell, S. M., & Kaluzny, A. D. (2006). *Health Care Management* (5th ed.). Clifton Park, NY: Delmar Cengage Learning.

Shortell, S. M., & Zajac, E. J. (1990). Health care organizations and the development of the strategic management perspective. In S. S. Mick and Associates, *Innovations in health care delivery: Insights for organization theory* (pp. 144–180). Ann Arbor, MI: Health Administration Press.

Stodgill, R. M. (1948). Personal factors associated with leadership: A survey of the literature. *Journal of Psychology, 25,* 35–71.

Stodgill, R. M. (1974). *Handbook of leadership: A survey of theory and research.* New York: Free Press.

Strasser, S. (1983, winter). The effective application of contingency theory in health settings: Problems and recommended solutions. *Health Care Management Review,* 15–23.

Taylor, F. (1947). *Scientific management.* New York: Harper & Row.

Thompson, J. D. (1967). *Organization in action.* New York: McGraw-Hill.

Tichy, N., & Devanna, D. (1986). *Transformational leadership.* New York: Wiley.

Upenieks, V. (2003). Nurse leaders' perceptions of what comprises successful leadership in today's acute inpatient environment. *Nursing Administration Quarterly, 27*(2), 140–152.

Uzzi, B. (1997). Social structure and competition in interfirm networks: The paradox of embeddedness. *Administrative Science Quarterly, 42*(1), 35–67.

Uzzi, B. (1999). Embeddedness in the making of financial capital: How social relations and networks benefit firms seeking financing. *American Sociological Review, 64,* 481–505.

Weber, M. (1964). *The theory of social and economic organization.* Glencoe, IL: Free Press.

Wheatley, M. J. (1999). *Leadership and the new science: Learning about organization from an orderly universe.* San Francisco: Berrett-Koehler.

Wheatley, M. J. (2005). *Finding our way: Leadership for an uncertain time.* San Francisco, CA: Berrett-Koehler Publishers.

Williamson. O. E. (1981).The economies of organization: The transaction cost approach. *The American Journal of Sociology, 87,* 548–577.

Wolf, G., Boland, S., & Aukerman, M. (1994). A transformational model for the practice of professional nursing. Part 1. *Journal of Nursing Administration, 24*(4), 51–57.

Young, S. (1992). Educational experiences of transformational nurse leaders. *Nursing Administration Quarterly, 17*(1), 25–33.

Yukl, G. (1998). *Leadership in organizations* (4th ed.). Upper Saddle River, NJ: Prentice Hall.

Yukl, G., Wall, S., & Lepsinger, R. (1990). Preliminary report on validation of the managerial practices survey. In K. E. Clarke & M. B. Clark (Eds.), *Measures of leadership* (pp. 223–238). West Orange, NJ: Leadership Library of America.

SUGGESTED READINGS

Cummings, G., Lee, H., Macgregor, T., Davey, M., Wong, C., Paul, L., & Stafford, E. (2008). Retrieved from: www.ncbi.nlm.nih.gov/pubmed/18806183?ordinalpos=24&itool=EntrezSystem2.PEntrez.Pubmed.Pubmed_ResultsPanel.Pubmed_DefaultReportPanel.Pubmed_RVDocSum. Factors contributing to nursing leadership: a systematic review. *Journal of Health Services Research Policy, 13*(4), 240–8.

Davenport, T. H. (2005). *Thinking for a living: How to get better performances and results from knowledge workers.* Cambridge, MA: Harvard School Press.

Donley, R. (2005). *Reflecting on 30 years of nursing leadership: 1975–2005.* Indianapolis, IN: Sigma Theta Tau International.

Houser, B., & Player, K. (2004). *Pivotal moments in nursing: Leaders who changed the path of a profession.* Indianapolis, IN: Sigma Theta Tau International.

Hyrkäs, K., & Dende, D. (2008). Retrieved from: www.ncbi.nlm.nih.gov/pubmed/18558919?ordinalpos=35&itool=EntrezSystem2.PEntrez.Pubmed.Pubmed_ResultsPanel.Pubmed_DefaultReportPanel.Pubmed_RVDocSum. Clinical nursing leadership—perspectives on current topics. *Journal of Nursing Management, 16*(5), 495–8.

Institute of Medicine Committee on the Work Environment for Nurses and Patient Safety. (2004). *Keeping patients safe: Transforming the work environment of nurses.* Washington, DC: The National Academies Press.

CHAPTER 2

The Health Care Environment

Consumers can guess the price of a Honda Accord within $1,000 of the cost, but they're off by $12,000 for a four-day hospital stay.

(Great-West Health Care, 2006)

OBJECTIVES

Upon completion of this chapter, the reader should be able to:

1. Discuss the history and current influences on U.S. health care.
2. Describe how the American health care system is organized and financed.
3. Critique the quality of American health care as compared to other industrialized countries.
4. Describe the role of the nurse and other stakeholders in the health care system.
5. Discuss health care disparities that affect how people are advantaged or disadvantaged in accessing the health care system and the outcomes they experience as a result.

Janice, a 32-year-old woman, lives with her 31-year-old husband and two children, ages 8 and 10. Janice is employed as a nursing assistive personnel in a long-term care facility. Her husband is recently unemployed, having been forced to quit his part-time job due to an exacerbation of his multiple sclerosis (MS). Janice is overweight and is coping with Type II diabetes and hypertension. She cannot afford the health care insurance plan offered by her employer. After paying for housing, groceries, utilities, car, gasoline, heating fuel, clothing, and school supplies, Janice says there is little left to pay the approximately $200 a month for her employer's health insurance plan. Instead, she and her family obtain health care as they need it through a free clinic in their community, where they also purchase their medications at a reduced cost. Janice says she often cuts back on her meds to make them last longer. She says her husband quit smoking when he was diagnosed with MS about two years ago, but she is concerned that he might start smoking again because of the stress of the family's financial situation.

With no insurance, what outcome can Janice and her family anticipate?

What stories could you add to this one describing the difficulties your patients experience with the U.S. health care system?

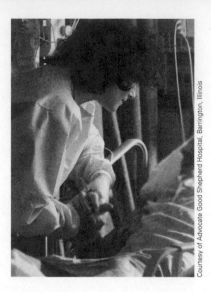

Courtesy of Advocate Good Shepherd Hospital, Barrington, Illinois

Over 300 million Americans depend on the U.S health care system to assist them in improving or maintaining their health. The high costs of this health care system presents obstacles for a growing number of Americans who lack access to what is otherwise a superior system (National Coalition on Health Care [NCHC], 2008a). Because of these high costs, 47 million Americans under the age of 65 lack access to health care because they do not have any form of health insurance (NCHC, 2008a).

Countries such as France, Canada, Japan, Germany, and the United Kingdom provide Universal Health Care (UHC) programs to their citizens. In these countries, per capita spending is considerably less than in the U.S., yet health care outcomes for such things as infant mortality, immunization rates, and life expectancy in the U.S. are poorer by comparison (Nolte & McKee, 2008).

Throughout the history of the U.S., efforts to implement a UHC program have been resisted, with costly social and economic consequences. Americans who lack health coverage are not likely to benefit from the care needed for health promotion, illness prevention, early detection, and health restoration programs. To avoid the financial burden of health care costs, Americans who lack health insurance often delay obtaining care. Their contact with the health care system is episodic and usually in acute care settings. Even after their symptoms have progressed and are well-advanced, uninsured Americans are more likely to obtain only irregular, sporadic care. This means that they lack consistent care from a health care provider whom they see regularly, whether for health promotion, illness prevention, or treatment. Inability to pay for recommended treatments and medications also compromises their adherence to health care recommendations, which in turn affects their recovery. A cascading effect then occurs, with soaring costs and progressively worsening health outcomes. A growing number of working Americans is affected by this dilemma, putting health for all into sharp focus on the national agenda.

This chapter provides a brief overview of historical and current influences on the U.S. health care system. The organization, funding, and quality of health care is reviewed. Comparisons with other high-income industrialized nations, e.g., France, Canada, and Japan are made. The role of the nurse and other stakeholders in the health care system is explored. Finally, health care access, primary care, quality, outcomes, and health care disparities are discussed.

HISTORY OF U.S. HEALTH CARE

One hundred years ago, illnesses such as tuberculosis or pneumonia required lengthy hospitalizations and were often catastrophic for individuals and families. Today, such illnesses are preventable and are often easily treated. Handwashing and vaccination programs have been used extensively to prevent the spread of communicable diseases. Additionally, surgical interventions in hospitals, for example, tonsillectomies, appendectomies, and reproductive procedures, have improved to treat otherwise debilitating or mortal conditions (Mayo, 2007). Health care is delivered by professional nursing and medical practitioners who are science-based and use evidence-based practice. It is primarily directed at preventing and treating chronic and behavioral diseases. Health care advances have extended life expectancy with the consequence of more elderly people requiring more health care for chronic and complex health problems. The majority of clinical care is still provided in hospitals, but length of stays are much shorter and a variety of innovative models of care are now used to provide cost-effective care for people with acute, community, and long-term clinical needs (Health Workforce Solutions LLC, & Robert Wood Johnson Foundation, 2008).

Yet generations after the insights of Florence Nightingale were first set forth, some problems continue to challenge us, including preventing the spread of disease, structuring organizations to benefit both clinicians and patients, collecting and using data and information to encourage improvement, and understanding how external and political forces influence care delivery. Based on her observations, Nightingale was convinced that noise, food, rest, light, fresh air, and cleanliness were instrumental in health and illness patterns. Thus, she maintained, the aim of nursing was to put the patient in the best condition for nature to act upon her or him (Nightingale, 1865/1970).

Nightingale also discovered the link between adverse patient outcomes and a lack of cleanliness and hand-washing. The surprising lack of adherence by health care providers to hand-washing accounts for 2 million hospital-acquired infections, is attributable for up to 90,000 deaths, and burdens the health care system with a cost of up to $29 billion annually (Jarvis, 2006). The most prevalent and preventable hospital-acquired infections are bloodstream infections, pneumonia, and surgical site and urinary tract infections (Gaynes et al., 2001). The highest rates of infection have been found to occur in Burn Intensive Care Units (ICUs), Neonatal ICUs, and Pediatric ICUs; areas where infections can easily be fatal (National Nosocomial Infections Surveillance [NNIS], 1998). (Agency for Healthcare Research and Quality [AHRQ], 2007b; Center for Health Design, 2005; Hamilton, 2003).

STRUCTURING HOSPITALS AROUND NURSING CARE

Nightingale also described the importance of structuring hospitals around nursing care. The initial design of hospitals followed that advice by building large wards where nurses could easily monitor and observe their patients. Later, hospital design evolved so that patient rooms surrounded centrally located nursing stations. Then, as today, the physical environment of hospitals could create stress for patients, their families, and clinical staff. In 1946, the Hospital Survey and Construction Act was enacted by Congress, which accelerated the building of hospitals and public health centers nationwide ("Hospital Survey and Construction Act," 1946). This legislation, also known as the Hill-Burton Act, solidified the corporatization of health care delivery. Today, research is finding links between the physical environment and patient outcomes, patient safety, and patient and staff satisfaction (Hamilton, 2003). Studies show that elements of hospital design such as exposure to natural light, private rooms, and facilities that are staff friendly and have less noise contribute to improved patient outcomes (Ulrich, Quan, Zimring, Joseph, & Choudhary, 2004).

Although little is known about how to best design the hospital environment to facilitate clinical advances and care delivery, an estimated $200 billion will be expended for new hospital construction across the United States during the next 10 years (Institute of Medicine [IOM], 2004a). The Robert Wood Johnson Foundation, the nation's largest philanthropy devoted exclusively to health and health care, has provided funding to the Center for Health Design, a nonprofit research organization, for the Designing the 21st Century Hospital Project, which is the most extensive review of the evidence-based approach to hospital design ever conducted. See www.healthdesign.org.

COLLECTING DATA

Nightingale also astutely recognized the importance of collecting and using data to assess the quality of health care. She employed coxcomb diagrams to present visual images of the number of preventable deaths during the Crimean war and then later in London hospitals.

Today, data is collected from numerous sources—patient records, surveys, clinical trials and other health research, administrative systems, government agencies, and policy institutes. A focus on clinical performance, outcome measures, and quality improvement brought about the beginning of formalized measurement in the 1970s (Dunefsky, 2008). From this measurement, reports are developed, such as the Centers for Disease Control and Prevention (CDC) National Vital Statistics Reports (Martin, Hamilton, Sutton, & Ventura, 2006); The National Healthcare Disparities Report (NHDR) (Agency for Healthcare Research and Quality [AHRQ], 2007a); and other reports from the Institute of Medicine (IOM, 1999, 2001) and the Surgeon General's office.

Additionally, private philanthropic organizations such as the Commonwealth Fund, the Kaiser Family Foundation, and the Robert Wood Johnson Foundation also analyze health care data and publish reports related to the health care needs of America. Locally, data is available from each state department of health. Internationally, organizations such as the World Health Organization and the Pan American Health Organization report on global health trends and issues.

To make informed decisions and set goals, health policy makers rely on the data and findings documented by such organizations. Table 2-1 lists several health data Web sites.

INFLUENCE OF EXTERNAL FORCES ON HEALTH CARE

Recognizing the influence of external forces on care delivery and scope of practice, Nightingale also kept informed of the activities of practitioners and government policy makers (Dossey, Selanders, & Beck, 2005). With health care being the largest sector of our economy, insurance companies, pharmaceutical companies, and health care technology and equipment companies, as well as employers, clinicians, managers, and patients all have a vested interest in proposed changes to health care financing, organization, and the responsibilities and scope of practice for clinicians.

POLITICAL INFLUENCES ON HEALTH CARE

In 1912, considerations by President Theodore Roosevelt's administration to adopt a modified workers' health insurance plan were swept aside when President Woodrow Wilson took office. Physicians and the life insurance industry supported this move through the early 1930s, as they were opposed to government regulation and were motivated to avoid any restraint on the fees and premiums they charged. The need for more equitable health insurance was highlighted with the onset of the Depression in the 1930s. At this

TABLE 2-1	WEBSITES FOR HEALTH DATA SOURCES

Agency for Healthcare Research and Quality: www.ahrq.gov

Centers for Disease Control and Prevention: www.cdc.gov

Commonwealth Fund: www.commonwealthfund.org

The Institute for Healthcare Improvement: www.ihi.org

Institute of Medicine: www.iom.edu

Joint Commission: www.jointcommission.org

Kaiser Family Foundation: www.kff.org

Robert Wood Johnson Foundation: www.rwjf.org

Surgeon General's Office: www.surgeongeneral.gov

World Health Organization: www.who.int

time, growing medical costs associated with hospital care, technological advances, and increased physician fees meant that vast numbers of previously well-to-do people could no longer afford to pay for the medical attention they required. In response to this national dilemma, the American Medical Association organized the Committee on the Cost of Medical Care, which attempted to organize the health care system and curb its costs. The work completed by this Committee was fraught with social and political divisions, and, in response, President Franklin Roosevelt formed the Committee on Economic Security. The "New Deal" program was implemented at this time and included federal relief programs, social services, and aid for the elderly. The Social Security Act of 1935 was also introduced, which defined the role of the federal government in the delivery and financing of health care (Maville & Huerta, 2007; Ross, 2002).

In 1965, an amendment to the Social Security Act was signed by President Lyndon Johnson, which introduced Medicare, a health insurance program for the elderly, and Medicaid, a health insurance program for the needy, both paid for with government funds. Due to rising health care costs in the 1990s, health care reform was again on the national agenda and President Bill Clinton introduced the Health Security Act. Although this Act failed to achieve the necessary political approval, health care has been a priority issue with each successive year and is high on the agenda as President Barack Obama takes office in 2009.

Health care continues to operate within a free market system, which means that it is a health care system controlled by private individuals and corporations rather than by a government. This free market system exerts control over health care delivery and financing. Payment for health care in this system stems primarily from multiple third party payers. Health care services are provided to the patient (first party) by the health care provider and hospital (second party). These clinicians and hospitals (second party) bill their services to multiple insurance companies and health care programs (third party). This third party payer system leads to high administrative costs in the U.S. system (Figure 2-1).

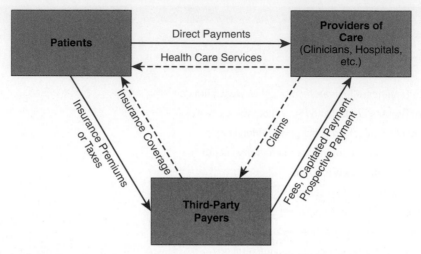

Figure 2-1 Economic relationships in the health care delivery system. (*Source:* Adapted from Jönsson B. (1989) What can Americans learn from Europeans? *Health Care Financing Review.* Dec; Spec No: 79-93; discussion 93-110.).

ORGANIZATION OF HEALTH CARE

Health care systems have three simple components: structure, process, and outcome (Donabedian, 2005). The **structure** component of health care includes resources or structures needed to deliver quality health care, for example, human and physical resources, such as nurses and nursing and medical practitioners, hospital buildings, medical records, and pharmaceuticals. Providing a mechanism whereby access to health care is made possible is also a necessary structural component. The **process** component of health care includes the quality activities, procedures, tasks, communication, and processes performed within the health care structures, such as hospital admissions, surgical operations, and nursing and medical care delivery following standards and guidelines to achieve quality outcomes. Referrals to specialized providers, treatments, and the provision of evidence-based care from health care providers, as well as discharge procedures, are also illustrations of health care processes. The **outcome** component of health care refers to the results of good care delivery achieved by using quality structures and quality processes and includes the achievement of outcomes such as patient satisfaction, good health and functional ability, and the absence of health care-acquired infections and morbidity. Measuring patient length of stay and the factors contributing to increasing or decreasing patient admissions and recruitment and retention of the health care workforce are also important outcome measures. Table 2-2 offers examples of structure, process, and outcome performance measures in clinical care, financial management, and human resources management.

It would be naïve to consider health care in the United States as it is currently being delivered as an effective system of care. If that were true, it would imply that health care is based on shared values and goals; is organized around the patient; utilizes all pertinent information; ensures value-based and quality-based care; rewards quality care; is universally standardized and simplified; is available to everyone regardless of income, race, ethnicity, or education; is affordable; and reflects effective collaboration among clinicians and with patients (Davis, 2005; World Health Organization [WHO], 2000, p. 35).

TABLE 2-2	EXAMPLES OF PERFORMANCE MEASURES BY CATEGORY

	Clinical Care	Financial Management	Human Resources Management
Structure	*Effectiveness* ■ Percent of nurses and physicians who are certified ■ JC (formerly JCAHO) accreditation ■ Presence of Magnet recognition	*Effectiveness* ■ Qualifications of administrators in finance department ■ Presence of an integrated financial and clinical information system and clinical decision-making technology	*Effectiveness* ■ Ability to attract desired nursing and medical practitioners ■ Competitive salary and benefits ■ Quality staff education
Process	*Effectiveness* ■ Ratio of medication errors ■ Ratio of complications *Productivity* ■ Ratio of total patient days to total full-time equivalent (FTE) nursing and medical practitioners *Efficiency* ■ Average cost per admission ■ Average cost per surgery	*Effectiveness* ■ Days in accounts receivable ■ Market share *Productivity* ■ Ratio of collections to FTE financial staff ■ Ratio of new capital acquisitions to fund-raising staff *Efficiency* ■ Debt/equity ratio	*Effectiveness* ■ Number and type of staff grievances ■ Organizational climate *Productivity* ■ Ratio of front-line staff to managers *Efficiency* ■ Recruitment costs
Outcome	*Effectiveness* ■ Severity-adjusted mortality ■ Patient satisfaction ■ Patient functional health status ■ Medical errors	*Effectiveness* ■ Return on assets ■ Operating margins	*Effectiveness* ■ Staff turnover rate ■ Staff satisfaction

Source: Compiled with information from Shortell, S. M., & Kaluzny, A. D. (2006). *Health Care Management* (5th ed.). Clifton Park, NY: Delmar Cengage Learning.

U.S. HEALTH CARE RANKINGS

Although state-of-the art health care is available in the U.S., access is limited to those who can afford the high costs associated with such care. The U.S. spends more money on health care than any other nation, yet health status and outcomes are significantly lower than in other industrialized or high income countries. When compared to five other high income nations—Australia, Canada, Germany, New Zealand, and the United Kingdom—the U.S. ranked last with respect to healthy lives, access, patient safety, efficiency, and equity (Davis et al., 2007). An overall score of 66% was recently given to the U.S. for its achievement across 37 core health indicators related to long, healthy, and productive lives; quality; access; efficiency; and equity of health care (Commonwealth Fund, 2008) (Figure 2-2).

Some major findings from the U.S. Scorecard include the following:

- The U.S. infant mortality rate is 7.0 deaths per 1,000 live births, compared with 2.7 deaths in the top 3 countries.
- 49% of U.S. adults received preventive and screening tests according to guidelines for their age and sex.
- 34% of U.S. adults under age 65 have problems paying their medical bills or have medical debt they are paying off over time.
- U.S. insurance administrative costs were more than three times the rates of other countries.
- The U.S. lags well behind other nations in use of electronic medical records.
- There is a wide gap between low-income or uninsured populations and those with higher incomes and insurance.
- Hispanics are at particularly high risk of being uninsured, lacking a regular source of primary care, and not receiving essential preventive care.
- It would require a 24% or greater improvement in African American mortality, quality, access, and efficiency indicators to approach benchmark rates for Whites.
- Blacks are much more likely to die at birth or from conditions such as heart disease, diabetes, and cancer (Commonwealth Fund National Scorecard on U.S. Health System Performance, 2008).

UNIVERSAL HEALTH CARE

Universal Health Care (UHC) is a government-sponsored system that ensures health care coverage for all eligible residents of a nation regardless

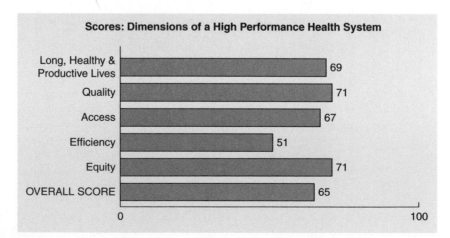

Scores: Dimensions of a High Performance Health System

	Score
Long, Healthy & Productive Lives	69
Quality	71
Access	67
Efficiency	51
Equity	71
OVERALL SCORE	65

Figure 2-2 U.S. scorecard on health system performance. (*Source:* Commonwealth Fund National Scorecard on U.S. Health System Performance. [2008]. Retrieved September 11, 2008, from www.commonwealthfund.org/usr_doc/site_docs/slideshows/NatlScorecard/NatlScorecard.html).

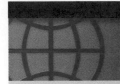

REAL WORLD INTERVIEW

As a nurse practitioner, there are many things about the American health care system that I really value. There are minimal wait times and there are lots of specialties. I like that a patient whom I refer with a serious diagnosis can be seen by a specialist within two weeks. We develop and make top-notch technology available and we have great health care standards. For all of these reasons, we keep the world on track and it follows our lead. I'm also aware every day of the shortcomings of the health care system. It's far too expensive, there are too many special interest groups, and it's all going to collapse under its own weight, a classic example of capitalism gone amuck. For example, health insurance companies have too much power, and I hate how all the insurance hoops prevent me and my colleagues from giving the best care to our patients.

We need a national health policy, and if the American people make enough noise, politicians will get behind it, too. I'm in favor of a national health plan, one that will ensure that all Americans have access to care. It needs to be one that incorporates what we already do best with what's useful from other countries such as Japan and Canada. We have a lot to learn from what they do well that we don't do.

Nadine Lamoreau, RN, MSN, FNP, APRN-C
Fort Fairfield, Maine

of income level or employment status. UHC varies widely in its structure and funding mechanisms, particularly the degree to which it is publicly funded. Typically, most UHC costs are met by the population via compulsory health insurance or taxation or a combination of both. In some cases, government involvement in UHC also includes being the single payer and directly managing the health care system, though many countries use mixed public-private payment systems to deliver universal health care. According to the Institute of Medicine (Insuring America's Health: Principles and Recommendations, 2004b), the United States is the only wealthy, industrialized nation that does not provide universal health care. Access to health care for most Americans is tied directly to having health insurance. As a result, serious gaps in health care coverage leaves millions of people in the U.S. uninsured, thus placing them at risk of being sicker and dying younger than the insured. (Muenning et al., 2005, pp. 2–34). In 2007, fifty three percent of the U.S. has employer health insurance. Four percent has individual health insurance, thirteen percent has Medicaid, twelve

percent has Medicare, and fifteen percent has no insurance (Kaiser Family Foundation 2008a, available at www.statehealthfacts.org/comparecat.jsp?cat=3).

EMPHASIS ON HOSPITAL CARE

The number of acute care hospital beds in the U.S. is 2.7 per 1,000 people. This number is lower than the average of 3.9 acute care hospital beds per 1,000 people in other countries such as France, Canada, and Japan. Since 1980, hospital bed use and length of stay have decreased in the U.S., which corresponds to an increase in the use of outpatient and day-surgery facilities (Health System Change, 2006; Organisation for Economic Co-operation and Development, 2008). In the United States, the emphasis on acute care health care services has driven health care costs higher, but has not necessarily improved the quality of care or patient outcomes (Werner & Bradlow, 2006; Jeffrey & Newacheck, 2006). Considering what health care services are needed by patients to improve their health status, only 8 out of 1,000 people will benefit from hospitalization, something that seems odd when considering where the research dollars are targeted and where the majority of health care dollars are devoted, that is, acute care settings in hospitals. When you look at a group of 1,000 people, it is estimated that 800 of them will experience symptoms of some disease or condition. Of this group of 800, 265 will be seen in a practitioner's office, hospital outpatient department or emergency department, or use home health care. Only eight will eventually be hospitalized. The majority don't need hospitalization and would benefit from more resources available for primary health care delivery outside the hospital (Green, Gryer, Yawn, Lanier, & Dovery, 2000). Note that a consistent focus on illness and injury, often referred to as a downstream focus, means fewer dollars are invested in upstream efforts. A focus on upstream efforts directed at keeping the population well through health promotion and illness prevention strategies would be less costly.

CRITICAL THINKING 2-1

Dalen and Alpert (2008) maintain that the U.S. needs only to follow its own Medicare model to implement a viable national health care program. They state, "Medicare pays the private sector to deliver quality health care to more than 44 million Americans. Those who stick with traditional Medicare have free choice of physicians and hospitals. Nearly every U.S. physician and nearly every hospital in the U.S. has elected to participate in Medicare. The administrative costs of Medicare are only 2% compared to costs of 12% with for-profit health insurers" (p. 554).

Is a national health care plan the solution to our health care problems?

What is the position of your state board of nursing and the American Nurses Association on this? Visit their web sites to compare their position statements.

NEED FOR PRIMARY HEALTH CARE

Thirty years ago, **Primary Health Care** (PHC) was declared an international goal and was defined as "the first level of contact of individuals, the family, and community with the national health system, bringing health care as close as possible to where people live and work, and constituting the first element of a continuing health care process" (WHO, 1978). PHC includes health promotion and prevention, diagnosis, and treatment of illness and injury (International Council of Nurses [ICN], 2008). In the U.S., PHC is provided by clinicians who provide entrance to the health care system, for example, nursing and medical practitioners, physician assistants, and optometrists and chiropractors.

PUBLIC HEALTH VERSUS MEDICAL CARE

The health care system in America has been described as an industry consisting of a "sprawling set of activities and enterprises" (Knickman & Kovner, 2008, p. 4), with "profit-making as its objective" (Demaro, 2008). Use of the term, "health care system" is misleading, as it suggests an organized system with knowledgeable individuals and concerned agencies working together to achieve health goals for the population through appropriate public health and medical care—ideal, but not the case in the U.S. The difference between public health care for the entire population and medical care for individuals is an important distinction to understand with respect to the organization and delivery of health care in the U.S.

Public health care activities are directed toward keeping communities and the population healthy. Medical care consists of activities that assist in restoring health of individuals after the onset of symptoms of an illness or injury. Public health care, which receives less than 4% of national health spending (Hunt & Knickman, 2008), is provided by a diverse group of health care professionals such as public health nursing and medical practitioners. Public health care promotes and protects public health through programs directed toward healthier lifestyles, immunization, disease prevention,

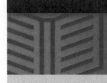

EVIDENCE FROM THE LITERATURE

Citation: Coddington, J. A., & Sands, L. P. (2008). Cost of health care and quality outcomes of patients at nurse-managed clinics. *Nursing Economics, 26*(2), 75–83.

Discussion: Lack of health insurance is a critical factor in access to appropriate health services and is directly associated with increased morbidity and mortality, lack of continuity of care, and rising health care costs. Nurse-managed clinics (NMCs) can serve as an important safety net in the health care delivery system by offering needed health services to populations of people affected by poverty and lack of insurance. NMCs remove barriers to care, improve health care access, and foster therapeutic relationships with nurse practitioners who provide primary care to vulnerable people. Much evidence also exists that nurse-managed clinics improve the use of preventative services, aid in the promotion of health, increase compliance with treatment, improve patient satisfaction, and reduce emergency room visits and re-hospitalizations.

Implications for Practice: The opportunity to provide quality care to vulnerable populations through NMCs is excellent. Overcoming the challenge of policies that restrict third-party reimbursement for nurse practitioners would allow an increased number of patients to be seen at NMCs.

environmental protection, and ensuring safe food and water; this can be provided in clinics, work sites, and other public forums. Conversely, medical care, provided after the onset of symptoms primarily by medical practitioners, is available in clinics and hospitals. With a focus on short-term acute care treatment, medical care costs much more than public health care. A persistent emphasis on short-term medical care fails at keeping the population well through ongoing disease prevention efforts and demonstrates where American health care priorities rest (Figure 2-3).

The U.S. health care system is defined by other features as well (Knickman & Kovner, 2008). The role of institutions in delivering care includes the organization of acute, long-term, and community health care. Each respective institution has evolved with its own roles and traditions to meet different health care needs. A diverse group of health professionals is responsible for organizing and delivering health care. Physicians, nurses, administrators, policy makers, business leaders, physical therapists, social workers, researchers, and technicians all hold vested interests in how care is delivered, and the differing ideologies may pose tensions between groups.

THE FEDERAL GOVERNMENT

The federal government provides for the general welfare of the population through the collection and allocation of money for the oversight and

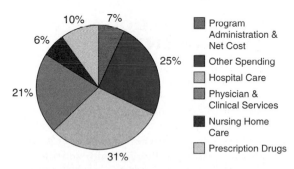

**Other Spending includes dentist services, other professional services, home health, durable medical products, over-the-counter medicines and sundries, public health, other personal health care, research, and structures and equipment.

Figure 2-3 The nation's health dollar, calendar year 2006: where it went. (*Source:* Centers for Medicare & Medicaid Services, Office of the Actuary National Health Statistics Group. [2008]. Retrieved August 4, 2008, from www.cms.hhs.gov/NationalHealth ExpendData/downloads/PieChartSourcesExpenditures2006.pdf).

administration of health care programs. Several organizations and divisions of the federal government are specifically involved in health care programs. The U.S. Department of Health and Human Services is the largest such organization. A visit to the Web site of the U.S. Department of Health and Human Services (USDHHS) (www.hhs.gov/about/index.html) demonstrates that this federal body oversees the functioning of several subdivisions and agencies, including:

- Agency for Healthcare Research and Quality
- Centers for Disease Control and Prevention (CDC)
- Centers for Medicare and Medicaid Services (CMS)
- Food and Drug Administration (FDA)
- Health Resources and Services Administration (HRSA)
- Indian Health Services (IHS)
- National Institutes of Health (NIH)
- Substance Abuse and Mental Health Services Administration (SAMHSA)

Other arms of the federal government and other departments such as the Department of Housing and Urban Development, the Department of Justice, the Department of Labor, and the Department of Defense also assume some responsibility for the health and wellbeing of the population.

STATE AND LOCAL GOVERNMENTS

The role of state governments with respect to health care is wide ranging. State government oversight includes the administration of Medicaid programs for low-income and disabled residents, the regulation of health care facilities such as state mental hospitals, and the licensure of professional health care providers. Public health activities at the state and local level include responsibility for activities administered through boards of health, as well as state and local health departments.

HOME HEALTH CARE

Currently, health care is provided in the homes of 7.6 million individuals in the U.S. Home health agencies, home aide organizations, and hospices provide care that is estimated to cost approximately $53 billion per year.

Care in the home is cost-effective and reduces the costs associated with hospitalization or admission to nursing homes, hospices, or other skilled facilities. Perhaps best of all, home care is a humane and compassionate way to deliver health care and provide supportive services in ways that keep the recipient's dignity and independence intact (National Association for Home Care & Hospice, 2007).

HEALTH CARE DISPARITIES

Social inequalities have been recognized as great influences on health (Figure 2-4). Socioeconomic status is the number one predictor of poor health. The poor are more than three times as likely as the wealthy to die prematurely or have a disability from illness (Lantz et al., 1998). Not enough health care delivery and attention are directed toward the top underlying causes of death in the United States, i.e., tobacco, poor diet and physical inactivity, alcohol consumption, microbial agents, toxic agents, motor vehicle accidents, firearms, sexual behavior, and illicit drug use (Mokdad, Marks, Stroup, & Gerberding, 2004).

Analysis of large data sets illustrates that as one ages, more health care services are utilized; women use health care services more frequently then men; and whites have greater health care access, and therefore higher utilization rates, than do patients of color (National Healthcare Disparities Report [NHDR], 2005); (National Healthcare Quality Report [NHQR], 2005).

A disproportionate number of racial and ethnic minority groups are uninsured. Injury and illness are more common among Black, Asian, American Indian, Hispanic, and socioeconomically poor people, due in part to the lower level of care they receive as compared with Whites (AHRQ, 2008a). For example, disparities in infant morbidity and mortality, cardiovascular and pulmonary disease, diabetes, communicable disease, cancer, and disease prevention, i.e., immunization and health screening, are more

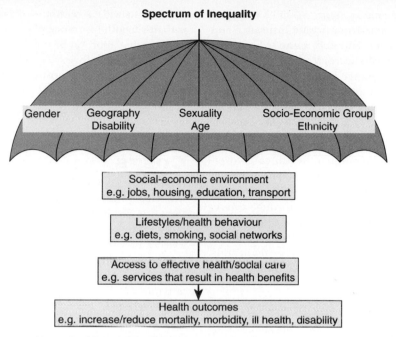

Figure 2-4 The spectrum of inequality. (*Source:* BMJ Health Intelligence [2007]. Health Inequalities. Retrieved August 5, 2008, from healthintelligence.bmj.com/hi/do/public-health/topics/content/inequalities-in-health/definition.html).

likely to be experienced by people disadvantaged by poverty, age, skin color, or ability to speak English. Such differences are further aggravated by miscommunication and misunderstanding, stereotyping, discrimination, and prejudice between patients and providers. Lifestyle behaviors that contribute to illness are higher among vulnerable groups. Because of their financial difficulties and other difficulties in accessing the health care system, vulnerable people often postpone health care. They are more likely to use the acute care system when their illness symptoms are advanced. Use of emergency departments and other acute care facilities for treatment is the most expensive way to obtain health care. In countries with a national health care system, health disparities also exist but virtually everyone in those countries regardless of socioeconomic background is assured of equal access to quality health care. In a recent study, health status, access to health care, and use of the health care system in the U.S and Canada compared disparities such as race, income, and immigration status. Health care was determined to be less accessible in the U.S., and disparities related to health care access were minimized in Canada because of universal health care (Lasser, Himmelstein, & Woolhandler, 2006).

HEALTH CARE SPENDING

Currently, the U.S. health care system consists of a mix of health care providers from either nonprofit or for-profit organizations in both the public and private sectors. Reimbursement for health care services is paid in one or a combination of these four ways:

- private insurers,
- publicly funded payers,
- charitable entities, or
- direct payment by consumers.

In 2006, as indicated in Figure 2-5, 53% of health care financing came from private insurance and individual payment, and 46% came from public programs such as Medicare, Medicaid, State Children's Health Insurance Program (SCHIP), and other public programs such as the Department of Veterans Affairs (Centers for Medicare & Medicaid Services, 2008).

Many gaps exist in these private and public programs, including incomplete health care coverage, need for copayments and deductibles, lack of provider choice, need for pre-authorizations, and other difficulties in maneuvering through the requirements. **Co-payments** are a fixed health care fee paid by the patient to the health care provider at the time of service; this amount is paid in addition to the money the health care provider will receive from the insurance company. **Deductibles** are a predetermined out-of-pocket fee paid by a patient for health care services before reimbursement through health insurance begins to be paid. For example, if an insurance plan has a $50 co-payment and a $1,000 deductible, the patient is responsible for paying the $50 at each health care visit plus paying the first $1,000 of health care costs, after

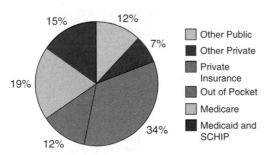

*Other Public includes programs such as workers' compensation, public health activity, Department of Defense, Department of Veterans Affairs, Indian Health Service, state and local subsidies, and school health.
**Other Private includes industrial in-plant, privately funded construction, and non-patient revenues, including philanthropy.
NOTE: Numbers shown may not add to 100.0 because of rounding.

Figure 2-5 The nation's health dollar, calendar year 2006: where it came from. (*Source:* Centers for Medicare & Medicaid Services, Office of the Actuary National Health Statistics Group. [2008]. Retrieved August 4, 2008, from www.cms.hhs.gov/NationalHealthExpendData/downloads/PieChartSources Expenditures2006.pdf).

which costs will be reimbursed as allowed by the patient's health insurance plan. Pre-authorization requires that approval be obtained from the insurance company before care or treatment such as hospitalization or diagnostic testing is initiated if such services are to be reimbursed by the patient's health insurance plan.

RISING HEALTH CARE COSTS

Health care costs are measured as part of the U.S. Gross Domestic Product (GDP). The **Gross Domestic Product (GDP)** is an economic measure of a country's national income and output within a year and reflects the market value of goods and services produced within the country. The GDP is used as a barometer of the national economy. Internationally, the U.S. spends more of its GDP on health care than any other wealthy country, all of which provide health care insurance for all their citizens. Health care costs in the U.S. are increasing 2.5 percentage points faster than the annual U.S. GDP. Employer-based health care premiums have doubled since 2000, yet those who are insured incur greater financial burdens as they pay for more out-of-pocket expenses. U.S. national health care expenditures were $1.9 trillion in 2004 (KFF & Health Research and Education Trust, 2006). A staggering 16% of the GDP was spent on health care. From 1960 to 2000, the GDP for health care grew nearly 15-fold, from approximately $526 billion to the trillions of dollars spent today. It is projected that health care spending will rise to $4 trillion by 2015 (Borger et al., 2006). Health care spending continues to increase faster than the overall U.S. economy. This is 2.5 percentage points faster than the growth of the GDP (Centers for Medicare and Medicaid Services [CMS], 2006). In 2000, the percentage of GDP for health care was 15.3%, and analysts project this number to keep rising to 20% (Borger et al., 2006).

Medical debt is now the number one reason for personal bankruptcy. The majority of people declaring bankruptcy because of medical debt are employed and have health insurance (Himmelstein, Warren, Thorne, & Woolhander,

2005). Spending on health care services is concentrated in disproportionate ways, which adds to the inflation of health care costs. For example, 10% of people account for 60% of spending on health care services; 20% of health care expenditures are spent on 1% of the population, indicating that a small percentage of the population absorbs a tremendous amount of health care services and spending. On the other side of the health care spectrum, 50% of the population contributes to 3% of health care expenditures. From another perspective, 44% of health care expenses are concentrated in the treatment of five predominant health problems: heart conditions, cancer, trauma, mental health disorders, and pulmonary conditions (Kaiser Family Foundation, 2007a; Stanton, 2006).

HEALTH CARE INSURANCE

The majority of Americans have some level of either public or private health care insurance coverage.

Publicly funded health insurance programs such as Medicare, Medicaid, and SCHIP provide health care coverage to people who qualify on the basis of low income, disability, or age (children and the elderly), leaving an estimated 46 million people, or 15.3% of the population, uninsured. This estimate includes 9 million children (Robert Wood Johnson Foundation, 2008). The Kaiser Family Foundation (2008b) estimates that this figure increases to 77 million people when factoring in the number of people who go without health insurance coverage for all or part of the year.

Because of the high costs of private health insurance premiums, only 60% of U.S. employers offer health insurance coverage to at least some of their employees (National Coalition on Health Care, 2008b). Note that the likelihood that a low paid employee will accept and buy an employer's health care plan is largely dependent on what is manageable to pay based on his or her income.

On average, the annual cost for family health care insurance premiums is approximately $12,000 annually, with employers contributing approximately $3,000 per year. By 2012, this figure is projected to increase by 60%, suggesting that most Americans will struggle financially to obtain adequate health care coverage (Kaiser Family Foundation, 2007b; NCHC, 2008b).

STATE REGULATION OF HEALTH INSURANCE

Three key pieces of federal legislation set forth national standards that the individual states use to regulate health insurance. First, the Employee Retirement Income Security Act (ERISA) of 1974 provides a framework for states to regulate health insurers. Second, the Consolidated Omnibus Budget Reconciliation Act (COBRA) of 1985 ensures that employees who resigned, were laid off, were terminated, or lost their job due to family-related reasons can retain their health insurance coverage for up to 18 months and, in some cases, up to a maximum of 36 months if they are deemed qualified and pay the full premium. A third piece of legislation, the Health Insurance Portability and Accountability Act (HIPAA) of 1996 imposed restrictions on limitations and exclusions of insurance coverage for those with preexisting conditions and restricted other attempts to exclude employees from insurance coverage. It also provides protection of insurance coverage as employees change employers, and it provides tax exclusions for medical savings accounts.

INTERNATIONAL PERSPECTIVE

To the extent that the U.S. is similar economically and sociopolitically to countries such as France, Canada, and Japan, an examination of the health systems in those countries is useful. The differences between allocation of health care spending in the U.S. as compared to other countries are graphically displayed in Figure 2-6.

FRANCE

France, ranked as having the best health care system in the world (Nolte & McKee, 2008), spends 11.1% of its gross domestic product on health care (Organisation for Economic Co-operation and Development, 2008). This is approximately one-half of what the U.S. spends on health care

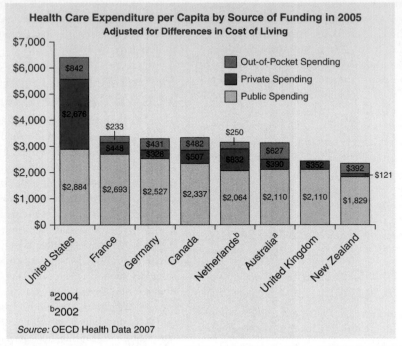

Figure 2-6 International health care spending per capita by source of funding (2005). (*Source:* Osborn, R. [2008]. Comparing health care systems performance: Opportunities for learning from abroad [slide #4]. Commonwealth Fund. Retrieved October 4, 2008, from www.allhealth.org/briefingmaterials/osborn-1189.ppt).

per person. Comprehensive health care is guaranteed for all citizens and legal residents in France. Similar to the U.S., health care in France is provided through private and government insurance. Unlike Canada and Britain, there are no lengthy wait times in France. Unlike the U.S., everyone is insured in France and there are no additional patient charges for health insurance plan deductibles (Shapiro, 2008).

Employed residents are covered by a national health insurance plan, referred to as Securite Sociale, which includes spouses and children. Another plan, Couverture Maladie Universelle (CMU), provides coverage for those people who do not qualify for the securite sociale program and is free to some people whose income is below a certain level. The national health insurance plan is funded through private and public means, with employees paying up to 21% of their income to the national health care system and employers making similar contributions. By

comparison, Americans pay fewer taxes, but pay more for health care, e.g., through paying health insurance premiums and other out-of-pocket expenses not covered by their insurance plan. In France, costs are dependent upon the type of provider seen; for example, a general practitioner is less expensive than a specialist. Likewise, it is more expensive to seek treatment at night, on the weekend, or on public holidays. Hospital care is reimbursed through the national health plan, and a percentage of the cost of prescription drugs is also reimbursed to the patient. Essentially, the sicker a person is, the more coverage is allowed, including for expensive drugs and experimental cancer treatments. Reducing cost and improving efficiency are the challenges for this system. Waste, such as "doctor shopping," whereby a patient seeks treatment from more than one health care provider for the same ailment, and overuse of prescription drugs are partly responsible for high health care costs in France (National Coalition on Health Care, 2008c; Shapiro, 2008).

CANADA

Annually, the Canadian government spends 10% of its gross domestic product on its national health care system. Canada has the eighth largest global health care budget in the world (Organisation for Economic Co-operation and Development, 2008). The Canadian health care system is administered by each Canadian provincial or territorial government. Seventy percent of health spending is publicly funded through federal and provincial taxation of individuals and corporations, and the remaining thirty percent is paid through private and out-of-pocket sources for additional services such as prescription medications or dental and vision care (Canadian Institute for Health Information, 2006). All Canadians have equal access to the same quality and quantity of health care. Under the Canada Health Act of 1984, comprehensive health care is publicly administered, portable between provinces, and accessible to all. Primary care is provided by physicians and nurse practitioners, who may work in private clinics or public institutions. These health care providers are reimbursed on a fee-for-service basis, which allows them to be reimbursed by each provincial or territorial health plan for each health care service rendered to a patient.

Unlike the privatized health care system in the U.S., extra billing, deductibles, and co-payments are not allowed. The health care provider bills the provincial or territorial health plan and is reimbursed with an agreed upon amount for each health service given. No additional charges or costs can be billed to or recovered from the patient. With only one insurance payer, referred to as a single payer system, many of the problems embedded within the American health care system are eliminated. The problem currently facing the Canadian health care system is the lengthy wait times to access family practitioners, specialists, emergency room services, diagnostic tests, and surgical procedures (National Coalition on Health Care, 2008c). Same-day access to the health care system is lowest in Canada (23%). The U.S. is slightly better (30%), but considerably lower than Germany (56%) (Commonwealth Fund, 2006). Wait times in Canada are circumvented based on

the gravity of a patient's condition, but this solution aggravates the waiting time for less urgent cases. In a geographically vast country with a small population compared to the U.S., some Canadians in rural or isolated locales often travel long distances to obtain specialized services.

As an example of the comprehensiveness and affordability of the Canadian health care service, a 51-year-old Canadian nurse working in the U.S. recently returned with her spouse and 15-year-old child to her home province of Alberta for one year. During that time, the family enrolled in the Alberta Health Care Insurance Plan for a cost of $88 per month (Alberta Health and Wellness, 2004). Health care for the nurse included an annual physical examination, lab tests, mammogram, bone density testing, and a routine colonoscopy. The colonoscopy required a five-month wait. Her husband underwent elective day surgery, which was booked seven months in advance. Her daughter was immunized at school, and she was once treated at a community health center for a persistent respiratory infection. Beyond payment of their monthly premium, the family was issued no bills for the health care they received.

JAPAN

To pay for its national health care system, Japan spends 8.2% of its gross domestic product on health care. This is less than France, Canada, or the U.S., and Japan enjoys the longest life expectancy of all, i.e., 82.4 years (Organisation for Economic Co-operation and Development, 2008). Membership in either of two broad health insurance programs is mandatory in Japan. The Employee Health Insurance Program provides health care coverage for people employed by medium to large companies, national or local government, or private schools. The National Health Insurance Program covers self-employed and unemployed persons, as well as those employed in agriculture, forestry, or the fisheries industry. Payment toward each health insurance plan varies, but in both programs, patients share in paying for their health care costs up to a certain level, after which the insurance plan provides full coverage (National Coalition on Health Care, 2008c).

CRITICAL THINKING 2-2

In 2007, Maine's immunization rate among children up to 35 months of age fell to the lowest among New England states (CDC, 2008; Huang, 2008). This rate is expected to drop further after January 1, 2009, when free immunization will be provided only to those children who qualify on the basis of low family income. Immunization reimbursement for other children will need to be obtained through family health insurance plans. Families who lack health insurance and who do not meet the income criteria for free immunizations will be required to pay the costs of vaccinating their children against communicable diseases such as whooping cough, diphtheria, measles, mumps, and rubella. These immunizations could cost a family hundreds of dollars per child. Children in families that cannot afford such a fee will likely be forced to forgo vaccination. Declining vaccination rates in Maine and other states such as Alaska, Idaho, and Nevada pose a serious threat to public health from vaccine-preventable illnesses.

How do immunization rates in countries with national health care compare to the U.S., which does not have a national health care plan? What percentage of immunizations are funded by federal or state grants in your state? Check your state at this site, www.cdc.gov/mmwr/preview/mmwrhtml/mm5735a1.htm.

The Japanese health care system provides comprehensive care and is one of the most advanced in the world. Physicians and hospitals are predominantly run as private businesses, and costs for care are reimbursed through the national health care system. Patients' health care costs are reimbursed at a fixed amount determined by the government. Refusal of coverage by insurers is impossible, and personal medical debt is nonexistent. Because health care providers are reimbursed for the number of services provided, Japan leads other countries in the number of drugs prescribed, the number of tests ordered per patient, and patient length of stay in a hospital. The Japanese average 16 consultations with a health care provider per year, 3 to 4 times the rate of consultations in the U.S.

Factors contributing to lower health care costs in Japan include healthier diets and lifestyles with a lower incidence of chronic diseases. Reimbursement rates for health care services are low, but reimbursement strategies for quantity rather than quality of services erodes the advantage a healthier lifestyle might have in terms of curbing costs. Despite cost containment efforts, health care expenses are increasing. A shortage of physicians also means the wait time to access the health system is an issue. Additionally, with an aging population and shrinking workforce, concerns as to how access, affordability, and quality will continue in the future are being voiced (National Coalition on Health Care, 2008c; Reid, 2008).

FACTORS CONTRIBUTING TO RISING HEALTH CARE COSTS

Many factors contribute to the rising costs of health care. Some of these key factors include the aging of the population with growth in the demand for health care, increased utilization of pharmaceuticals, expensive new technologies, rising hospital care costs, practitioner behavior, cost shifting, and administrative costs (Thorpe, Woodruff, & Ginsburg, 2005).

AGING AND PHARMACEUTICAL USE

Americans 65 years and older make up 13% of the population but incur 36% of health care expenses (Stanton, 2006). The number of beds in nursing homes has increased from 1.298 million to 1.839 million (Kramarow et al., 1999). Increased need to manage and treat chronic illnesses and long-term care needs with increasing age for patients aged 75 and older has incurred per capita health expenditures that are five times higher than those of people between 25 and 34 years of age (Boddenheimer, 2005a). On average, annual per capita expenditures on those patients aged 65 and older is $11,089, significantly higher than the annual expenditure of $3,352 for those aged 19 to 64 (Keehan, 2004).

Prescription medications are used by 92% of seniors and 61% of nonelderly adults (Woo, Ranji, Lundy, & Chen, 2007). These medication cost add 10% to national health care expenditures. Prescription drug use increased among the elderly after Medicare Part D, a prescription drug benefit plan, was introduced in 2006 (Catlin, Cowan, Hartman, Heffler, & National Health Expenditure Accounts Team 2008).

TECHNOLOGY AND RISING HOSPITAL COSTS

Although technological advances have facilitated earlier diagnoses and better treatment of disease, factors such as the greater availability of new technology drive per capita expenditures higher (Boddenheimer, 2005b). Treatment for the five most expensive health conditions, heart disease, cancer, trauma, mental disorders, and pulmonary conditions (Stanton, 2006), requires the use of expensive medications and technologies. While use of some technologies such as electronic record keeping may reduce costs, the presumed success of sophisticated drugs and technologies shapes consumer expectations of what the health care system can deliver. Health care consumers, including both patients and providers, also contribute to the cost of health care. These consumers' demands for intense services despite the lack of definite clinical need or evidence of efficacy strains health care spending. As an example, the U.S. performs more than three times (83) the number of magnetic resonance imaging (MRI) scans per person than does Canada (25.5) or Great Britain (19) (Canadian Institute for Health Information, 2006). Yet the U.S. lags behind these same countries with respect to patient care outcomes (Commonwealth Fund, 2006; Commonwealth Fund, 2008).

Today, there are almost 6,000 hospitals nationwide. Hospital services contribute to the rise in health care costs due to the increased utilization of expensive technologies, high labor costs, rising malpractice premiums, and increased costs of hospitalization. Given the aging hospital infrastructure and increases in hospital reimbursements, future building of new hospital beds will also increase health care costs (Bazzoli, Gerland, & May, 2006).

PRACTITIONER BEHAVIOR

A shortage of frontline health care providers, most noticeably among registered nurses (RNs), also adds to the cost of health care. With 10.5 nurses per 1,000 members of the population, the number of RNs in the U.S. is slightly greater than among other wealthy countries, which average 9.7 nurses per 1,000 members of the population (Organisation for Economic Co-operation and Development, 2008). Regardless, the number of nurses is insufficient to meet the needs of the American population. See ftp://ftp.hrsa.gov/bhpr/workforce/behindshortage.pdf.

The number of physicians per person in the U.S. is less than in other wealthy countries such as France, Canada, or Japan (Organisation for Economic Co-operation and Development, 2008). This shortage is most pronounced in certain practice specialties, for example, family practice physicians and geriatric physicians. Physician shortages are also apparent in rural areas. In addition, American physicians earn more than their counterparts in other countries. A physician specialist who makes $300,000 in the U.S. or a family physician whose income is $175,000 per year in the U.S. would, on average, earn approximately 25%–50% less in Canada (Eisenberg, 2006). Defensive medicine and the high cost of medical malpractice insurance all add to increasing physician costs. Malpractice claims in the U.S. are filed 50% more often than in Great Britain and 350% more often than in Canada (Anderson, Hussey, Frogner, & Waters, 2005). Two-thirds of claims in the U.S. are dropped, which results in a similar distribution of claim settlements among these countries. Regardless, the need for medical malpractice insurance to protect American physicians against such claims contributes to the cost of physician care.

COST SHIFTING AND ADMINISTRATIVE COSTS

The practice of **cost shifting**, whereby health care providers raise prices for the privately insured to offset the lower health care payments from both

Medicare and Medicaid as well as the often non-payment of health care premiums from the uninsured, continues to raise the cost of health care. Medicare and Medicaid payments are less than 50% of what private insurers pay. Health care providers shift charges for health care costs to the private insurance sector. Some estimates of the cost shift are being valued at $6 billion annually. Costs to the public for these programs continue to increase. While the intent of the Medicaid program has been to ensure access to health care for mainly low-income pregnant women and children, over 72% of Medicaid's $295.9 billion dollars in expenditures in 2004 went toward care of the disabled and dual-eligibles. Dual-eligibles are the elderly who are eligible for both Medicaid and Medicare, and they are the fastest growing proportion enrolled in Medicaid (Holahan & Cohen, 2006).

According to Boddenheimer (2005a), the cost of administration of U.S. health care in 1999 was 24% of the nation's health care expenditures. In an attempt to reduce these costs, providers such as practitioner's offices, clinics, and hospitals have invested in Information Technology (IT). Because of the increased demand for such systems, the administrative cost of implementation has gone up though efficient use of these systems in the future has the potential to decrease costs.

Finally, note that ongoing attention to healthy lifestyles, such as eating healthy foods, engaging in regular exercise, maintaining a healthy weight, living smoke-free, and limiting alcohol intake, reduces the health care required to manage the chronic disease conditions associated with the absence of such behaviors. However, as indicated by Knickman and Kovner (2008), these healthy lifestyle strategies have failed to reduce overall health care costs.

OTHER FACTORS CONTRIBUTING TO RISING HEALTH CARE COSTS

Because rising health care costs are based on utilization, it is important to understand other factors that can both increase and decrease utilization, as listed in Table 2-3.

HEALTH CARE QUALITY

The health care report, *To Err Is Human,* confronted health care clinicians and managers with concerns about the poor quality of health care attributable to misuse, overuse, and underuse of resources and procedures, which was responsible for thousands of deaths (IOM, 1999). The health care report *Crossing the Quality Chasm* (IOM, 2001) and several large studies (McGlynn et al., 2003; Thomas et al., 2000) have shown that the quality of health care in the United States is at an unexpected low level given the amount of money the United States spends on health care and needs to set goals and guidelines for health care improvement. (Table 2-4).

The next phase of the IOM quality initiative focuses on operationalizing the vision of a future health system described in the *Quality Chasm* report. This phase has generated several publications, including *Preventing Medication Errors* (2006), *Performance Measurement: Accelerating Improvement* (2005), *Patient Safety: Achieving a New Standard for Care* (2003), *Keeping Patients Safe: Transforming the Work Environment of Nurses* (2003), *Health Professions Education: A Bridge to Quality* (2003), and *Priority Areas for National Action: Transforming Health Care Quality* (2003).

HEALTH CARE VARIATION

Groundbreaking research beginning in the 1970s has demonstrated that significant variation in utilization of specific health care services associated with geographic location, provider preferences and training, type of health insurance, and patient-specific factors such as age and gender exists (Wennberg & Gittelsohn, 1973; Leape, 1992; Adams, Fraser, & Abrams, 1973; Safran, Rogers, Tarlov, McHorney, & Ware, 1997; Greenfield et al., 1992; Williams, L.S. et al., 2003). Utilization rates of health care services have been found to be associated with availability of services and technologies, for example, MRIs, hospital beds, practitioners (Joines, Hertz-Picciotto, Carey, Gesler, &

TABLE 2-3	FORCES THAT AFFECT OVERALL HEALTH CARE UTILIZATION	
Force	**Factors That May Decrease Health Services Utilization**	**Factors That May Increase Health Services Utilization**
Financial incentives that reward practitioners and hospitals for performance (e.g., pay for performance [P4P] programs that reward quality practice)	■ Changes in clinician practice patterns (e.g., encouraging patient self-care and healthy lifestyles; reduced length of hospital stay)	■ Changes in clinician practice patterns (e.g., more aggressive treatment of the elderly)
Increased accountability for performance	■ Consensus documents or guidelines that recommend decreases in utilization	■ Consensus documents or guidelines that recommend increases in utilization
Technological advances in the biological and clinical sciences	■ Better understanding of the risk factors of diseases and prevention initiatives (e.g., smoking-prevention programs, cholesterol-lowering drugs)	■ New procedures and technologies (e.g., hip replacement, stent insertion, magnetic resonance imaging [MRI]) ■ New drugs, expanded use of existing drugs ■ Increased supply of services (e.g., ambulatory surgery centers, assisted living residences)
Increase in chronic illness	■ Discovery/implementation of treatments that cure or eliminate diseases ■ Public health/sanitation advances (e.g., quality standards for food and water distribution)	■ More functional limitations associated with aging ■ More illness associated with aging ■ More deaths among the increased number of elderly
Increased ethnic and cultural diversity of the population	■ Lack of insurance coverage ■ Low income	■ Growth in national population ■ Efforts to eliminate disparities in access and outcomes
Changes in the supply and education of health professionals	■ Decreased supply (e.g., hospital closures, large numbers of nursing and medical and nursing practitioners retiring) ■ Shifts to other sites of care may cause declines in utilization of staff at the original sites, e.g., ambulatory surgery, assisted living	■ Increase in chronic conditions ■ Growth in national population

(continues)

TABLE 2-3	**FORCES THAT AFFECT OVERALL HEALTH CARE UTILIZATION (CONTINUED)**	

Force	Factors That May Decrease Health Services Utilization	Factors That May Increase Health Services Utilization
Social morbidity (e.g., drugs, violence, disasters)	■ Disparities in access to health services and outcomes	■ New health problems (e.g., HIV/AIDS, bioterrorism)
Access to patient information	■ Changes in consumer preferences (e.g., home birthing, more self-care, alternative medicine)	■ Changes in consumer demand
Globalization and expansion of the world economy	■ Growth in uninsured population	■ Growth in national population
Cost control and competition for limited resources	■ Insurance payer pressures to reduce costs	■ Increased health insurance coverage
		■ Consumer/employee pressures for more comprehensive insurance coverage
		■ Changes in consumer preferences and demand (e.g., cosmetic surgery, hip and knee replacements, direct marketing of pharmaceuticals)

Source: Adapted from Bernstein, A. B., Hing, E., Moss, A. J., Allen, K. F., Siller, A. B., & Tiggle, R. B. (2003). *Health care in America: Trends in utilization.* Hyattsville, MD: National Center for Health Statistics; and Shortell, S. M., & Kaluzny, A. D. (2006). *Health care management* (5th ed.). Clifton Park, NY: Delmar Cengage Learning.

Suchindran, 2003), prevalence and severity of morbidities (Dunn, Lyman, & Marx, 2005; National Healthcare Quality Report, 2005), race/ethnicity (National Healthcare Quality Report, 2005), patient adherence, health-seeking behaviors of patients (Calvocoressi et al., 2004), and many other factors. Variation in the delivery and quality of health services is also associated with socio-demographics; hospital types, e.g., urban/rural, teaching/non-teaching; and clinical areas,

e.g., heart disease, diabetes, pneumonia, and clinical preventive services. According to Fisher, Goodman, & Chandra (2008), hospitalization for medical conditions such as worsening diabetes or heart failure increases the risk of medical error and complications, both of which entail more costs. Findings from a study by the Dartmouth Atlas Project revealed that the supply of services, not how sick people were, was more likely to determine the resources used (Fisher, Goodman, &

TABLE 2-4	GOALS AND GUIDELINES FOR HEALTH CARE IMPROVEMENT

6 Goals for Improved Health Care System

1. Safe: Avoid injuries from care intended to help patients.

2. Effective: Provide services based on scientific knowledge to all who could benefit and refrain from providing services to those not likely to benefit (Avoid Overuse and Underuse).

3. Patient Centered: Provide respectful and responsive care to individuals; Patient preferences, needs, and values must guide clinical decision-making.

4. Timely: Reduce wait time and harmful delays for those who receive and give care.

5. Efficient: Avoid waste, for example, of equipment, supplies, ideas, energy, and other costly resources.

6. Equitable: Provide care consistent in quality irrespective of gender, ethnicity, geographical, and socioeconomic factors.

Guidelines for Redesigning Care

1. Offer care based on continuous healing relationships: Make care available every day through face-to-face visits, telephone, Internet, and other means.

2. Customize care based on patient needs and values: Provide care responsive to patient needs and preferences.

3. Have patient as source of control: Foster patient empowerment and autonomy through information and shared decision-making.

4. Share knowledge and free flow of information: Facilitate patient access to his or her own medical information and to available clinical knowledge.

5. Use evidence-based decision making: Provide consistent quality of care based on best available scientific knowledge.

6. Develop safety as a systems property: Develop systems of safety that mitigate error, promote patient safety, and reduce risk of injury.

7. Be transparent: Make information available to patients and families about health plans, hospitals, clinical practice, and alternative treatment options, including performance related to their safety, evidence-based practice, and patient satisfaction.

8. Anticipate needs: Anticipate patient needs rather than respond to events.

9. Continuously decrease waste: Use limited resources wisely.

10. Cooperate among clinicians: Collaborate and coordinate care between clinicians and institutions.

Source: Compiled from the Institute of Medicine. (2001). Crossing the quality chasm: A new health system for the 21st century. Washington, DC: National Academy Press; and Berwick, D. M. (2002). A user's manual for the IOM's 'Quality Chasm' report. *Health Affairs, 2*(3), 80–90.

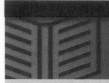

EVIDENCE FROM THE LITERATURE

Citation: Lankshear, A. J., Sheldon, T. A., & Maynard, A. (2005). Nurse staffing and healthcare outcomes: A systematic review of the international research evidence. *Advances in Nursing, 28*(2), 163–174.

Discussion: The relationship between quality of care and the cost of the nursing workforce is of concern to policymakers. This study assesses the evidence for a relationship between the nursing workforce and patient outcomes in the acute sector through a systematic review of international research produced since 1990 involving acute hospitals and adjusting for case mix. Twenty-two large studies of variable quality were included. They strongly suggest that higher nurse staffing and richer skill mix (especially of RNs) are associated with improved patient outcomes, such as failure to rescue and mortality, although the effect size cannot be estimated reliably.

In the United States, the California Department of Health Services has set absolute minimum ratios for licensed nurses (RNs and licensed vocational nurses) at 1:6 (4 Care Hours Per Patient Day [CHPPD]), day and night for medical and surgical areas, although the introduction of the 1:5 (4.8 CHPPD) ratio has recently been postponed to 2008. In Australia, the state of Victoria has recommended that RN ratios should be 1:4/5 (4.8–6 CHPPD) for day shifts in general medical and surgery units, depending on the type of hospital. However, the research evidence presented here does not support a precise recommendation on staffing levels, and evidence of diminishing returns implies that the cost-effectiveness of using nurse staffing as a quality improvement lever must fall as levels increase. More research is needed to investigate the resource implications alongside the impact on patient outcomes.

Implications for Practice: Overall, there is accumulating evidence of a relationship between nurse staffing, especially higher nursing skill mix, and patient outcomes. However, the estimates of the nurse staffing effects are likely to be unreliable. There is emerging evidence of a curvilinear relationship that suggests that the cost-effectiveness of using RN levels as a quality improvement tool will gradually become less cost-effective. The research is not yet clear.

Chandra, 2008). Regions of the country and health care providers with more resources had higher rates of use and cost. Efforts to decrease the variation of health care practices through standardization of care with quality, evidence-based guidelines are important to improve clinical decision-making, care delivery, health outcomes, and cost efficiency. Achieving transparency or truth in reporting practice preferences and medical error is often hampered by the fear of litigation or reprisal against the health care provider. The Patient Safety and Quality Improvement Act of 2005 (see www.ahrq.govqual/psoact.htm) addresses such concerns by encouraging health care providers to participate in developing and implementing evidence-based improvement initiatives. The Act also highlights the importance of recognizing and responding to the underlying hazards

and risks to patient safety. Establishing national health benchmarks, such as those in Healthy People 2010 (USDHHS, 2000) is another strategy by which to achieve and measure quality improvement. Performance is monitored between states and reflects the health trends and improvements among groups demonstrated to be disadvantaged or vulnerable (AHRQ, 2008b).

IMPROVEMENTS IN THE PROCESS OF CARE

Using the example of the management of hypertension, recent research findings illustrate the need for significant improvements in the process of health care delivery. Blood pressure control is strongly linked to the delivery of evidence-based quality care for those with hypertension

(Goldstein, Lavori, Coleman, Advani, & Hoffman, 2005). Each year, uncontrolled high blood pressure contributes to more than 68,000 deaths (Woolf, 1999). When 61% of patients with a myocardial infarction were appropriately given aspirin, which has been shown to reduce the risk of death by 15%, the risk of nonfatal myocardial infarction was reduced by 30%, and the risk of nonfatal stroke was reduced by 40% (Antman, Lau, Kupelnick, Mosteller, & Chalmers, 1992). When simple evidence-based changes of administering aspirin and beta-blockers are made, thus changing the processes of care for patients who have had a myocardial infarction, health care dollars can be lowered and lives saved. This is true even if it is because aspirin use is being measured to assess provider performance (Williams, Schmaltz, Morton, Koss, & Loeb, 2005). Such change in the processes of care delivery could change the list of the top ten causes of death, i.e., heart disease, cancer, cerebrovascular disease, chronic pulmonary disease, accidents, diabetes mellitus, influenza and pneumonia, alzheimer's disease, kidney disease, and septicemia (CDC, 2005).

PERFORMANCE AND QUALITY MEASUREMENT

When the quality of care is measured, it improves (Brook, Kamberg, & McGlynn, 1996; Chassin & Galvin, 1998) possibly largely due to the Hawthorne effect, which has illustrated that observed activity shows improvement. Unfortunately, those aspects of care not being measured may not improve. Nursing leaders have also recognized the need to establish indicators that can be used to measure nursing care. Selected quality indicators are listed in Table 2-5.

Note that setting standards for appropriate care and guideline development should have a basis in validated measures of quality, using reliable performance data, and making appropriate adjustments in care delivery. However, it is important to know that the majority of quality care is not measurable

TABLE 2-5	SELECTED CLASSIFICATION SYSTEMS

North American Nursing Diagnosis Association (NANDA): www.nanda.org

Home Health Care Classification (HHCC): www.sabacare.com

PeriOperative Nursing Data Set: www.aorn.org

National Quality Forum-endorsed Nursing-sensitive Consensus Standards: www.qualityforum.org

Omaha System: www.omahasystem.org

ABC Codes: www.alternativelink.com

Logical Observation Identifiers Names and Codes: www.loinc.org

Patient Care Data Set: e-mail: judy.ozbolt@vanderbilt.edu

SNOMED CT: www.snomed.org

International Classification of Nursing Practice: www.icn.ch

Nursing Interventions Classification: www.nursing.uiowa.edu

Nursing Outcomes Classification: www.nursing.uiowa.edu

National Database of Nursing Quality Indicators (NDNQI): www.nursingworld.org. Search for NDNQI.

using current methods (Epstein, 1995; Smith, Atherly, Kane, & Pacala, 1997). Reliable methods and measures need to be developed and tested. Also, practitioners have been resistant to their care delivery being measured because they have believed that it would interfere with their professionalism and autonomy. If this belief persists, the majority of health care delivery will not be measured.

MALCOLM BALDRIDGE NATIONAL QUALITY AWARD

Health care organizations are eligible to apply for the Malcolm Baldridge National Quality Award. The Baldridge Award highlights the importance of leadership; strategic planning; and a focus on patients, other customers, and markets in building a quality health care system. The award also stresses the importance of measurement, analysis and knowledge management; workforce focus; process management; and results (Baldridge National Quality Program, 2007).

OUTCOME MEASUREMENT

Outcome measurements can be made indicating an individual's clinical state, such as his severity of illness, course of illness, and the effect of interventions on his clinical state. Outcome measures involving a patient's functional status evaluate his ability to perform activities of daily living (ADLs). These can include measures of physical health in terms of function, cost of care, health care access, and general health perceptions. The measures can distinguish the concepts of physical and mental health and identify the five indicator categories of clinical status, functioning, physical symptoms, emotional status, and patient/family evaluation and perceptions about quality of life. Selected quality-of-life measures include quality-adjusted life years (QALY), quality-adjusted life expectancy (QALE), and quality-adjusted healthy life years (QUALY) (Drummond, Stoddart, & Torrance, 1994).

The Medical Outcomes Study (MOS) "Short Form 36" Health Survey is one of the many health indices that have been developed since 1950. The SF-36, as it is commonly known (Ware & Sherbourne, 1992), measures physical functioning, role limitations due to physical health, bodily pain, social functioning, general mental health, role limitations due to emotional problems, vitality, and general health perceptions.

Other health status measurement surveys in use today include the Quality of Life Index (Spitzer, 1998), developed to measure the general health and well-being of terminally ill individuals; the COOP Charts for primary care practice patients; the functional status questionnaire (Jette & Cleary, 1987), a self-administered general health and social well-being survey for ambulatory patients; the Duke Health Profile (Parkerson, Broadhead, & Tse, 1990), which evaluates health status in primary care patients; the Sickness Impact Profile (Bergner, Bobbit, Carter, & Gilson, 1981), which was developed to measure changes in an individual's behavior as a result of illness; and the Nottingham Health Profile (Hunt, McKenna, McEwen, Williams, & Papp, 1981), developed as a measure of perceived general health status for primary care patients and general population health surveys.

PUBLIC REPORTING OF HEALTH CARE OUTCOMES

Transparency of health care outcome performance through public reporting based on national standards and methods is integral to reforming health care to improve patient outcomes, cost efficiency, and access to health care, particularly for vulnerable populations. Public reporting of health care outcomes encourages consumers to make informed choices about the quality and cost of health services. Likewise, health care practitioners, who are often reimbursed for the volume of patients that they see rather than the quality of care that they provide, may be motivated and rewarded to improve quality. Public reporting can be used to determine where inefficient and ineffective care exists. It can also influence reimbursement policies in which payment is linked to the ability to achieve standards and benchmarks, for example, payment for quality performance (Dudley & Rosenthal, 2006).

OTHER NATIONAL PUBLIC QUALITY REPORTS

Several key national public quality reports of interest for health care and nursing leaders and managers are as follows:

- *AHRQ National Healthcare Quality Report (2005):* Available at www.ahrq.gov/qual/nhqr05/nhqr05.htm.
- *AHRQ National Healthcare Disparities Report (2005):* Available at www.ahrq.gov/qual/nhdr05/nhdr05.htm.
- *Healthy People 2010:* Accessible at www.healthypeople.gov.
- *Health Grades for Hospitals and Physicians:* Available at www.healthgrades.com.
- *Leapfrog:* Available at www.leapfroggroup.org.

Public reporting of quality performance has been shown to influence declines in cardiac surgery mortality (Peterson, DeLong, Jollis, Muhlbaier, & Mark, 1998); improvements in the processes of obstetrics care (Bost, 2001); and employee enrollment and desire to switch health care providers (Beaulieu, 2002). While providers and policymakers do seek out these public quality reports, the general public typically does not search them out, does not understand them, distrusts them, and fails to make use of them (Marshall, Hiscock, & Sibbald, 2002).

In many respects, hospitals are providing quality care. Data to assess clinical performance from the Joint Commission (JC), formerly known as the Joint Commission on Accreditation of Healthcare Organizations (JCAHO), core measures program, which uses standardized, evidence-based measures, and data from the Medicare program show improvements in the quality of care in hospitals (Williams et al., 2005; Jencks, Huff, & Cuerdon, 2003). Yet at hospitals that do not meet the sample-size requirement for national comparisons, quality performance remains mediocre (Jha, Li, Orav, & Epstein, 2005).

DISEASE MANAGEMENT

A key challenge for health care is the numerous deficiencies in the delivery of care to patients with chronic conditions (IOM, 2001). The amount and breadth of knowledge about the effectiveness of regular disease management for improving care across populations and disease states is building (Ofman et al., 2004). **Disease management** is a systematic population-based approach to identifying persons at risk, intervening with specific programs of care, and measuring clinical and other outcomes (Epstein & Sherwood, 1996). What makes caring for patients with chronic diseases problematic is that usually multiple chronic conditions are involved. In the elderly, nine out of ten patients with ischemic heart disease or congestive heart failure had three or more chronic conditions, including hypertension, diabetes, urinary incontinence, and chronic pain; the majority of these patients had an average of five chronic conditions (Bierman, 2004). Because of this, condition-specific disease management will not be successful given the likelihood of disease comorbidities, that is, other diseases. Documented widespread variation in disease management and treatment interventions have led health care payors to consider the option of paying-for-performance (P4P). These types of financial incentives may be an effective way of changing professional behavior (Robinson, 2001; Chaix-Couturier, Durand-Zaleski, Jolly, & Durieux, 2000) and the quality of care delivered.

PATIENT SAFETY

One of the greatest forces driving quality-improvement efforts in hospitals is the Joint Commission's (JC) patient safety requirements, in large part due to hospital's fears of possibly losing accreditation if the JC standards are not achieved and sustained (Devers, Pham, & Liu, 2004). Because of patterns of medical error that became apparent through JC and other national reporting mechanisms, National Patient Safety Goals (NPSG) were established by the JC in 2003. The 2009 National Patient Safety Goals for Hospitals, Ambulatory Health Care, Behavioral Health Care, Critical Access Hospitals, Disease-Specific Care, Home Care, Laboratories, Long Term Care, Office-Based Surgery, and others, are available at www.jointcommission.org/patientsafety/nationalpatientsafetygoals.

MAGNET PROGRAM

The Magnet Recognition Program of the American Nurses Credentialing Center can be a tool for establishing an environment that recognizes excellence in nursing services in a health care system (Magnet Recognition Program [MRP], 2005). Research continues to demonstrate positive implications of the magnet program, relating magnet characteristics to nurse job satisfaction and retention, prevention of job burnout, and improvement in perceived quality of care (Aiken, Havens, & Sloane, 2000; Friese, 2005; Lake & Friese, 2006).

IMPROVING QUALITY THROUGH HEALTH PROFESSIONS EDUCATION

To begin to realize the quality agenda set forth by the IOM (IOM, 2001), a subsequent report, *Health Professions Education: A Bridge to Quality* (IOM, 2003), delineates a needed "overhaul" of the curriculum of health professionals' education to transform current skills and knowledge (IOM, 2003, p. 1). The five IOM Health Professions competencies are identified as:

1. *Ability to provide patient-centered care*
2. *Ability to effectively work in interdisciplinary teams*
3. *Ability to understand evidence-based practices*
4. *Ability to measure the quality of care*
5. *Ability to use health information technology*

CHALLENGES AND OPPORTUNITIES FOR NURSES

Eight principles are integral to health care reform as envisioned by the Institute of Medicine (2008). These eight principles are accountability, efficiency, objectivity, scientific rigor, consistency, feasibility, responsiveness, and transparency. These principles are consistent with a professional nursing agenda, which states that all persons are entitled to affordable, quality health care services (American Nurses Association [ANA], 2008).

CRITICAL THINKING 2-3

As more is learned about quality improvement, including the prevention of health care error or risk and using research findings in daily practice, organizations must make shifts in how they practice. For example, organizations must recruit and retain a qualified workforce, make quality improvements, and assess and reward performance.

What can the clinical nurse do to improve quality of care, patient outcomes, and patient and staff satisfaction, and also minimize health care error?

What are the contributing and inhibiting factors in your workplace in identifying errors and reporting them?

CASE STUDY 2-1

Review the ratings of hospitals in your area of the country at www.healthgrades.com, www.solucient.com, www.100tophospitals.com, www.leapfroggroup.org, and one of the July issues of *US News and World Report,* published annually.

What kinds of ratings are given to hospitals in your area?

Review the criteria and evaluation system used to rate the hospitals. Are they valid and reliable?

Will you choose a hospital for your own family's care using a rating system like this?

Individual nurses can influence a renewed health care system by doing the following:

- Keep abreast of current issues affecting patients and their access to affordable, quality health care. Newspaper, television, radio, and Internet sources publicize numerous items related to health care.
- Dispel the myths and opinions that often shape the misguided beliefs about health care, its consumers, and the direction the system needs to take. Decipher what is reliable and valid information from what is biased, shocking, or fear-filled. Clarify such matters with colleagues, family, and friends who may be less informed.
- Pay attention to the quality measures employed at your workplace. Speak up about what is working well, where safety is risked, or where waste is occurring.
- Heighten awareness of the health care issues you encounter in your practice related to the health care crisis. Craft letters to newspapers or legislators and write opinion editorials or blogs to convey why health care reform is needed.
- Get involved professionally. Become a member of your state nursing association and determine what is being done at the state and national level to address health care reform.

- Health care and health care reform are political issues. Be informed about the political process, with all of its stakeholders and vested interests. Identify what your elected representatives are doing at the state and national level to address concerns about the health care system. Are their efforts sustainable and moving toward a national health plan, or do they add to the patchwork approach that currently characterizes the health care system?
- Talk about nursing and the work you do as a health care provider. Be vocal about the expertise nurses have as affordable, caring, and competent clinicians and as agents for health care renewal.
- Support colleagues and promote their talent. Prompt others who show interest and aptitude to pursue nursing as a career. Encourage colleagues to consider advanced nursing roles, whether as clinicians, educators, administrators, researchers, or perhaps even as potential legislators.
- Volunteer in the ways you can to assist the leaders in health care whom you trust and respect.

This list is but a beginning of the many opportunities in which all nurses can be involved. Change in the health care system is ongoing and inevitable, but with more nurses actively engaged, the process is far more likely to meet the goal of providing health care for all.

KEY CONCEPTS

- Health care reports provide invaluable information that emphasizes the successes and failures of health care throughout our nation.
- Evidence of significant disparities and low quality continue to demonstrate the need for significant health care improvement.
- Health care systems have three simple components: structure, process, and outcome.
- The United States is one of only a few large countries in the world without a universal system of health care.

- In the United States, the emphasis on acute care health care services has successfully driven health care costs higher, but has not necessarily improved the quality of care or patient outcomes.
- Primary care provides integrated, accessible health care services by clinicians who are accountable for addressing a large majority of personal health care needs, developing a sustained partnership with patients, and practicing in the context of family and community.

- The federal government is a major driver of health care organization and delivery.

- Inequalities in income, insurance coverage, gender, race or ethnicity, and geography affect a person's ability to have access to health care.

- Many factors contribute to the rising costs of health care. The key factors include the aging of the population with growth in the demand for health care, increased utilization of pharmaceuticals, expensive new technologies, rising hospital care costs, practitioner behavior, cost shifting, and administrative costs.

- The health care report *Crossing the Quality Chasm* (IOM, 2001) and several large studies (McGlynn et al., 2003; Thomas et al., 2000) have shown that the quality of health care in the United States is at an unexpected low level given the amount of money the United States spends on health care and that it needs improvement in many dimensions.

- Groundbreaking research beginning in the mid-1980s demonstrated that there was significant variation in utilization of specific health care services associated with geographic location, provider preferences and training, type of health insurance, and patient-specific factors such as age and gender.

- Health care performance and quality are measured to determine resource allocation, organize care delivery, assess clinician competency, and improve health care delivery processes and outcomes.

- Several key reports of interest for health care and nursing leaders and managers for purposes of performance measurement and benchmarking are available.

- Evidence-based practice involves supplementing clinical expertise with the judicious and conscientious implementation of the most current and best evidence along with patient values and preferences to guide health care decision making.

- Health care accreditation is a mechanism used to identify if organizations meet certain national standards.

- The Magnet Recognition Program of the American Nurses Credentialing Center can be a tool for establishing an environment that recognizes excellence in nursing services in a health care system.

- There is a need to focus on retooling the health care workforce with new knowledge and requisite skills to function in better, redesigned health care systems.

- Health professionals' education to transform current skills and knowledge includes training clinicians to effectively work in interdisciplinary teams; have an educational foundation in informatics; and deliver patient-centered care that fully exploits evidence-based practice, quality improvement approaches, and informatics.

- The Institute of Medicine's 2004 *Report on Patient Safety* was one of the first in a series of reports published to emphasize the connections among nursing, patient safety, and quality of care.

KEY TERMS

Co-payments
Cost shifting
Deductibles
Disease management
Fee for service
Gross Domestic Product

Health disparities
Outcome
Primary Health Care
Process structure
Universal Health Care (UHC)

REVIEW QUESTIONS

1. People who lack health insurance or who are underinsured are more likely to do which of the following? Select all that apply.
   A. use less costly alternative therapies and treatments
   B. seek health care as soon as illness symptoms occur
   C. postpone health care, resulting in higher morbidity, mortality, and cost
   D. obtain free health care through the emergency department
   E. buy organic produce to improve health through nutrition

2. When asked to describe the advantages of a universal health care system, the nurse explains that such systems are typically characterized by which of the following? Select all that apply.
   A. lower costs
   B. comprehensive care for all
   C. access to care regardless of ability to pay
   D. access to care regardless of employment
   E. improved health promotion and disease prevention care
   F. reduced administrative costs
   G. unanticipated out-of-pocket expenses

3. Knowledge of the structure and function of the health care system is important for nurses as a way to do which of the following?
   A. help themselves negotiate the health care system should they become ill
   B. become knowledgeable and skilled leaders in health care reform
   C. focus on significant issues such as social justice within the health system
   D. assist patients to obtain the best health insurance plan possible

4. The largest purchaser of health care in America is which of the following?
   A. private individuals
   B. private insurance companies
   C. Health Maintenance Organizations
   D. Medicare, Medicaid, and other governmental programs

5. What is the top underlying cause of health care disparity in the United States?
   A. Socioeconomic status
   B. Race
   C. Ethnicity
   D. Gender

REVIEW ACTIVITIES

1. Although it is difficult to modify the structure of health care, what could you do to implement a system to continually modify the process of health care delivery to improve health care quality in your organization?

2. What are strategies to ensure patient access to appropriate health care services in public and private health care agencies?

3. How can the five IOM health professions competencies for quality care be achieved in the current workplace?

EXPLORING THE WEB

Federal Government:

- Alliance for Health Reform:
  www.allhealth.org
- Single Payer.com:
  www.calnurses.org
- Centers for Medicare and Medicaid Services (CMS):
  www.cms.gov
- Department of Defense (DOD) TRICARE program:
  www.tricare.mil
- Health Resources and Services Administration (HRSA):
  www.hrsa.gov
- National Center for Health Statistics:
  www.cdc.gov
  Search for *National Center for Health Statistics*.
- National Institutes of Health (NIH):
  www.nih.gov

- Substance Abuse and Mental Health Services Administration (SAMHSA):
  www.samhsa.gov
- Veterans Health Administration (VHA):
  www.va.gov

Private Foundations and Organizations:

- Joint Commission (JC):
  www.jointcommission.org
- National Committee for Quality Assurance (NCQA):
  www.ncqa.org
- National Quality Forum (NQF):
  www.qualityforum.org
- Malcolm Baldridge Quality Award (MBQA):
  www.quality.nist.gov
- Press Ganey Patient Satisfaction Surveys:
  www.pressganey.com

REFERENCES

Adams, D. F., Fraser, D. B., & Abrams, H. L. (1973). The complications of coronary arteriography. *Circulation, 48*(3), 609–618.

Agency for Healthcare Research and Quality (AHRQ). (2007a). National Healthcare Quality & Disparities Report. Rockville, MA.

Agency for Healthcare Research and Quality (AHRQ). (2007b). Transforming hospitals: Designing for safety and quality. Retrieved July 28, 2008, from www.ahrq. gov/qual/transform.pdf.

Agency for Healthcare Research and Quality (AHRQ). (2008a). National Healthcare Disparities Report. Rockville, MD: Author. Retrieved August 4, 2008, from www.ahrq.gov/qual/qrdr07.htm.

Agency for Healthcare Research and Quality (AHRQ). (2008b). National Healthcare Quality Report. Rockville, MD: Author. Retrieved August 4, 2008, from www.ahrq.gov/qual/qrdr07.htm#toc.

Aiken, L. H., Havens, D. S., & Sloane, D. M. (2000). The Magnet Nursing Services Recognition Program. *American Journal of Nursing, 100*(3), 26–36.

Alberta Health and Wellness. (2004). Health care insurance plan. Edmonton, Alberta. Retrieved August 2, 2008, from www.health.alberta.ca.

American Nurses Association (ANA). (2008). Health System Reform Agenda. Retrieved September 11, 2008, from www.nursingworld.org/MainMenuCategories/HealthcareandPolicyIssues/HSR/ANAsHealthSystemReformAgenda.aspx.

Anderson, G. F., Hussey, P. S., Frogner, B. K., & Waters, H. R. (2005). Health spending in the United States and the rest of the industrialized world. *Health Affairs, 24*(4), 903–914.

Antman, E. M., Lau, J., Kupelnick, B., Mosteller, F., & Chalmers, T. C. (1992). A comparison of results of meta-analyses of randomized control trials and recommendations of clinical experts: Treatments for myocardial infarction. *The Journal of the American Medical Association, 268,* 240–258.

Baldridge National Quality Program. (2007). *Health care criteria for performance excellence.* Gaithersburg, MD: Baldridge National Quality Program.

Bazzoli, G. J., Gerland, A., & May, J. (2006). Construction activity in U.S. hospitals. *Health Affairs, 25*(3), 783–791.

Beaulieu, N. D. (2002). Quality information and consumer health plan choices. *Journal of Health Economics, 21*(1), 43–63.

Bergner, M., Bobbit, R. A., Carter, W. B., & Gilson, B. S. (1981). The Sickness Impact Profile: Development and final revision of a health status measure. *Medical Care, 19*(8), 787–805.

Berwick, D. M. (2002). A user's manual for the IOM's "Quality Chasm" report. *Health Affairs, 21*(3), 80–90.

Bierman, A. S. (2004). Coexisting illness and heart disease among elderly Medicare managed care enrollees. *Health Care Financing Review, 25*(4), 485–488.

Bernstein, A.B., Hing, E., Moss, A.J., Allen, K.F., Siller, A.B., Tiggle, R.B. (2003). Health care in America, trends in utilization. U.S. Department of Health and Human Services. Centers for disease control and prevention. National center for health statistics. Hyattsville, MD. Available at www.cdc.gov/nchs/data/misc/healthcare.pdf.

BMJ Health Intelligence. (2007). Health Inequalities. Retrieved August 5, 2008, from healthintelligence.bmj.com/hi/do/public-health/topics/content/inequalities-in-health/definition.html.

Boddenheimer, T. (2005a). High and rising health care costs. Part 1: Seeking an explanation. *Annals of Internal Medicine, 142*(10), 847–854.

Boddenheimer, T. (2005b). High and rising health care costs. Part 2: Technologic innovation. *Annals of Internal Medicine, 142*(11), 932–937.

Borger, C., Smith, S., Truffer, C., Keehan, S., Sisko, A., Poisal, J., et al. (2006). Health spending projections through 2015: Changes on the horizon. *Health Affairs, 25*(2), 61–73.

Bost, J. (2001). Managed care organization publicly reporting 3 years of HEDIS data. *Managed Care Interface, 14,* 50–54.

Brook, R. H., Kamberg, C. H., & McGlynn, E. A. (1996). Health system reform and quality. *The Journal of the American Medical Association, 276,* 476–480.

Calvocoressi, L., Kasl, S. V., Lee, C. H., Stolar, M., Claus, E. B., & Jones, B. A. (2004). A prospective study of perceived susceptibility to breast cancer and nonadherence to mammography screening guidelines in African American and white women ages 40 to 79 years. *Cancer Epidemiology Biomarkers Preview, 13*(12), 2096–2105.

Canadian Institute for Health Information. (2006). CIHI looks at how Canada measures up in health spending. Ottawa, Ontario: Author. Retrieved August 4, 2008, from www.cihi.ca/cihiweb/en/downloads/Dir_Wint06_ENG.pdf.

Catlin, A., Cowan, C., Hartman, M., Heffler, S., & National Health Expenditure Accounts Team. (2008). National health spending in 2006: A year of change for prescription drugs. *Health Affairs, 27*(1), 14–29.

Center for Health Design. (2005). Scorecards for evidence based design. Retrieved July 28, 2008, from www.healthdesign.org/research/reports/documents/scorecard_12_05.pdf.

Centers for Disease Control and Prevention (CDC). (2005). Leading causes of death. Atlanta, GA. Available at www.cdc.gov/nchs/FASTATS/lcod.htm.

Centers for Disease Control and Prevention (CDC). (2007). Tobacco use among adults: United States, 2006. *Morbidity and Mortality Weekly Report, 56*(4), 1157–1161.

Centers for Disease Control and Prevention (CDC). (2008). National, state, and local area vaccination coverage among children aged 19–35 months: United States, 2007. *Morbidity and Mortality Weekly Report, 57*(35), 961–966.

Centers for Medicare & Medicaid Services (CMS). (2006). Historical National Health Expenditure Data. Retrieved June 4, 2006, from www.cms.hhs.gov/NationalHealthExpendData/02_NationalHealthAccountsHistorical.asp#TopOfPage.

Centers for Medicare & Medicaid Services (CMS). (2008). The nation's health dollar, calendar year 2006. Retrieved August 4, 2008, from www.cms.hhs.gov/NationalHealthExpendData/downloads/PieChartSourcesExpenditures2006.pdf.

Chaix-Couturier, C., Durand-Zaleski, I., Jolly, D., & Durieux, P. (2000). Effects of financial incentives on medical practice: Results from a systematic review of the literature and methodological issues. *International Journal on Quality Health Care, 12,* 133–142.

Chassin, M. R., & Galvin, R. W. (1998). The urgent need to improve health care quality: Institute of Medicine National Roundtable on Health Care Quality. *The Journal of the American Medical Association, 280,* 1000–1005.

Coddington, J. A., & Sands, L. P. (2008). Cost of health care and quality outcomes of patients at nurse-managed clinics. *Nursing Economics, 26*(2), 75–83.

Commonwealth Fund. (2006). International comparison: Access and timeliness. New York: Author. Retrieved July 23, 2008, from www.commonwealthfund. org/snapshotscharts/snapshotscharts_show. htm?doc_id=409110.

Commonwealth Fund. (2008). Why not the best? Results from the National Scorecard on U.S. Health System Performance, 2008. The Commonwealth Fund Commission on a High Performance Health System. Retrieved July 30, 2008, from www.commonwealthfund.org/ publications/.

Commonwealth Fund National Scorecard on U.S. Health System Performance. (2008). Available at www.commonwealthfund.org/Content/Publications/ Fund-Reports/2008/Jul/Why-Not-the-Best--Results- from-the-National-Scorecard-on-U-S-Health- System-Performance--2008.aspx

Dalen, J. E., & Alpert, J. S. (2008). National health insurance: Could it work in the U.S.? *American Journal of Medicine, 121*(7), 553–554.

Davis, K. (2005). Ten points for transforming the U.S. health care system. Retrieved October 4, 2006, from www.cmwf.org/aboutus/aboutus_show. htm?doc_id=259233.

Davis, K., Schoen, C., Schoenbaum, S. C., Doty, M. M., Holmgren, A. L., Kirss, J. L., & Shea, K. K. (2007). Mirror, mirror on the wall: An international update on the comparative performance of American health care. New York: The Commonwealth Fund.

Demaro, R.A. (2008). Posted in Bill Moyers Journal. Available at www.pbs.org/moyers/journal/05092008/profile.

Devers, K. J., Pham, H. H., & Liu, G. (2004). What is driving hospitalsí patient-safety efforts? *Health Affairs, 23*(2), 103–115.

Donabedian, A. (2005). Evaluating the quality of medical care. *Milbank Quarterly, 20*(1) 137–141.

Dossey, B., Selanders, L., & Beck, D. (2005). *Florence Nightingale today: Healing, leadership, global action*. Washington, DC: American Nurses Publishing.

Drummond, M. F., Stoddart, F. L., & Torrance, G. W. (1994). *Methods for the economic evaluation of health care programmes*. Oxford, England: Oxford University Press.

Dudley, R. A., & Rosenthal, M. B. (2006). *Pay for performance: A decision guide for purchasers*. Rockville, MD: Agency for Healthcare Research and Quality. AHRQ Pub. No. 06-0047.

Dunefsky, F. (2008). Quality health care. In R. Kearney- Nunnery (Ed.), *Advancing Your Career* (4th ed.). Philadelphia: Davis.

Dunn, W. R., Lyman, S., & Marx, R. G. (2005). Small area variation in orthopedics. *Journal of Knee Surgery, 18*(1), 51–56.

Eisenberg, M. J. (2006). An American physican in the Canadian health care system. *Archives of Internal Medicine, 166,* 281–282.

Epstein, A. M. (1995). Performance reports on quality—prototypes, problems, and prospects. *New England Journal of Medicine, 333,* 57–61.

Epstein, R. S., & Sherwood, L. M. (1996). From outcomes research to disease management: A guide for the perplexed. *Annuals of Internal Medicine, 124*(9), 832–837.

Fisher, E. S., Goodman, D. C., & Chandra, A. (2008). Disparities in health and health care among Medicare beneficiaries: A brief report of the Dartmouth Atlas Project. Dartmouth Institute for Health Policy and Clinical Practice/Robert Wood Johnson Foundation. Retrieved August 7, 2008, from www.dartmouthatlas.org/af4q/AF4Q_Disparities_ Report.pdf.

Friese, C. R. (2005). Nurse practice environments and outcomes: Implications for oncology nursing. *Oncology Nursing Forum, 32*(4), 765–772.

Gaynes, R., Richards, C., Edwards, J., Emori, T. G., Horan, T., Alonso-Eschanove, J., et al. (2001, Mar.–Apr.). Feeding back surveillance data to prevent hospital acquired infections. *Emerging Infectious Diseases, 7*(2), 295–298.

Goldstein, M. K., Lavori, P., Coleman, R., Advani, A., & Hoffman, B. B. (2005). Improving adherence to guidelines for hypertension drug prescribing: Cluster-randomized controlled trial of general versus patient-specific recommendation. *American Journal of Managed Care, 11*(11), 677–685.

Great-West Health Care. (2006). 2006 Consumer attitudes survey. Retrieved October 5, 2008, from www.greatwesthealthcare.com/C5/StudiesSurveys/Document%20Library/m5031-gwh-consumer-attud-survy-06.pdf.

Green, L. A., Gryer, G. E., Yawn, B. P., Lanier, D., & Dovery, S. M. (2000). The ecology of medical care revisited. *New England Journal of Medicine, 344,* 2021–2025.

Greenfield, S., Nelson, E. C., Zubkoff, M., Manning, W., Rogers, W., Kravitz, R. L., et al. (1992). Variations in resource utilization among medical specialties and systems of care. Results from the medical outcomes study. *Journal of the American Medical Association, 267*(12), 1624–1630.

Hamilton, D. K. (2003). The four levels of evidence based practice. *Healthcare Design, 3,* 18–26.

Health System Change. (2006). Tracking health care costs: Spending growth remains stable at high rate in 2005. *Data Bulletin, 33.* Retrieved August 3, 2008, from www.hschange.org.

Health Workforce Solutions LLC, & Robert Wood Johnson Foundation. (2008). Innovative care models. Retrieved July 25, 2008, from www.innovativecaremodels.com/about/about.

Himmelstein, D. U., Warren, E., Thorne, D., & Woolhandler, S. (2005, Feb. 2). Illness and injury as contributors to bankruptcy. Health Affairs Web Exclusive, pp. W5–63. Retrieved July 28, 2008, from content.healthaffairs.org/cgi/content/abstract/hlthaff.w5.63v1.

Holahan, J., & Cohen, M. (2006). Understanding the recent changes in Medicaid spending and enrollment growth between 2000–2004. Issue Paper. Kaiser Commission on Medicaid and the Uninsured. Retrieved October 4, 2006, from www.kff.org/medicaid/upload/7499.pdf.

Hospital Survey and Construction Act. (1946). *Canadian Medical Association Journal, 55,* 616.

Huang, J. (2008, Oct. 2). Health groups say childhood vaccination rates unacceptable. Maine Public Broadcasting Network. Retrieved October 4, 2008, from www.mpbn.net/radio/mainenews/081002vaccinations.htm.

Hunt, K. A., & Knickman, J. R. (2008). Financing health care. In A. R. Kovner & J. R. Knickman (Eds.), *Jonas and Kovner's Health Care Delivery in the United States* (9th ed.). New York: Springer.

Hunt, S. M., McKenna, P., McEwen, J., Williams, J., & Papp, E. (1981). The Nottingham Health Profile: Subjective health status and medical consultations. *Social Science and Medicine, 15*(3, Pt. 1), 221–229.

Institute of Medicine (IOM). (1999). To err is human: Building a safer healthcare system: Washington, DC: National Academy Press.

Institute of Medicine (IOM). (2001). *Crossing the quality chasm: A new health system for the 21st century.* Washington, DC: National Academy Press.

Institute of Medicine (IOM). (2003, Jan. 7). Priority Areas for National Action: Transforming Health Care Quality. Available at, www.iom.edu/?id=35961.

Institute of Medicine (IOM). (2003, Apr. 8). Health Professions Education: A Bridge to Quality. Available at, www.iom.edu/?id=35961.

Institute of Medicine (IOM). (2003, Nov. 4). Keeping Patients Safe: Transforming the Work Environment of Nurses. Available at www.iom.edu/?id=35961.

Institute of Medicine (IOM). (2003, Nov. 20). Patient Safety: Achieving a New Standard for Care. Available at, www.iom.edu/?id=35961.

Institute of Medicine (IOM). (2004a). *Evidence-based hospital design improves healthcare outcomes for patients, families, and staff.* Washington, DC: National Academy Press.

Institute of Medicine (IOM). (2004b). Insuring America's health: Principles and recommendations. Washington, DC: National Academy Press.

Institute of Medicine (IOM). (2005, Dec. 1). Performance Measurement: Accelerating Improvement. Available at www.iom.edu/CMS/2955.aspx?show=0;3#LP3.

Institute of Medicine (IOM). (2006, July 20). Preventing Medication Errors: Quality Chasm Series. Available at www.iom.edu/?id=35961.

International Council of Nurses (ICN). (2008). Delivering quality, serving communities: Nurses leading primary health care. Geneva: Author.

Jarvis, W. R. (2006). The state of the science of health care epidemiology, infection control, and patient safety. Infection Control Association (Singapore). Retrieved July 25, 2008, from www.icas.org.sg/images/StateofScience.pdf.

Jeffrey, A. E., & Newacheck, P. W. (2006). Role of insurance for children with special health care needs: A synthesis of the evidence. *Pediatrics, 118*(4), 1027–1038.

Jencks, S. F., Huff, E. D., & Cuerdon, O. (2003). Change in the quality of care delivered to Medicare beneficiaries. *Journal of the American Medical Association, 289,* 305–312.

Jette, A. M., & Cleary, P. D. (1987). Functional disability assessment. *Physical Therapy, 67,* 1854–1859.

Jha, A. K., Li, Z., Orav, E. J., & Epstein, A. M. (2005). Care in U.S. hospitals: The Hospital Quality Alliance program. *New England Journal of Medicine, 353*(3), 265–274.

Joines, J. D., Hertz-Picciotto, I., Carey, T. S., Gesler, W., & Suchindran, C. (2003). A spatial analysis of count-level variation in hospitalization rates for low back problems in North Carolina. *Social Science and Medicine, 56*(12), 2541–2553.

Joint Commission (JC). (2009). National patient safety goals. Retrieved October 5, 2008, from www.jointcommission.org/GeneralPublic/NPSG/09_npsgs.htm.

Jönsson B. (1989) What can Americans learn from Europeans? *Health Care Financing Review.* Dec; Spec No: 79-93; discussion 93-110.

Kaiser Family Foundation (KFF). (2007a). Trends in health care costs and spending. Menlo Park: Kaiser Family Foundation. Retrieved September 28, 2008, from www.kff.org/insurance/upload/7692.pdf.

Kaiser Family Foundation (KFF). (2007b). Insurance premium cost-sharing and coverage take-up. Menlo Park: Author. Retrieved September 27, 2008, from www.kff.org/insurance/snapshot/chcm020707oth.cfm.

Kaiser Family Foundation (KFF). (2008a). Health Coverage for the Uninsured. Available at www.statehealthfacts.org/comparecat.jsp?cat=3.

Kaiser Family Foundation (KFF). (2008b). Covering the uninsured in 2008: Key facts about current costs, sources of payment, and incremental costs. Menlo Park: Author. Retrieved September 24, 2008, from www.kff.org/uninsured/upload/7810.pdf.

Kaiser Family Foundation (KFF) & Health Research and Education Trust. (2006). Employer Health Benefits: 2006 Annual Survey. Publication number 7527. Retrieved October, 2006, from www.kff.org.

Keehan, S. (2004). Health spending by age. *Health Affairs, 23*(6), 280–281.

Knickman, J. R., & Kovner, A. R. (2008). Overview: The state of health care delivery in the United States. In A. R. Kovner & J. R. Knickman (Eds.), *Jonas and Kovner's Health Care Delivery in the United States* (9th ed.). (pp. 3–11). New York: Springer.

Kramarow, E., Lentzner, H., Rooks, R., Weeks, J., & Sayday, S. (1999). *Health and aging chartbook: Health,* United States, 1999. Hyattsville, MD: National Center for Health Statistics, U.S. Department of Health and Human Services.

Lake, E. T., & Friese, C. R. (2006). Variations in nursing practice environments: Relation to staffing and hospital characteristics. *Nursing Research, 55*(1), 1–9.

Lankshear, A. J., Sheldon, T. A., & Maynard, A. (2005). Nurse staffing and healthcare outcomes: A systematic review of the international research evidence. *Advances in Nursing, 28*(2), 163–174.

Lantz, P., House, J. S., Lepkroski, J. M., Williams, D. R., Mero, R. P., & Chen, J. (1998). Socioeconomic factors, health behaviors, and mortality. *Journal of the AMA, 279,* 1703.

Lasser, K. E., Himmelstein, D. U., & Woolhandler, S. (2006). Access to care, health status, and health disparities in the United States and Canada: Results of a cross-national population-based survey. *American Journal of Public Health, 96*(7), 1300–1307.

Leape, L. L. (1992). Unnecessary surgery. *Annual Review Public Health, 13,* 363–383.

Magnet Recognition Program (MRP). (2005). *Force of magnetism statement of evidence* (pp. 32–45). Silver Spring, MD.

Marshall, M. N., Hiscock, J., & Sibbald, B. (2002). Attitudes to the public release of comparative information on the quality of general practice care: A qualitative study. *British Medical Journal, 325*(7375), 1278.

Martin, J. A., Hamilton, B. E., Sutton, P. D., & Ventura, S. J. (2006). Births: Final data for 2004. *National vital statistics reports* (Vol. 55, No. 1). Hyattsville, MD: National Center for Health Statistics.

Maville, J. A., & Huerta, C. G. (2007). *Health promotion in nursing* (2nd ed.). Clifton Park, NY: Delmar Cengage Learning.

Mayo, T. W. (2007). U. S. Health Care Timelines. Southern Methodist University, Dedman School of Law. Retrieved July 25, 2008, from faculty.smu.edu/tmayo/health%20care%20timeline.htm.

McGlynn, E. A., Asch, S. M., Adams, J., Keesey, J., Hicks, J., DeCristofaro, A., & Kerr, A. (2003). The quality of health care delivered to adults in the United States. *New England Journal of Medicine*, 348, 2635–2645.

Mokdad, A. H., Marks, J. S., Stroup, D. F., & Gerberding, J. L. (2004). Actual causes of death in the United States, 2000. *Journal of American Medical Association*, 291(10), 1238–1245.

Muenning, P., Franks, P., Jia, H., Lubetkin, E., & Gold, M. R. (2005). The income-associated burden of disease in the United States. *Social Science Medicine*, 61(9), 2018–2026.

National Association for Home Care & Hospice. (2007). Basic statistics about home care. Washington, DC: Home Care & Hospice. Retrieved August 4, 2008, from www.nahc.org/facts/08HC_Stats.pdf.

National Coalition on Health Care (NCHC). (2008a). Facts on health care costs. Retrieved July 28, 2008, from www.nchc.org/facts/costs.shtml.

National Coalition on Health Care (NCHC). (2008b). The impact of rising health care costs on the economy. Retrieved September 27, 2008, from www.nchc.org/facts/Economy/effects_on_business_operations.pdf.

National Coalition on Health Care (NCHC). (2008c). World health care data. Retrieved August 2, 2008, from www.nchc.org/facts/world/shtml.

National Healthcare Disparities Report (NHDR). (2005). Agency for Healthcare Research and Quality, Rockville, MD. Retrieved November 4, 2006, from www.ahrq.gov/qual/nhdr05/nhdr05.htm.

National Healthcare Quality Report (NHQR). (2005). Agency for Healthcare Research and Quality, Rockville, MD. www.ahrq.gov/qual/nhqr05/nhqr05.htm.

National Nosocomial Infections Surveillance (NNIS) System Report. (1998, Oct.). Data summary from October 1986–April 1998, issued June 1998. *American Journal of Infectious Control*, 26(5), 522–533.

Nightingale, F. (1865/1970). *Notes on nursing*. Princeton: Vertex.

Nolte, E., & McKee, C. M. (2008). Measuring the health of nations: Updating an earlier analysis. *Health Affairs*, 27(1), 58–71.

Ofman, J. J., Badamgarav, E., Henning, J. M., Knight, K., Gano, A. D., Jr., Levan, R. K., et al. (2004). Does disease management improve clinical and economic outcomes in patients with chronic diseases? A systematic review. *American Journal of Medicine*, 117(3), 182–192.

Organisation for Economic Co-operation and Development. (2007). Health at a glance 2007: OECD indicators (chapter 6). Retrieved October 4, 2008, from fiordiliji.sourceoecd.org/pdf/health2007/812007051-6-9.pdf.

Organisation for Economic Co-operation and Development. (2008). OECD Health Data 2008: How does Japan compare. Paris: Author. Retrieved September 28, 2008, from www.oecd.org/document/46/0,3343,en_2649_33929_34971438_1_1_1_1,00.html.

Osborn, R. (2008). Comparing health care systems performance: Opportunities for learning from abroad (slide #4). Commonwealth Fund. Retrieved October 4, 2008, from www.allhealth.org/BriefingMaterials/Osborn-1189.ppt.

Parkerson, G. R., Jr., Broadhead, W. E., & Tse, C.-K. J. (1990). The Duke health profile: A 17 item measure of health and dysfunction. *Medical Care, 28*, 1056–1072.

Peterson, E. D., DeLong, E. R., Jollis, J. G., Muhlbaier, L. H., & Mark, D. B. (1998). The effects of New York's bypass surgery provider profiling on access to care and patient outcomes in the elderly. *Journal of the American College of Cardiology, 32*(4), 993–999.

Reid, T. R. (2008). Japanese pay less for more health care. Washington: National Public Radio. Retrieved August 5, 2008, from www.npr.org/templates/story/story.php?storyId=89626309.

Robert Wood Johnson Foundation. (2008). Cover the uninsured. Retrieved August 7, 2008, from covertheuninsured.org/.

Robinson, J. C. (2001). Theory and practice in the design of physician payment incentives. *Milbank Quarterly, 79,* 149–177.

Ross, J. S. (2002). The Committee on the Costs of Medical Care and the history of health insurance in the United States. *Einstein Quarterly Journal of Biological Medicine, 19,* 129–134.

Safran, D. G., Rogers, W. H., Tarlov, A. R., McHorney, C. A., & Ware, J. E., Jr. (1997). Gender differences in medical treatment: The case of physician-prescribed activity restrictions. *Social Science Medicine, 45*(5), 711–722.

Shapiro, J. (2008). Health care lessons from France. Washington: National Public Radio. Retrieved August 2, 2008, from www.npr.org/templates/story/story.php?storyId=91972152.

Shortell, S. M., & Kaluzny, A. D. (2006). Health Care Management (5th ed., p. 9). Clifton Park, NY: Delmar Cengage Learning.

Smith, M. A., Atherly, A. J., Kane, R. L., & Pacala, J. T. (1997). Peer review of the quality of care: Reliability and sources of variability for outcome and process assessment. *The Journal of the American Medical Association, 278,* 1573–1578.

Spitzer, W. O. (1998). Quality of life. In D. Burley & W. H. W. Inman (Eds.), *Therapeutic risk: Perception, measurement, and management.* New York: Wiley.

Stanton, M. W. (2006). The high concentration of U.S. health care expenditures. *Research in Action, 19,* 1–11. Retrieved July 31, 2008, from www.ahrq.gov/research/ria2019/expendria.pdf.

Thomas, E. J., Studdert, D. M., Burstin, H. R., Orav, E. J., Zeena, T., Williams, E. J., et al. (2000). Incidence and types of adverse events and negligent care in Utah and Colorado. *Medical Care, 38,* 261–271.

Thorpe, K., Woodruff, R., & Ginsburg, P. (2005). Factors driving cost increases. Retrieved on June 6, 2006, from www.ahrq.gov/ news/ulp/costs/ulpcosts1.htm.

U.S. Department of Health and Human Services. (2000). *Healthy People 2010: Understanding and Improving Health* (2nd ed.). Washington, DC: U.S. Government Printing Office.

Ulrich, B., Quan, X., Zimring, C., Joseph, A., & Choudhary, R. (2004). *The role of the physical environment in the hospital of the 21st Century.* Concord, CA: Center for Health Design. Retrieved July 28, 2008, from www.rwjf.org/files/publications/other/RoleofthePhysicalEnvironment.pdf.

Ware, J. E., & Sherbourne, C. D. (1992). The MOS 36-item short form health survey I: Conceptual framework and item selection. *Medical Care, 30,* 473–478.

Wennberg, J. E., & Gittelsohn, A. M. (1973). Small area variations in health care delivery. *Science, 182*(117), 1102–1108.

Werner, R. M., & Bradlow, E. T. (2006). Relationship between Medicare's hospital compare performance measures and mortality rates. *Journal of American Medical Association, 296*(22), 2694–2702.

Williams, L.S., Eckert, G.J., L'italien, G.J., Lapucrta, P., & Weinberger, M. (2003). Regional Variation in Healthcare Utilization and Outcomes in Ischemic Stroke, *Journal of Stroke and Cerebrovascular Disease, 12*(6) 259–265.

Williams, S. C., Schmaltz, S. P., Morton, D. J., Koss, R. G., & Loeb, J. M. (2005). Quality of care in U.S. hospitals as reflected by standard measures, 2003–2004. *New England Journal of Medicine, 353*(3), 255–264.

Woo, A., Ranji, U., Lundy, J., & Chen, F. (2007). Prescription drug costs. Menlo Park: Kaiser Family Foundation. Retrieved August 4, 2008, from www.kaiseredu.org/topics_im.asp?id=352&parentID=68&imID=1.

Woolf, S. H. (1999). The need for perspective in evidence-based medicine. *Journal of the American Medical Association, 282,* 2358–2365.

World Health Organization (WHO). (1978). Declaration of Alma-Ata: International conference on primary health care. Geneva: Author.

World Health Organization (WHO). (2000). The World Health Report 2000—Health systems: Improving performance. Geneva: Author.

SUGGESTED READINGS

American Association for Accreditation of Ambulatory Surgery Facilities (AAAASF). (2001). About AAAASF. Retrieved October 4, 2006 from www.aaaasf.org/aboutAAAAst/about.cfm.

American Association of Colleges of Nursing (AACN). (2008). Nursing shortage fact sheet. Washington: Author. Retrieved August 4, 2008, from www.aacn.nche.edu/Media/pdf/NrsgShortageFS.pdf.

American College of Physicians. (2008). Achieving a high-performance health care system with universal access: What the United States can learn from other countries. *Annals of Internal Medicine, 148*, 55–75.

An, J., Saloner, R., & Ranji, U. (2008). U.S. health care costs. Menlo Park: Kaiser Family Foundation. Retrieved August 4, 2008, from www.kaiseredu.org/ topics_im.asp?imID=1&parentID=61&id=358.

Anderson, R. M., Rice, T. H., & Kominski, G. F. (2007). Changing the U.S. health care system: Key issues in health services policy and management (3rd ed.). San Francisco: Jossey-Bass.

Anell, A., & Willis, M. (2000). International comparison of health care systems using resource profiles. *Bulletin of the World Health Organization, 78*(6), 770–778.

Baker, S. (2008). U.S. National Health Spending, 2006. University of South Carolina, Arnold School of Public Health, Department of Health Services Policy and Management, HSPM J712. Retrieved October 6, 2008, from hspm.sph.sc.edu/Courses/Econ/Classes/nhe06/hspm.sph.sc.edu/Courses/Econ/Classes/nhe06/.

Berwick, D. M. (1994). Eleven worthy aims for clinical leadership of health system reform. *Journal of the American Medical Association, 272*, 797–802.

Buerhaus, P. I., & Staiger, D. O. (1999, Jan.–Feb.). Trouble in the nurse labor market? Recent trends and future outlook. *Health Affairs,* 214–222.

Coalition for Patients Rights. (2008). Retrieved September 11, 2008, from www.patientsrightscoalition.org/.

Cooper, R. A., Getzen, T. E., McKee, H. M., & Laud, P. (2002). Economic and demographic trends signal an impending physician shortage. *Health Affairs, 21*(1), 140–154.

Cover the Uninsured. (2008). Robert Woods Johnson Foundation. Retrieved September 11, 2008, from covertheuninsured.org/.

Department of Defense (DOD). (2003). TRICARE: The Basics. Retrieved October 4, 2006, from www.tricare.mil/Factsheets/viewfactsheet.cfm?id=127.

DMAA. (2008). DMAA definition of disease management. Washington, DC: DMAA: The Care Continuum Alliance. Retrieved August 8, 2008, from www.dmaa.org/contact_us.asp.

Donaldson, L. (2001). Safe high-quality health care: Investing in tomorrow's leaders. *Quality in Health Care, 10*(suppl II), ii8 ii12.

Gabel, J., Claxton, G., Holve, E., Pickreign, J., Whitmore, H., & Dhont, K., et al. (2003). Health benefits in 2003: Premiums reach thirteen-year high as employers adopt new forms of cost sharing. *Health Affairs, 22*(5), 117–126.

Gilmer, T., & Kronick, R. (2005). It's the premiums stupid: Projections of the uninsured through 2013. *Health Affairs, 24*, w143–w151, (published online April 5, 2005).

Ginsburg, P. B. (2003). Can hospitals and physicians shift the effects of cuts in Medicare reimbursement to private payers? *Health Affairs, W3*, 472–479.

Gordon, S. (2005). *Nursing against the odds: How health care cost cutting, media stereotypes, and medical hubris undermine nurses and patient care.* Ithaca, NY: Cornell.

Green, L. A., Yawn, B. P., Lanier, D., & Dovey, S. M. (2001). The ecology of medical care revisited. *New England Journal of Medicine, 344*(26), 2021–2025.

Ho, K., Brady, J., & Clancy, C. M. (2008). Improving quality and reducing disparities: The role of nurses. *Journal of Nursing Care Quality, 23*(3), 185–188.

Hohlen, M. M., Manheim, L. M., Fleming, G. V., Davidson, S. M., Yadkowsky, B. K., Weiner, S. M., et al. (1990). Access to office-based physicians under capitation reimbursement and Medicaid case management: Findings from the Children's Medicaid Program. *Medical Care, 28*, 59–68.

Indian Health Service (IHS). (2006). Indian Health Service Fact Sheet. Retrieved October 4, 2006, from info.ihs.gov/Files/IHSFacts-June2006.pdf.

Institute for Healthcare Improvement. (2008). Retrieved September 11, 2008, from www.ihi.org/ihi.

Institute of Medicine (IOM). (1996). Primary care: America's health in a new era. Washington, DC: National Academy Press.

Institute of Medicine (IOM). (2008). Knowing what works in health care: A roadmap for the nation. Washington, DC: National Academy Press.

Kahn, C. N., Ault, T., Isenstein, H., Potetz, L., & Van Gelder, S. (2006). Snapshot of hospital quality reporting and pay-for-performance under Medicare. *Health Affairs, 25*(1), 148–162.

Kaiser Family Foundation (KFF). (2004). Trends and Indicators in the Changing Health Care Marketplace. Publication number: 7031. Retrieved October 4, 2006, from www.kff.org/insurance/ 7031/ti2004–1-1.cfm.

Kaiser Family Foundation (KFF). (2005). Navigating Medicare and Medicaid, 2005: Medicaid. Washington, DC: Kaiser Family Foundation. Accessible at www.kff.org/medicare/7240/medicaid.cfm.

Kaiser Family Foundation (KFF). (2007). The uninsured, a primer: Key facts about Americans without health insurance. Washington, DC: Kaiser Family Foundation. Accessible at www.kff.org/uninsured/upload/7451-03.pdf.

Kleinpell, R. M. (2007). Advanced practice nurses: Invisible champions? *Nursing Management, 38*(5), 18–22.

Knox, R., & Poole, J. W. (2008, Aug. 2). Health care for all: Massachusetts steps forward on health coverage. Washington: National Public Radio. Retrieved August 2, 2008, from www.npr.org/templates/story/story.php?storyId=92758148.

Lansky, D. (2002, July–Aug.). Improving quality through public disclosure of performance information. *Health Affairs,* 52–62.

Lapetina, E. M., & Armstrong, E. M. (2002, July–Aug.). Preventing errors in the outpatient setting: A tale of three states. *Health Affairs,* 26–39.

Laschinger, H. K. S., & Leiter, M. P. (2006). The impact of nursing work environments on patient safety outcomes: The mediating role of burnout/engagement. *Journal of Nursing Administration, 36*(5), 259–267.

Leape, L .L., Park, R. E., Solomon, D. H., Chassin, M. R., Kisecoff, J., & Brook, R. H. (1990). Does inappropriate use explain small area variations in the use of health care services? *Journal of the American Medical Association, 263,* 669–672.

Lohr, K. N., Brook, R. H., Kamberg, C. J., Goldberg, G. A., Leibouitz, A., Keesey, J., et al. (1986). Use of medical care in the Rand Health Insurance Experiment. *Medical Care,* Supplement 24, S1.

Lurie, N., Manning, G. W., Peterson, C., Goldberg, G. A. Phelps, C. A., & Lillard, L. (1987). Preventive care: Do we practice what we preach? *New England Journal of Medicine, 329,* 478.

Massachusetts Nurses Association. (2008). Single payer health care. Retrieved September 11, 2008, from www.massnurses.org/single_payer/singlepay.htm.

McGinnis, J. M., & Foege, W. H. (1993). Actual causes of death in the United States. *Journal of the American Medical Association, 270*(18), 2207–2212.

Miller, K. (Producer) (2008, May 9). Bill Moyers Journal: California Nurses Association. Washington, DC: Public Broadcasting Service. Retrieved September 11, 2008, from www.pbs.org/moyers/journal/05092008/profile.html.

Montalvo, I. (2007). The National Database of Nursing Quality Indicators (NDNQI). *Online Journal of Issues in Nursing, 12*(3). Retrieved August 8, 2008, from www.nursingworld.org/MainMenuCategories/ANAMarketplace/ANAPeriodicals/OJIN/TableofContents/Volume122007/No3Sept07/NursingQualityIndicators.aspx.

Murry, J. P., Greenfield, S., Kaplan, S. H., & Yano, E. M. (1992). Ambulatory testing for capitation and fee-for-service patients in the same practice setting: Relationship to outcomes. *Medical Care, 30,* 252–261.

Norman, L. D., Donelan, K., Buerhaus, P. I., Willis, G., Williams, M., Ulrich, B., et al. (2005). The older nurse in the workplace: Does age matter? *Nursing Economics, 23*(6), 279, 282–289.

Nurses for a Healthier Tomorrow. (n.d.). Retrieved October 4, 2008, from www.nursesource.org/.

O'Neil, E. (2008). Centering on...a nursing leadership agenda for a new health care age. The Center for the Health Professions, University of California, San Francisco. Retrieved July 24, 2008, from www.futurehealth.ucsf.edu/from_the_director_0308.html.

Scherer, F. M. (2004). The pharmaceutical industry: Prices and progress. *New England Journal of Medicine, 351*(9), 927–932.

Schoen, C., Collins, S. R., Kriss, J. L., & Doty, M. M. (2008). How many are underinsured? Trends among U.S. adults, 2003 and 2007. New York: Commonwealth Fund. Retrieved July 28, 2008, from www.commonwealthfund.org/publications/publications_show.htm?doc_id=688615.

Schwartz, B. (1995, July 16). The best medicine. *Boston Globe Magazine*. Retrieved September 5, 2008, from www.theschwartzcenter.org/story/best_medicine.html.

Starfield, B. (1998). *Primary care: Balancing health needs, services, and technology*. New York: Oxford University Press.

States take on national health insurance crisis. (2007, Jan.) *USA Today,* 12A.

Teenier, P. (2008). 2008 refinements to the Medicare home health Prospective Payment System. *Home Healthcare Nurse, 26*(3), 181–184.

U.S. Department of Health and Human Services. (2004). What is behind HRSA's projected supply, demand, and shortage of registered nurses? Retrieved October 5, 2008, from ftp.hrsa.gov/bhpr/workforce/behindshortage.pdf.

U.S. Department of Health and Human Services. (2008). Annual update of the HHS poverty guidelines. Accessible at aspe.hhs.gov/poverty/08Poverty.shtml.

U.S. Department of Health and Human Services. (2008). Medicare and You 2008. Centers for Medicare and Medicaid Services. Baltimore, MD: Author. Retrieved August 7, 2008 from www.cms.hhs.gov

U.S. Office of Management and Budget. (1998). *The Budget for Fiscal Year 1999, Analytical Perspectives*.

CHAPTER 3

Nursing Today

For us who Nurse, our Nursing is a thing, which, unless in it we are making progress every year, every month, every week, take my word for it, we are going back.

(Florence Nightingale, 1872)

OBJECTIVES

Upon completion of this chapter, the reader should be able to:

1. Discuss the evolution of nursing.
2. Review elements of a profession.
3. Identify professional nursing organizations and languages.
4. Review major subcultures of health care professionals.
5. Discuss evidence-based practice.
6. Identify nursing indicators and health care ratings.
7. Review Joint Commission (JC) accreditation standards.

You are at the annual Nurses' Day luncheon. The nursing manager of your unit stops to chat. She voices her concern about the variability in the use of nursing interventions on the units, as this may negatively affect the patient outcomes in the institution. She would like to see your unit incorporate evidence in patient-care processes, and she wants to appoint you to a task force to incorporate evidence-based care (EBC) into unit practices to reduce variability and improve patient outcomes. This scenario is becoming more and more common in health care institutions as nurses explore new ways to improve the quality of care.

What do you know about evidence-based care?

Is serving on a task force an appropriate nursing role?

How will you prepare yourself for the role?

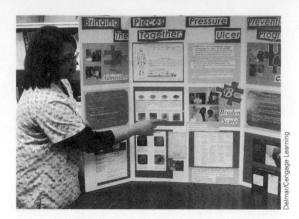

Registered nurses are the major professional group providing citizens with health care today. There are more than 2.5 million licensed RNs, and approximately 2 million are employed in the profession. Nurses deliver expert, highly skilled yet caring, evidence-based nursing services to patients to avoid the development of nursing-sensitive patient outcomes. Nursing practice has evolved for thousands of years with a long history of serving society, and nursing theorists continue to give direction to the profession of nursing. Nurses are often members of professional nursing organizations and have developed nursing languages, quality indicators, and health care systems to deliver, document, and measure nursing practice delivered to individuals and groups or populations of patients.

This chapter addresses these topics and methods designed to improve the quality of health care, including the movement to measure and rate quality and provide care according to evidence-based clinical practice guidelines.

EVOLUTION OF NURSING

The evolution of nursing dates back to 4000 BC to primitive societies in which mother-nurses worked with priests. Modern nursing was founded by Florence Nightingale, with the opening of the first Training School of Nurses, St. Thomas's Hospital, London, in 1860. Table 3-1 outlines some significant events in the history of nursing.

NURSING THEORISTS

Many nursing theorists contributed to the development of modern nursing; refer to Table 3-2.

PROFESSION OF NURSING

Nursing is recognized as a profession in most circles today, although in the 2000s, some nurses still report that they know the right thing to do but have little support or authority to carry it out.

Experts in the social sciences are considered the authorities on what makes an occupation a profession. Although there is some variation in actual criteria, there is general agreement in several areas:

- Professional status is achieved when an occupation involves a unique practice that carries individual responsibility and is based on theoretical knowledge.
- The privilege to practice is granted only after the individual has completed a standardized program of highly specialized education and has demonstrated an ability to meet the standards for practice.

TABLE 3-1	**SELECTED EVENTS INFLUENCING THE EVOLUTION OF NURSING**

Date	Event
1859	*Nightingale's Notes on Nursing* published in England
1860	First Nightingale School of Nursing, St. Thomas's Hospital, London
1871	New York State Training School for Nurses, Brooklyn Maternity, Brooklyn, New York
1872	New England Hospital for Women: one year program for nurses
1873	First three Nightingale schools in United States: Bellevue (New York City), Connecticut, and Massachusetts General
1893	Founded: first American Nursing Society, American Society of Superintendents of Training Schools for Nurses (Superintendents' Society)
1896–1911	Founded: Nurses' Associated Alumnae of the United States and Canada (Associated Alumnae)
1899	Founded: International Council of Nurses (ICN)
	First postgraduate courses for nurses at Teachers College, Columbia University
1900	*American Journal of Nursing (AJN)*
1901–1912	Founded: American Federation of Nurses
1903	North Carolina: passed first state nurse registration law
	Founded: Army Nurse Corps
1905	Federation joined ICN
1908	National Association of Colored Graduate Nurses (NACGN)
	Founded: Navy Nurse Corps
1909	Founded: first 3-year diploma school in a university setting at University of Minnesota
1911	Founded: American Nurses Association (ANA), formerly the Associated Alumnae
1912	Founded: National League of Nursing Education (NLN), formerly the Superintendents' Society
	ANA represented American nurses at ICN
	Nutting Report: Educational Status of Nursing
1920	Congress passed the federal suffrage amendment
1921	Women earned right to vote
1922	Studies of institutional nursing
1923	Studies of nursing education
	Founded: Yale University School of Nursing
1940	Cost studies of nursing education and service
1943	Founded: Federal Cadet Nurse Corps

(continues)

TABLE 3-1	SELECTED EVENTS INFLUENCING THE EVOLUTION OF NURSING (CONTINUED)

Date	Event
1948	Brown report: *Future of Nursing*
1953	U.S. Public Health Services Studies in Nursing Education
1955	Practical Nursing (Title III) Health Amendment Act
1956	Hughes study: *20,000 Nurses Tell Their Stories*
1964	Nurse Training Act
1965	First nurse practitioner program, pediatric
	ANA position paper on entry into practice
1966	Educational opportunity grants for nurses
1970	Secretary's commission to study extended roles for nurses
1983	Institute of Medicine Committee on Nursing and Nursing Education study
1987	HHS Secretary's Commission on Nursing
1997	Agency for Health Care Policy and Research, now known as the Agency for Healthcare Research and Quality, established 12 evidence-based practice centers

Source: Adapted from DeLaune, S.C. & Ladner, P.K. (2006). *Fundamentals of Nursing* (3rd ed.). Clifton Park, NY: Delmar Cengage Learning.

TABLE 3-2	SELECTED NURSING THEORISTS AND THEIR MODEL

Theorist–Model

Nightingale (1859)–Environmental Theory	Orem (1971)–Self-Care Deficit Theory
Peplau (1952)–Interpersonal Process	Roy (1976)–Adaptation Model
Henderson (1955)–Basic Needs	Paterson & Zderad (1976)–Humanistic Nursing
Levine (1969)–Conservation Theory	Neuman (1972/1995)–Systems Model
Rogers (1970)–Science of Unitary Beings	Watson (1979/1989)–Human Caring Theory
King (1971)–Goal Attainment Theory	Parse (1981/1995)–Human Becoming Theory

Source: Adapted from DeLaune, S.C. & Ladner, P.K. (2006). *Fundamentals of Nursing* (3rd ed.). Clifton Park, NY: Delmar Cengage Learning.

- The body of specialized knowledge is continually developed and evaluated through research.

- The members are self-organizing and collectively assume the responsibility of establishing standards for education in practice. They continually evaluate the quality of service provided in order to protect the individual members and the public.

In recent years, a trend has arisen to call every occupation a profession. Have you heard of "professional baseball players" or "professional automobile mechanics"? There has been a tendency to confuse *professionalism* and *profession*. The term *professionalism* generally refers to an individual's commitment and dedication to the occupation. Professionalism often also refers to the attitude, appearance, and conduct of the individual. Whether an occupation is a profession requires more analysis. Table 3-3 refers to some studies about the characteristics of a profession. Table 3-4 lists some of the various values, behaviors, and attributes that may be exhibited by a "professional" (Mitchell & Grippando, 1994).

TABLE 3-3	CHARACTERISTICS OF A PROFESSION

Flexner, 1915

- Intellectual activities
- Activities based on knowledge
- Activities can be learned
- Activities must be practical
- Techniques are teachable
- A strong organization exists
- Altruism motivates the work

Bixler and Bixler, 1959

- Specialized body of knowledge
- Growing body of knowledge
- New knowledge used to improve education and practice
- Education takes place in higher education institutions
- Autonomous practice
- Service above personal gain
- Compensation through freedom of action, continuing professional growth, and economic security

Pavalko, 1971

- Work based on systematic body of theory and abstract knowledge
- Work has social value
- Length of education required for specialization
- Service to public
- Autonomy
- Commitment to profession
- Group identity and subculture
- Existence of a code of ethics

Public Law 93-360 on Collective Bargaining

- Predominantly intellectual work
- Varied work requirements
- Requires discretion and judgment
- Results cannot be standardized over time
- Requires advanced instruction and study

Source: From Mitchell, G. M. & Grippando, P. R. (1994). *Nursing Perspectives and Issues* (5th ed.). Clifton Park, NY: Delmar Cengage Learning.

TABLE 3-4 | CHARACTERISTICS OF A PROFESSIONAL

Professional Values:

Caring	Freedom	Justice
Altruism	Esthetics	Truth
Equality	Human dignity	Ethical
Nonjudgmental		

Professional Behaviors and Attributes:

Appearance	
Time-management skills	
Self-discipline	Stress management
Maintenance of licensure/certification	Self-evaluation
Participation in institutional/community activities	Initiative
Participation in continuing education	Motivation
Political awareness	Creativity
Reading professional journals	Effective communication
Participation in nursing research	

Source: From Mitchell, G. M. & Grippando, P. R. (1994). *Nursing Perspectives and Issues* (5th ed.). Clifton Park, NY: Delmar Cengage Learning.

CASE STUDY 3-1

Note the professional values in Table 3-4. Do you agree with them? Now note the professional behaviors and attributes characteristic of a professional in the same Table. Which professional behaviors and attributes do you have? Make a one-year and a five-year plan for any goals you feel that you need to work on. Identify an experienced nursing mentor and review your goals with your mentor. Does your behavior agree with your goals?

PROFESSIONAL NURSING ORGANIZATIONS

Nursing professionals can belong to many different nursing organizations. These organizations often develop standards and offer continuing education to their members; refer to Table 3-5.

SUBCULTURES OF HEALTH PROFESSIONALS

Individual professionals within several subcultures of health care work in various health care settings—nursing, medicine, physical therapy,

TABLE 3-5	PROFESSIONAL NURSING ORGANIZATIONS
Academy of Medical Surgical Nursing	www.medsurgnurse.org
Air and Surface Transport Nurses Association	www.astna.org
American Academy of Ambulatory Care Nursing	www.aaacn.org
American Academy of Nurse Practitioners	www.aanp.org
American Academy of Nursing	www.nursingworld.org/aan
American Assembly of Men in Nursing	aamn.org
American Assisted Living Nurses Association	www.alnursing.org
American Association of Colleges of Nursing	www.aacn.nche.edu
American Association of Continuity in Care	www.continuityofcare.com
American Association of Critical-Care Nurses	www.aacn.org
American Association of Diabetes Educators	www.aadenet.org
American Association for the History of Nursing	www.aahn.org
American Association of Legal Nurse Consultants	www.aalnc.org
American Association of Neuroscience Nurses	www.aann.org
American Association of Nurse Anesthetists	www.aana.com
American Association of Nurse Attorneys	www.taana.org
American Association of Occupational Health Nurses	www.aaohn.org
American Association of Office Nurses	www.aaon.org
American Association of Spinal Cord Nurses	www.aascin.org
American Association of Nurse Midwives	www.acnm.org

(continues)

TABLE 3-5	PROFESSIONAL NURSING ORGANIZATIONS (CONTINUED)
American College of Nurse Practitioners	www.nurse.org/acnp
American Holistic Nurses Association	www.ahna.org
American Nephrology Nurses Association	anna.inurse.com
American Nurses Association	www.nursingworld.org
American Nurses Credentialing Center	www.nursingworld.org/ancc
American Nursing Informatics Association	www.ania.org
American Organization of Nurse Executives	www.aone.org
American Public Health Association	www.apha.org
American Psychiatric Nurses Association	www.apna.org
American Radiological Nurses Association	www.rsna.org
American Society of Ophthalmic Registered Nurses	webeye.ophth.uiowa.edu/asorn
American Society of Pain Management Nurses	www.aspmn.org
American Society of Perianesthesia Nurses	www.aspan.org
American Society of Plastic and Reconstructive Surgical Nurses	www.aspsn.org
Association of child and adolescent psychiatric nurses	www.ispn-psych.org
Association of Child Neurology Nurses	www.acnn.org
Association of Nurses in AIDS Care	www.anacnet.org
Association of Pediatric Oncology	www.apon.org
Association of Perioperative Registered Nurses	www.aorn.org
Association for Professionals in Infection Control and Epidemiology	www.apic.org
Association of Rehabilitation Nurses	www.rehabnurse.org
Association of Women's Health, Obstetrics and Neonatal Nurses	www.awhonn.org
Case Management Society of America	www.cmsa.org

(continues)

TABLE 3-5 — PROFESSIONAL NURSING ORGANIZATIONS (CONTINUED)

Dermatology Nurses Association	www.dnanurse.org
Developmental Disabilities Nurses Association	www.ddna.org
Emergency Nurses Association	www.ena.org
Endocrine Nurses Society	www.endo-nurses.org
Home Healthcare Nurses Association	www.hhna.org
Hospice and Palliative Nurses Association	www.hpna.org
Infusion Nurses Society	www.isn1.org
International Association of Forensic Nurses	www.forensicnurse.org
International Council of Nurses	www.icn.ch
National Association of Clinical Nurse Specialists	www.nacns.org
National Association of Hispanic Nurses	www.thehispanicnurses.org
National Association of Neonatal Nurses	www.nann.org
National Association of Nurse Massage Therapists	www.nanmt.org
National Association of Orthopedic Nurses	www.orthonurse.org
National Association of Pediatric Nurse Practitioners and Associates	www.napnap.org
National Association of School Nurses	www.nasn.org
National Black Nurses Association	www.nbna.org
National Council of State Boards of Nursing	www.ncsbn.org
National Gerontological Nursing Association	www.ngna.org
National League for Nursing	www.nln.org
National Nursing Staff Development Organization	nnsdo.org
National Organization for Associate Degree Nursing	www.noadn.org
National Organization of Nurse Practitioner Faculties	www.nonpf.com
National Student Nurses Association	www.nsna.org
Oncology Nursing Society	www.ons.org

(continues)

TABLE 3-5	PROFESSIONAL NURSING ORGANIZATIONS (CONTINUED)
Philippine Nurses Association of America	www.pnaa03.org
Sigma Theta Tau, International	www.nursingsociety.org
Society of Gastroenterology Nurses and Associates	www.sgna.org
Society of Pediatric Nurses	www.pedsnurses.org
Society of Urologic Nurses and Associates	suna.inurse.com
Society for Vascular Nursing	www.svnnet.org
Transcultural Nursing Society	www.tcns.org
Wound, Ostomy and Continence Nurses Society	www.wocn.org

social work, hospital administration, dietetics, and pharmacy, to name a few. These subcultures affect patient care delivered in the various settings. Table 3-6 lists generalized characteristics of three of these subcultures of health professionals. These characteristics are dynamic and constantly changing the culture of health care organizations and groups that nurses today work with to provide quality health care.

EVIDENCE-BASED PRACTICE

Evidence-based practice (EBP) is defined as the conscientious, explicit, and judicious use of current best evidence in making decisions about the care of individual patients (Sackett, Rosenberg, Gray, Haynes, & Richardson, 1996). EBP involves supplementing clinical expertise with the judicious and conscientious implementation of the most current and best evidence, along with patient values and preferences to guide health care decision making (Jennings & Loan, 2001). The body of evidence supporting clinical practice is

steadily growing. However, even when evidence-based quality care guidelines are available for numerous conditions, for example, diabetes, congestive heart failure, and asthma, they have not been fully implemented in actual patient care, and variation in clinical practice is abundant (Timmermans & Mauck, 2005; McGlynn et al., 2003; Kitson, 2007). EBP uses evidence-based resources to guide the development of appropriate strategies to deliver quality, cost-effective care (Table 3-7). Outcomes provide evidence about benefits, risks, and results of treatments so individuals can make informed decisions and choices to improve their quality of life. Select journal sources for evidence-based practice are listed in Table 3-8.

EVIDENCE-BASED PRACTICE MODEL

Nurses seeking to increase the use of evidence in their clinical practice may want to apply the model developed by the University of Colorado (Figure 3-1). This model highlights the elements of EBP, which can be measured.

TABLE 3-6	GENERALIZED CHARACTERISTICS OF THREE SUBCULTURES OF HEALTH PROFESSIONALS TODAY		
Characteristics	**Nursing**	**Medicine**	**Health Care Administration**
Major task	Use of nursing process to deliver patient care	Diagnosis and treatment of disease	Organizational stability and continuity
Membership	Historically female, white, middle class; caring, skilled, knowledgeable	Historically male, white, middle and upper class; scientific	Historically male-dominant,* problem solving
Leading role strength	Prevent nurse–sensitive patient outcomes, Comforter, promote health	Life-saver and treat disease	Keeper of the house
Role centrality	Coordinator of health services	Gatekeeper of health services	Proprietor of health services; holder of the purse strings
Relationships with other professional groups	Collaborative; work with team, hierarchy of supervision	Autonomy; directing the team	Negotiating, seeks cooperation
Perspective	Patient-centered, clinical unit/area	Patient- and practice-centered	Hospital's business and market relations
Conflict management	Interpersonal approach	Use leverage available, e.g., resources, patients, and authority, to maintain control	Structured, rational approach
Core dilemmas	Maintain professional safe care in time of staff shortages; build professional identity and respect for nursing	Choice of organizational and network affiliations, and the conditions and extent of agency affiliation; the future destiny of medical specialists	Where to invest strategic resources in an era of high future uncertainty
Major threats (current)	Decrease in job security; constraints on staffing levels and other resources; changes in role; nursing shortage	Health economics; changes in role; losses in authority and income; malpractice; potential for universal health care and funding changes	Organization survival, job security, funding changes

*The management of Catholic hospitals, typically run by orders of Catholic sisters, is a notable exception to the generalizations about male health care administrators.

TABLE 3-7 EVIDENCE-BASED RESOURCES

National guideline clearinghouse, Agency for Health Care Quality and Research	www.guideline.gov
Sigma Theta Tau International	www.nursingsociety.org
Global evidence	www.globalevidence.com
Cochrane collaboration	www.cochrane.org
Joanna Briggs Institute for Evidence-Based Nursing and Midwifery	www.joannabriggs.edu.au
Sarah Cole Hirsh Institute for Best Nursing Practices Based on Evidence	fpb.case.edu. Search for *Hirsh Institute.*
Centre for Evidence-Based Nursing	www.york.ac.uk. Search for *Evidence-Based Nursing.*
Registered Nurses' Association of Ontario	www.rnao.org
Gerontological Nursing Interventions Research Center (GNIRC)	www.nursing.uiowa.edu
Research Centre for Transcultural Studies in Health	www.mdx.ac.uk
Academic Center for Evidence-Based Nursing (ACE)	www.acestar.uthscsa.edu
Cumulative Index to Nursing and Allied Health (CINAHL)	www.cinahl.com
Evidence-Based Nursing Journal	www.evidencebasednursing.com
McGill University Health Centre, Clinical and Professional Staff Development, Research & Clinical Resources for Evidence-Based Nursing	www.muhc-ebn.mcgill.ca
MEDLINE via PubMed, free resource provided by the National Library of Medicine	www.ncbi.nlm.nih.gov
Netting the Evidence—A ScHARR Introduction to Evidence-based Practice on the Internet	www.shef.ac.uk
PubMed Tutorial (NLM), an in-depth tutorial from the National Library of Medicine	www.nlm.nih.gov
University of Minnesota evidence-based nursing site tutorial	evidence.ahc.umn.edu
Nursing Knowledge International	www.nursingknowledge.org
Virginia Henderson International Nursing Library	www.nursinglibrary.org

TABLE 3-8	SELECTED JOURNAL SOURCES FOR EVIDENCE-BASED PRACTICE

Advances in Nursing Science	Journal of Nursing Scholarship
American Journal of Nursing	Journal of Transcultural Nursing
American Journal of Public Health	New England Journal of Medicine
Applied Nursing Research	Nursing Clinics of North America
Clinical Nursing Research	Nursing Economics
Clinical Effectiveness in Nursing	Nursing Policy Forum
Hastings Report	Nursing Research
Health Affairs	Nursing Science Quarterly
Health Care Management Review	Oncology Nursing Forum
Health Services Research	Online Journal of Knowledge Synthesis for Nursing
Heart and Lung	Qualitative Health Research
Hospice Journal	Research in Nursing and Health
International Journal of Nursing Studies	Scholarly Inquiry in Nursing Practice
Journal of Advanced Nursing	Social Science and Medicine
Journal of Health Economics	Western Journal of Nursing Research
Journal of The American Medical Association	Worldviews on Evidence-Based Nursing

NURSE-SENSITIVE PATIENT OUTCOMES

The existence of professional nursing benefits patients who develop lower rates of nurse-sensitive outcomes, including lower death rates of patients from one of the following life-threatening complications: pneumonia, shock, cardiac arrest, urinary tract infection, gastrointestinal bleeding, sepsis, deep vein thrombosis, and "failure to rescue" (Needleman, Buerhaus, Mattke, Stewart, & Zelevinsky, 2002). Nurses combine caring with professional expertise to prevent these outcomes.

HEALTH CARE RATINGS

Thomson Reuters has reviewed the performance of hospitals of all types and sizes. It publishes a listing of the 100 top hospitals nationally. See www.100tophospitals.com/about100top/default. aspx. *U.S. News and World Report* annually publishes a list of the top hospitals nationally. See ucsfhr. ucsf.edu/index.php/general/article/ucsf-makes-us-news-world-report-americas-best-hospital-rankings-again. See also the health care ratings at Health Grades (www.healthgrades.com), Leapfrog Hospital Quality and Safety (www.leapfroggroup. org/cp), and at the Department of Health &

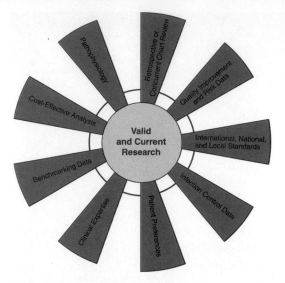

Figure 3-1 University of Colorado Hospital evidence-based multidisciplinary practice model. (*Source:* Used with permission of University of Colorado Hospital Research Council, Denver, CO).

CASE STUDY 3-2

Note the websites for evidence-based resources in Table 3-7. Search the National Guideline site for Diabetes. What information did you find there to apply to your patient care? Check some of the other websites in the Table. Did you find any good resources to help with your current patient care?

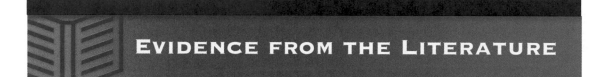

EVIDENCE FROM THE LITERATURE

Citation: Soukup, S. M. (2000). Preface to section on evidence-based nursing practice. *Nursing Clinics of North America, 35*(2), xvii–xviii.

Discussion: Author discusses a nurse's response to queries as to whether she has integrated evidence-based practice. The nurse responds, "Yes, I practice state-of-the-art nursing. My education and professional practice experiences have prepared me to care for more than 700 chronically ill patients annually, in the past 5 years. These patients have an average reported expected pain rating of 6.9 (using a scale of 1 to 10, with 10 being severe pain), and my pain management interventions have kept these patients, during my hours of care, at a reported actual pain rating of 4. Also, as a team member, these patients have not had any known pressure ulcers, skin tears, or catheter-related infections. On two occasions, for patients who were dying, I created a humanizing environment for these patients and their families when they were rapidly transferred from the critical care unit. My documentation has met organizational standards during monthly peer reviews; I have provided leadership for emergencies with positive outcomes; and physician and patient satisfaction rating for clinical practice on our unit is 9.5 on a scale of 10, with 10 being the highest. Our unit-based team has not had a needle-stick-related or back-related injury during the past 2 years. This has contributed to a significant cost avoidance and benefit to the organization.

Implications for Practice: Nurses practicing in the 21st century must embrace the principles of evidence-based practice as an approach to clinical care and professional accountability.

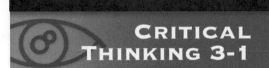

CRITICAL THINKING 3-1

Go to the Web site, www.sandiego.edu. Search for *nursing theorists*. How does nursing theory influence your practice as a professional? Pick one of the theories, and comment on how your practice of nursing may fit with the theory.

CRITICAL THINKING 3-2

Have you ever witnessed a "failure to rescue" or witnessed a nurse "rescuing" a patient? Would the patient have lived if the nurse did not prevent a nurse-sensitive outcome? How will you rescue your patients?

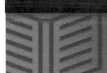

EVIDENCE FROM THE LITERATURE

Citation: Wu, Y., Larrabee, J. H., & Putman, H. P. (2006, Jan.–Feb.). Caring behaviors inventory. *Nursing Research,* *55*(1), 18–25.

Discussion: A short instrument for patient use is presented to measure the process of nurse caring. Elements of the patient instrument include patient assessment of the knowledge and skill, respectfulness, and connectedness, of the nurse. Some of the Caring Behaviors assessed include responding quickly to the patient's call; knowing how to give shots, IVs, and so on; attentively listening to the patient; and spending time with the patient. All twenty-four elements of the Caring Behaviors Inventory are presented.

Implications for Practice: Nurses interested in measuring the impact of their patient care can use this instrument to do so and improve their practice. The tool assesses the physical skill and caring behaviors of a nurse.

Human Services' Hospital Compare site (www. hospitalcompare.hhs.gov).

IMPORTANCE OF EVIDENCE, OUTCOMES, AND RATINGS

Why is evidence-based care (EBC), monitoring outcomes, and using rating systems important? It is estimated that many patients die each day because the current paper-based health care system introduces error or delays in treatment or limits what health care professionals know. Few clinician actions have been demonstrated to be supported by scientific evidence. Many actions are not

needed or are potentially harmful. Often, patients do not receive care which corresponds to present scientific evidence. Consequently, there is nothing more important to patients and professional nursing than evidence-based clinical interventions that can be linked to clinical outcomes and used as a basis for rating care. However, there has been a lack of generally agreed-upon standards or processes that are based on evidence. This lack of standards has been addressed of late with the development of EBC.

Generally speaking, nursing, medicine, health care institutions and health policy makers recognize EBC as care based on a method of collecting,

training in using tools to access evidence. Few regularly search for information from the evidence and many are not familiar with the term, EBC.

reviewing, interpreting, critiquing, and evaluating research and other relevant literature for direct application to patient care. EBC uses evidence from research; performance data; quality improvement studies such as hospital or nursing report cards, program evaluations, and surveys; national and local consensus recommendations of experts; rating systems; and clinical experience.

The EBC process further involves the integrating of both clinician-observed evidence and research-directed evidence. This then leads to state-of-the-art integration of available knowledge and evidence in a particular area of clinical concern that can be evaluated and measured through outcomes of care.

Applying the best available evidence does not guarantee good decisions, yet it is one of the keys to improving outcomes affecting health. EBC should be viewed as the highest standard of care so long as critical thinking and sound clinical judgment support it. Nurses and practitioners will always need to search for the best evidence available to support their clinical decisions. Sometimes, there is little research backing for clinical actions. In that case, nursing and medical practitioners should use their critical thinking skills and apply the consensus of experts. Institutions of care have a responsibility to provide nurses with an environment supportive of EBC. Currently, however, few nurses have received

POPULATION-BASED HEALTH CARE

Nurses today are working increasingly in population-based health care practices. **Population-based health care practice** is the development, provision, and evaluation of multidisciplinary health care services to population groups experiencing increased health risks or disparities, in partnership with health care consumers and the community, to improve the health of the community and its diverse population groups. Vulnerable population groups are subgroups of a community that are powerless, marginalized or disenfranchised, and experiencing health disparities. Figure 3-2 depicts the Minnesota Department of Health Public Health Intervention II Wheel. The Wheel identifies health care strategies to improve the care of individuals, communities, and systems. Research into health and illness has now recognized the contribution of social, economic, and environmental factors to health, and a critical body of evidence is beginning to document the influence of these factors on morbidity and mortality (American College of Physicians, 2004; Hartley, 2004; Institute of Medicine [IOM], 2002; Agency for Healthcare Research and Quality [AHRQ], 2005).

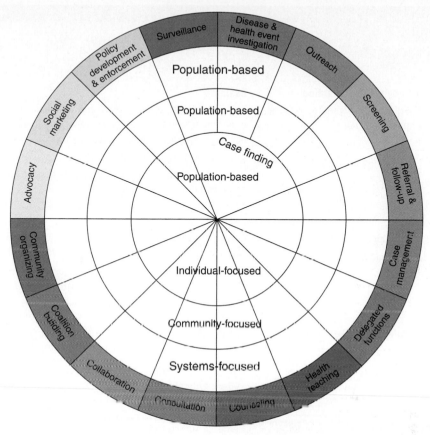

Figure 3-2 The Minnesota Department of Health public health interventions II wheel. (*Source:* Used with permission of the Section of Public Health Nursing, Minnesota Department of Health).

Population-based health care encourages society to direct resources toward strengthening five influences on health: health care system influences (e.g., access to medical care, cost, etc.); individual influences (lifestyle, genetics, etc.); interpersonal, social, and work influences (job satisfaction, social support, etc.); community influences (services, programs, etc.); and environmental influences (air, water, etc.). A society that spends so much on medical care that it cannot or will not spend adequately on other health-enhancing activities may actually be reducing the health of its population. Nursing today has begun to direct some of its efforts to population-based interventions designed to improve the health of populations (Table 3-9), Program evaluation of nursing efforts assesses patient access, quality, cost, and equity; refer to Table 3-10.

ACCREDITATION

Nurses today work in accredited health care organizations. The Joint Commission (JC) is the current national organization that develops standards and accredits health care organizations. This accreditation is important to hospitals because it is one of the ways hospitals can be certified to receive federal government Medicare and Medicaid reimbursement for delivery of patient care services.

As many as 50% of the JC's hospital accreditation standards were written to correspond

TABLE 3-9 — EXAMPLES OF POPULATION-BASED PUBLIC HEALTH INTERVENTION PROGRAMS*

Individual/Family Level of Practice

	Example
Referral and Follow-Up: Discharge referral from emergency department	Vulnerable older adults discharged from emergency department to home were referred for public health nursing home visits (Kelly, 2005).
Social Marketing: College campus initiative	Social marketing with a "grateful head" theme was used to increase helmet use among cyclists on a college campus (Ludwig, Buchholz, & Clarke, 2005).

Community Level of Practice

Coalition Building: Chicago southeast diabetes community action coalition	Coalition building was used as a strategy to reduce diabetic health disparities in a Chicago community (Giachello et al., 2003).
Screening: County of San Diego TB Control Program	County-level screening of recent immigrants and refugees for pulmonary tuberculosis was used to identify those with a positive Mantoux (LoBue & Moser, 2004).

Systems Level of Practice

Collaboration: Health disparities collaborative	Collaboration among health care providers improved diabetic care in community health centers (Chin et al., 2004).
Consultation and Delegated Functions: School-based health clinics	Use of POTS (plain old telephone system) to link school nurses with other health care providers improved school health services (Young & Ireson, 2003).

Source: Minnesota Department of Health, Section of Public Health Nursing. (2001). Public Health Interventions-Application for Public Health Nursing Practice. St. Paul, MN: Minnesota Department of Health.

TABLE 3-10 — PROGRAM EVALUATION OF POPULATION-BASED NURSING PRACTICE

Access	Did we find the high-risk, underserved, vulnerable population groups in the community/service area and provide timely and accessible services?
	Did we offer service regardless of age, gender, race, ethnicity, health care status, or location?
Quality	Did our services meet the greatest unmet health needs of the community or the at-risk, vulnerable, underserved population groups?
	Did their health status improve?
	Were their health risks reduced?

(continues)

TABLE 3-10	PROGRAM EVALUATION OF POPULATION-BASED NURSING PRACTICE (CONTINUED)
	Were they satisfied with the services they received?
Cost	Were patients able to afford what we had to offer?
	Did we manage to stay within our budget?
	Are we reducing the cost of care over time?
Equity	Did we use our resources in a way that met the priority health needs of all of our high-risk patient groups?
	Did we target our services and use our resources to improve the health status of those who were the most underserved?
	Did we have enough resources left over to meet the essential health needs of lower-risk population groups?

TABLE 3-11	HOSPITAL ACCREDITATION STANDARDS

Patient-focused functions	Organization-focused functions
■ Ethics, rights, and responsibilities	■ Improving organization performance
■ Provision of care, treatment and services	■ Leadership
■ Medication management	■ Management of the environment of care
■ Surveillance, prevention, and control of infection	■ Management of human resources
	■ Management of information
	■ Medical staff
	■ Nursing services

Source: © Joint Commission Resources. (2008). *CAMH: 2008 Comprehensive Accreditation Manual for Hospitals.* Oakbrook Terrace, IL: Joint Commission on Accreditation of Healthcare Organizations, available at www.jointcommission.org.

with Medicare's conditions of participation, a comprehensive set of criteria that hospitals and other care providers must meet to qualify for reimbursement. The JC's adherence to the conditions stems from its "deemed" status with Medicare, which means that JC-accredited hospitals are assumed to have met the Medicare participation standards. Hospitals pay an average of $20,000 for a JC survey (Lovern, 2001). Table 3-11 outlines the list of chapters in the accreditation manual. Each chapter highlights how quality is reviewed. All hospitals and long-term care organizations seeking JC accreditation monitor patient outcomes and use a performance measurement system to provide data about these patient outcomes and other indicators of care. Nurses today monitor accreditation standards and the other forces influencing health care; refer to Table 3-12.

TABLE 3-12	NINE FORCES INFLUENCING HEALTH CARE DELIVERY AND THEIR IMPLICATIONS FOR MANAGEMENT

External Force	Management Implication
1. Financial incentives that reward superior performance	■ Need for increased efficiency, productivity, and quality ■ Redesign of patient care delivery ■ Development of strategic alliances that add value ■ Increased growth of networks, systems, and physician groups
2. Increased accountability for performance	■ Information systems that facilitate patient-centered care across episodes of illness and "pathways of wellness" ■ Effective implementation of clinical practice guidelines and related care management processes ■ Ability to demonstrate continuous improvements of all functions and processes
3. Technological advances in the biological and clinical sciences	■ Expansion of the continuum of care, need for new treatment sites to accommodate new treatment modalities ■ Increased capacity to manage care across organizational boundaries ■ Need to confront new ethical dilemmas
4. Aging of the population and associated increase in chronic illness	■ Increased demand for primary care, wellness, and health promotion services and chronic care management ■ Challenge of managing ethical issues associated with prolongation of life
5. Increased ethnic and cultural diversity of the population	■ Greater difficulty in understanding and meeting patient expectations ■ Meeting the challenge of eliminating disparities in care provision and outcomes ■ Challenge of managing an increasingly diverse health services workforce
6. Changes in the supply and education of health professionals	■ Need for creative approaches in meeting the population's need for disease prevention, health promotion, and chronic care management services ■ Need to compensate for shortages in some categories of health professionals (i.e., physical therapy, pharmacy, and some areas of nursing) ■ Need to develop effective teams of caregivers across multiple treatment sites ■ Need to develop work settings conducive to recruitment and retention

(continues)

TABLE 3-12	NINE FORCES INFLUENCING HEALTH CARE DELIVERY AND THEIR IMPLICATIONS FOR MANAGEMENT (CONTINUED)

External Force	Management Implication
7. Social morbidity (AIDS, drugs, violence, bioterrorism "new surprises")	■ Ability to deal with unpredictable increases in demand ■ Need for increased social support systems and chronic care management ■ Need to work effectively with public health community agencies to address "preparedness" issues
8. Information technology	■ Training the health care workforce in new information technologies ■ Increased ability to coordinate care across sites ■ Challenge of managing an increased pace of change due to more rapid information transfer ■ Challenge of dealing with confidentiality issues associated with new information technologies
9. Globalization and expansion of the world economy	■ Need to manage cross-national and cross-cultural patient care referrals ■ Increasing the competitiveness and productivity of the American labor force ■ Managing global strategic alliances, particularly in the areas of biotechnology and new technology development ■ Meeting the challenge of new and reemerging infectious diseases

Source: From Shortell, S. M., & Kaluzny, A. D. (2006). *Health Care Management* (5th ed.) Clifton Park, NY: Delmar Cengage Learning.

KEY CONCEPTS

■ Nursing has evolved from early times into a highly skilled, educated discipline.

■ Caring, expert nursing practice is an important part of nursing's role in health care.

■ There is general agreement about the characteristics of a profession.

■ Nurses are members of many professional nursing organizations.

■ Health care professionals are divided into several major subcultures.

■ The focus on EBC can be expected to remain a driving force in the health care arena in the foreseeable future.

■ Quality nursing care avoids the development of nursing-sensitive patient outcomes.

- Nursing indicators have been developed to document and measure nursing.

- Nursing can make significant contributions to the advancement of evidence-based care.

- The focus of population-based health care is to reduce health disparities that exist among diverse population groups.

- The goals of population-based health care are access, quality, cost containment, and equity.

- The JC is the national organization that accredits health care organizations. This accreditation is one of the ways hospitals can be certified to receive federal government reimbursement for health care delivery to Medicare patients.

KEY TERMS

evidence-based practice

population-based health care practice

REVIEW QUESTIONS

1. What is the major purpose of evidence-based care (EBC)?
   A. To increase variability of care
   B. To cause a link to be missing in clinical care
   C. To determine what medical models can be applied by nursing
   D. To provide evidence-based care that supports clinical competency

2. Population-based nursing interventions are directed at
   A. all individuals who need health services.
   B. people without health care insurance.
   C. the health needs of the total community.
   D. only vulnerable groups within the community.

3. The four goals of population-based nursing practice are
   A. access, cost, empowerment, equity.
   B. access, cost, equity, resilience.
   C. access, cost, equity, quality.
   D. cost, equity, resilience, quality.

REVIEW ACTIVITIES

1. Compare and contrast individual-focused nursing practice with population-based nursing practice. What nursing knowledge and skills do you need to practice population-based nursing care?

2. Many believe that nurses should adopt a global framework for the empowerment of women to reduce health disparities. Discuss what you think this framework should include. How could you become a nursing advocate for this at the local, national, and international levels?

3. Review Pavalko's characteristics of a profession in Table 3-3. Is nursing a profession?

EXPLORING THE WEB

- Where could you find information to help serve the health care needs of immigrants? National Institutes of Health:
  www.nih.gov

- Visit the Oncology Nursing Society's Online Evidence-Based Practice Resource Area:
  www.ons.org

- What sites could you recommend to patients and families seeking information about self-help, hospital accreditation, research, and clinical practice guidelines, for example, the JC and the Agency for Healthcare Research and Quality?
  www.selfhelpweb.org
  www.jointcommission.org
  www.ahrq.gov
  www.centerwatch.com
  www.guideline.gov
  www.cdc.gov
  www.netdoctor.co.uk
  www.health.gov

- Go to the site for the Malcolm Baldridge National Quality Award. What information did you find there?
  www.quality.nist.gov

- Search the Web, checking these sites: Medicare, National Institutes of Health, American Nurses Association, National League for Nursing, American Cancer Society, American Heart Association, diabetes, Ellis Island records, and Delmar Learning. What did you find?
  www.medicare.gov
  www.nih.gov
  www.nursingworld.org
  www.nln.org
  www.cancer.org
  www.americanheart.org
  www.diabetes.org
  www.ellisislandrecords.org
  www.delmarhealthcare.com

- Go to PubMed. What did you find there? Can you access nursing and medical journals? Would you recommend this site to patients?
  www.ncbi.nlm.nih.gov

- What are some helpful sites for nurses?
  www.allnurses.com
  www.jointcommission.org
  www.continuingeducation.com
  www.hotnursejobs.com
  www.hospitalsoup.com

REFERENCES

Agency for Healthcare Research and Quality (AHRQ). (2005). *National Healthcare Disparities Report 2005.* USDHHS. Retrieved June 18, 2006, from www.ahrq.gov/qual/nhdr05/nhdr05.pdf

American College of Physicians (2004). Racial and ethnic disparities in health care. *Annals of Internal Medicine, 141*(3), 221–225.

Chin, M., Cook, S., Drum, M., Guillen, J., Humikowski, C., Koppert, J., Harrison, J., Lippold, S., Schaefer, C. (2004). *Improving diabetes care in midwest community health centers with the health disparities collaborative.* Diabetes Care, *27(1)*, 2–8.

Cochrane Library at McMaster University. (2000, March). *Using Medline to search for evidence.* Retrieved from www.londonlinks.ac.uk/evidence_strategies/coch_search.htm.

DeLaune, S. C. & Ladner, P. K. (2006). *Fundamentals of Nursing* (3rd ed.). Clifton Park, NY: Delmar Cengage Learning.

Giachello, A., Arrom, J., Davis, M., Sayad, J., Ramirez, D., Nandi, C., Ramos, C. (2003). Reducing diabetes health disparities through community-based participatory action research: the Chicago southeast diabetes community action coalition. *Public Health Reports, 118(4),* 309–323.

Hartley, D, (2004). Rural health disparities, population health, and rural culture. *American Journal of Public Health, 94*(10), 1675–1678.

Institute of Medicine (IOM). (2002). *Unequal treatment confronting racial and ethnic disparities in healthcare.* Institute of Medicine Report, Washington, DC: National Academy Press.

Jennings, B. M., & Loan, L. A. (2001). Misconceptions among nurses about evidence-based practice. *Journal of Nursing Scholarship, 33*(2), 121–127.

Joint Commission Resources. (2008). *CAMH: 2008 Comprehensive Accreditation Manual of Hospitals.* Oakbrook Terrace, IL: Joint Commission on Accreditation of Healthcare Organizations. Available at www.jointcommission.org.

Kelly, D. (2005). From the emergency department to home. *Journal of Clinical Nursing, 14,* 776–785.

Kitson, A. (2007). What influences the use of research in clinical practice? *Nursing Research, 56*(4), Supplement 1:S1–S3.

LoBue PA, Moser KS. (2004). *Screening of immigrants and refugees for pulmonary tuberculosis in San Diego County,* California. Chest. 2004 Dec;*126(6)*:1777–82.

Lovern, E. (2001, May 28). Oh no, not that type of review. JCAHO singling out more hospitals for noncompliance with standards. *Modern Healthcare, 31*(22), 4–5.

Ludwig, T., Buchholz, C., Clarke, S. (2005). Using social marketing to increase the use of helmets among bicyclists. Journal of American College Health, 4(1), 51–58.

McGlynn, E. A., Asch, S. M., Adams, J., Keesey, J., Hicks, J., DeCristofaro, A., et al. (2003). The quality of health care delivered to adults in the United States. *New England Journal of Medicine, 348,* 2635–2645.

Minnesota Department of Health, Section of Public Health Nursing. (2001). *Public Health Interventions-Application for Public Health Nursing Practice.* St. Paul, MN: Minnesota Department of Health.

Mitchell, G. M., & Grippando, P.R. (1994). *Nursing Perspectives and Issues* (5th ed.). Clifton Park, NY: Delmar Cengage Learning.

Needleman, J., Buerhaus, P., Mattke, S., Stewart, M., & Zelevinsky, K. (2002). Nurse-staffing levels and the quality of care in hospitals. *New England Journal of Medicine, 346*(22) 1715–1722.

Nightingale, F. (1914). Florence Nightingale to her nurses: A selection from Miss Nightingale's addresses to probationers and nurses of the Nightingale School at St. Thomas's Hospital [p. 1; Address in May 1872]. London: Macmillan.

Sackett, D. L., Rosenberg, W. M. C., Gray, J. A. M., Haynes, R. B., & Richardson, W. S. (1996). Evidence-based medicine: What it is and what it isn't. *British Medical Journal, 312*(7023), 71–72.

Shortell, S. M., & Kaluzny, A. D. (2006). *Health Care Management* (5th ed.). Clifton Park, NY: Delmar Cengage Learning.

Soukup, S.M. (2000). Evidence-based nursing practice [Preface]. *Nursing Clinics of North America, 35*(2) xvii–xviii.

Timmermans, S., & Mauck, A. (2005). The promises and pitfalls of evidence-based medicine. *Health Affairs, 24*(1), 18–28.

Young, T., Ireson, C., (2003). Effectiveness of school-based telehealth care in urban and suburban elementary schools. *Pediatrics, 112*(5), 1088–1094.

Wu, Y., Larrabee, J. H., & Putnam, H. P. (2006, Jan.–Feb.). Caring behaviors inventory. *Nursing Research, 55*(1), 18–25.

SUGGESTED READINGS

Kim S., Flaskerud, J., Koniak-Griffin, D., & Dixon, E. (2005). Using community-partnered participatory research to address health disparities in a Latino community. *Journal of Professional Nursing, 21*(4), 199–209.

Kolb, S., Gillilard, I., Deliganis, J., & Light, K. (2003). Ministerio de Salud: Development of a mission-driven partnership for addressing health disparities in a Hispanic community. *Journal of Multicultural Nursing & Health, 9*(3), 6–12.

Lavery, S., Smith, M., Esparza, A., Hrushow, A., Moore, M., & Reed, D. (2005). The community action model: A community-driven model designed to address disparities in health. *American Journal of Public Health, 95*(4), 611–616.

McNaughton, D. (2004). Nurse home visits to maternal-child clients: A review of intervention research. *Public Health Nursing, 23*(3), 207–219.

Reid, L, Hatch, J., & Parrish, T. (2003, Nov.). The role of a historically black university and the black church in community-based health initiatives: The project DIRECT experience. *Journal of Public Health Management Practice,* S70–S73.

Schoon, P. (2008). Population-Based Health Care Practice. In P. Kelly (Ed.), *Nursing leadership & management.* Clifton Park, NY: Delmar Cengage Learning.

Schultz, A., Senk, S., Odoms-Young, A., Hollis-Neely, T., Nwankwo, R., Lockett, M., et al. (2005). Healthy eating and exercising to reduce diabetes: Exploring the potential of social determinants of health frameworks within the context of community-based participatory diabetes prevention. *American Journal of Public Health, 95*(4), 645–651.

Welch, D., & Kneipp, S. (2005). Low-income housing policy and socioeconomic inequalities in women's health: The importance or nursing inquiry and intervention. *Policy, Politics, & Nursing Practice, 6*(4), 335–342.

CHAPTER 4

Decision Making, Critical Thinking, and Technology

When you have to make a choice and don't make it, that is in itself a choice.

(William James)

OBJECTIVES

Upon completion of this chapter, the reader should be able to:

1. Apply the decision-making process to patient care.
2. Explain how problem solving, critical thinking, reflective thinking, and intuitive thinking relate to decision making.
3. Examine tools to improve decision making.
4. Identify how technology can help with decision making.
5. Discuss individual vs. group decision making.
6. Discuss evaluation of information found on the Internet.

You are a new nurse on a medical-surgical unit and have just come from a unit meeting. At the meeting, your nurse manager reported the results of the patient satisfaction survey from the previous year. Patient satisfaction has steadily declined, and for the past 3 months, only 20% of patients were satisfied. The manager selected a task force to investigate potential solutions to this problem and appointed you to the committee. The survey identified some reasons for the dissatisfaction: long waiting periods after pushing the nurse call light, not being informed about tests and procedures being performed, and being treated in an impersonal manner.

What should be the first step of the task force?

How can critical thinking, the decision-making process, and technology help the group solve the situation?

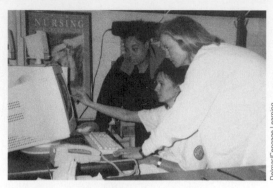

Delmar/Cengage Learning

Rapid changes in the health care environment have expanded the decision-making role of the nurse. Decision making and critical thinking by nurses is necessary for safe patient care. Patient care is becoming complex, and acuity is rising. Effective decisions using critical thinking about patient care must be made in a timely manner. Technology can help with this. Computers, technology, and the Internet have changed the way we communicate, obtain information, work, entertain, and make important health decisions. As documented in the PEW Report from April 19, 2006 (Horrigan & Rainie, 2006), some 21 million Americans rely on the Internet in a crucial or important way for career training, 17 million rely on it when helping someone else with a major illness or health care condition, and another 17 million rely on it when choosing a school for themselves or for a child. This chapter explores the decision-making process and the critical thinking process. It also examines advantages of and limitations to group decision making, as well as the use of technology in decision making.

DECISION MAKING

In everyday practice, nurses make decisions about patient care. DeLaune and Ladner (2006) define **decision making** as "considering and selecting interventions from a repertoire of actions that facilitate the achievement of a desired outcome" (p. 89). Problem solving and critical, reflective, and intuitive thinking (Table 4-1) may be used during the decision-making process, as illustrated in Figure 4-1.

Although decisions are unique to different situations, the same decision-making process can be applied to most all situations. The decision-making process consists of five steps (Table 4-2).

In the following clinical application, the decision-making process is applied to a clinical situation.

CLINICAL APPLICATION

You are the night shift nurse caring for Mr. Cintas. In the morning, Mr. Cintas is scheduled for a permanent pacemaker insertion to replace his

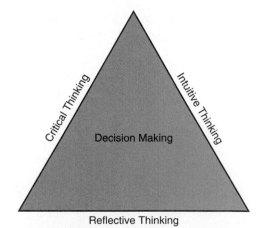

Figure 4-1 Critical thinking, intuitive thinking, and reflective thinking are incorporated throughout the decision-making process. (Delmar/Cengage Learning).

TABLE 4-1	REVIEW OF TERMS
Decision making	Considering and selecting interventions from a repertoire of actions that facilitate the achievement of a desired outcome (DeLaune & Ladner, 2006).
Critical thinking	Thinking about your thinking while you're thinking in order to make your thinking better (Paul, 1992).
Reflective thinking	Watching or observing ourselves as we perform a task or make a decision about a particular situation (Pesut & Herman, 1999). Journal writing assists with reflective thinking.
Intuitive thinking	An innate feeling that nurses develop that helps them to act in certain situations (Gardner, 2003). Intuitive thinking has been described as a "gut" feeling assessment that something is right or wrong.
Problem solving	An active process that starts with a problem and ends with a solution.

TABLE 4-2

THE DECISION-MAKING PROCESS

1. Identify the need for a decision and gather data. Identify key participants.

2. Determine the goal or outcome desired.

3. Identify alternatives.

   a. Identify consequences of each alternative.

   b. Identify benefits of each alternative.

4. Make the decision. Act on it.

5. Evaluate the decision.

temporary pacemaker, which is still functioning. Hospital policy states that no visitor may stay all night with a patient unless that patient is very critically ill. Mr. and Mrs. Cintas are both requesting that Mrs. Cinta stay all night in a chair beside Mr. Cintas' bed because both are anxious about his upcoming procedure. Use your decision-making and problem-solving skills to help you decide what to do.

- Step 1: Identify the need for a decision and gather data. Identify key participants. Should you let Mrs. Cintas spend the night? Consider all the information (hospital policy, the patient's and Mrs. Cintas' wishes, anxiety level, and so on).
- Step 2: Determine the goal or outcome. Questions to consider include the following: Can an exception to hospital policy be made? Is the goal to alleviate Mr. and Mrs. Cintas' anxiety? Will Mr. Cintas' level of anxiety adversely affect the outcome of the surgery? Will Mr. and Mrs. Cintas be satisfied? Are there other goals?
- Step 3: Identify all alternative actions and the benefits and consequences of each. If you enforce hospital policy, the benefits are that all patients are treated equally and the written policy supports the decision. Possible consequences are that Mr. Cintas' anxiety level increases, perhaps adversely affecting the outcome of his surgery, and Mr. and Mrs. Cintas will not be advocates for the health center. The other alternative is to allow Mrs. Cintas to stay all night. Potential

benefits are that Mr. Cintas' level of anxiety will decrease, and Mr. and Mrs. Cintas will be satisfied customers. The consequence is that a precedent is set that may make it difficult to enforce the existing hospital policy.

- Step 4: Make the decision and act on it. Consider the two alternatives and the benefits and consequences of each. Then implement the decision.
- Step 5: Evaluate the decision. Was the goal achieved?

From the beginning of their careers, new graduate nurses are faced with the responsibility of making decisions regarding patient care. When nurses are faced with a difficult clinical decision, they often benefit by consulting with others as early as possible. These may include other RNs on the unit or house supervisors.

LIMITATIONS TO EFFECTIVE DECISION MAKING

What are obstacles to effective decision making? Past experiences, values, personal biases, and preconceived ideas affect the way people view problems and situations. DeLaune and Ladner (2006) have identified criteria that may negatively affect the decision-making or problem-solving processes:

- Jumping to conclusions without examining the situation thoroughly
- Failing to obtain all of the necessary information
- Choosing decisions that are too broad, too complicated, or lack definition
- Failing to choose and communicate a rational solution
- Failing to intervene and evaluate the decision or solution appropriately

CRITICAL THINKING

What does it mean to be a critical thinker? Paul (1992) defines **critical thinking** as "thinking about your thinking while you're thinking in order to make your thinking better" (p. 7). A good critical

thinker is able to examine situations from all sides and make decisions, taking into account research and the best evidence and various points of view. A good critical thinker does not say, "We've always done it this way," and refuse to consider alternate ways. The critical thinker thinks "out of the box" and generates new ideas and alternatives when making decisions. The critical thinker asks "why?" questions about a situation to arrive at the best decision. Four basic skills—critical reading, critical listening, critical writing, and critical speaking—are necessary for the development of critical thinking skills. These skills are part of the process of developing and using thinking for decision making. Ability in these four areas can be developed by using the universal intellectual standards illustrated in Table 4-3.

TABLE 4-3

THE SPECTRUM OF UNIVERSAL INTELLECTUAL STANDARDS

Clear	Unclear
Precise	Imprecise
Specific	Vague
Accurate	Inaccurate
Relevant	Irrelevant
Logical	Illogical
Deep	Superficial
Detailed	General
Significant	Insignificant
Adequate	Inadequate
Fair	Unfair

Source: Adapted with permission from the Foundation for Critical Thinking. Please see Web site: www.criticalthinking.org.

CRITICAL THINKING 4-1

Use the decision-making process in Table 4-2 and ask yourself the critical thinking questions inspired by Table 4-3 when you are making decisions. Have I gathered the best, most up-to-date research and evidence to help with the decision? Is my information clear or unclear, precise or imprecise, specific or vague, accurate or inaccurate? Is it relevant or irrelevant, logical or illogical, deep or superficial, complete or incomplete, significant or insignificant, adequate or inadequate, and fair or unfair? Apply the critical thinking questions and review the research and best evidence at each step.

REAL WORLD INTERVIEW

I was in a situation where I just didn't think my patient looked good. I decided to go ahead and start two new IV sites, just in case. The patient arrested 2 hours later, and we really needed those IV sites. I felt good about my decision.

Cheryl Buntz, RN
New Graduate
Independence, Missouri

As you begin to apply critical thinking to nursing, use these universal intellectual standards when you are reading material from a textbook, listening to an oral presentation, writing a paper, answering test questions, or presenting ideas in oral form. Ask yourself whether the ideas are clear or unclear, precise or imprecise, specific or vague, accurate or inaccurate. Are they relevant or irrelevant, logical or illogical, deep or superficial, complete or incomplete, significant or insignificant, adequate or inadequate, and fair and unfair? You will improve your critical thinking skills over time with practice.

REFLECTIVE THINKING

Pesut and Herman (1999) describe **reflective thinking** as watching or observing ourselves as we perform a task or make a decision about a particular situation. We have two selves, the active self and the reflective self. The reflective self watches the active self as it engages in activities. The reflective self acts as observer and offers suggestions about the activities. To be a good critical thinker, one must practice reflective thinking. Reflection upon a situation or problem after a decision is made allows the individual to evaluate the decision. Students can become better reflective thinkers through the use of clinical journals.

INTUITIVE THINKING AND PROBLEM SOLVING

Intuition and **intuitive thinking** is described as an innate feeling that nurses develop that helps them to act in certain situations (Gardner, 2003). It has also been described as a gut feeling that something is wrong. Intuitive thinking may result from unconscious assessment and analysis of data based on an individual's past experience. Nurses may make decisions about patient care based, in part, on intuitive thinking. This may seem contrary to using the logical, evidenced-based reasoning that is so prevalent in nursing literature. Alfaro-LeFevre (2003) contends, however, that expert thinking is usually the result of using intuition and drawing on evidence at the same time to make well-reasoned decisions.

Ruth-Sahd and Hendy (2005) studied novice nurses and noted that older novice nurses, those with more social support, and those with more hospitalizations use intuition more often in decision making.

Problem solving is an active process that starts with a problem and ends with a solution. Nurses address multiple needs and problems of patients on a daily basis. Some problems are uncomplicated and require one simple solution. Other problems may be complex and require more analysis by the nurse.

DECISION-MAKING TOOLS AND TECHNOLOGY

Sometimes, when a decision is made, the outcome is certain. Other times, a nurse will need to make a decision without having all of the information needed to ensure a good outcome. Decision making in both certain and uncertain times can be improved by using various tools. Figure 4-2 shows a decision analysis tree for choosing whether to go

back to school. See Figure 4-3 for a decision analysis tree for a patient who smokes.

A decision-making grid may help to separate the multiple factors that surround a situation. Figure 4-4 illustrates use of a decision-making grid by a unit that was told it had to reduce the workforce by two full-time equivalents (FTEs). This grid is useful in this example to visually separate the factors of cost savings, effect on job satisfaction of remaining staff, and effect on patient satisfaction.

A decision-making grid is also useful when a nurse is trying to decide between two choices. Figure 4-5 is an example of a decision-making grid used by a nurse deciding between working at hospital A or hospital B.

The Program Evaluation and Review Technique (PERT) is useful in determining timing of decisions. The PERT flowchart provides a visual picture depicting the sequence of tasks that must take place to complete a project. Jones and Beck (1996) provide an example of a PERT flow diagram depicting

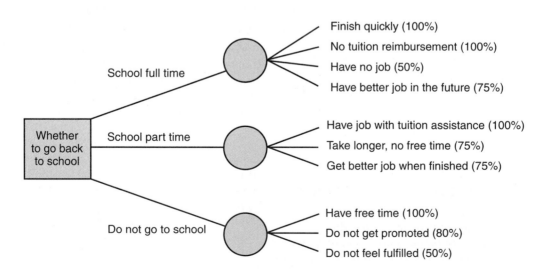

Key numbers represent percentage of possibility that event will occur

Figure 4-2 Decision tree for choosing whether to go back to school. (Delmar/Cengage Learning).

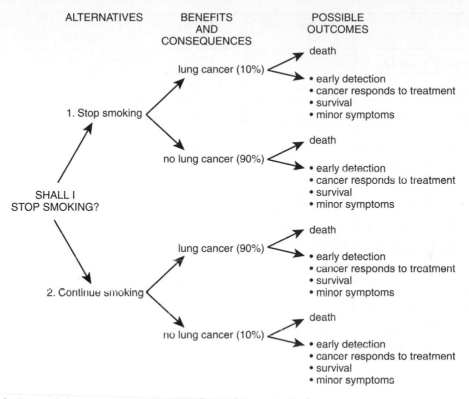

Figure 4-3 Decision analysis tree for a patient who smokes. (Delmar/Cengage Learning).

Methods of Reduction	Cost Savings	Effect on Job Satisfaction	Effect on Patient Satisfaction
Lay off the two most senior full-time employees	$93,500	Significant reduction	Significant reduction
Lay off the two most recently hired full-time employees	$63,200	Significant reduction	Moderate reduction
Reduce by staff attrition	$78,000	Minor reduction	Minor reduction

Figure 4-4 Sample decision-making grid. (Delmar/Cengage Learning).

Elements	Importance Score (out of 10)	Likelihood Score (out of 10)	Risk (multiply scores)
Work at hospital A			
Learning experience	10	10	100
Good mentor support	8	8	64
Financial reward	6	6	36
Growth potential	8	8	64
Good location	10	10	100
Total			364
Work at hospital B			
Learning experience	8	8	64
Good mentor support	7	7	49
Financial reward	8	8	64
Growth potential	9	9	81
Good location	6	6	36
Total			294

Figure 4-5 Sample decision-making grid. (Delmar/Cengage Learning).

from beginning to end an implementation of case management. See Figure 4-6. The chart shows the amount of time required to complete the project and the sequence of events necessary to complete the project. A Gantt chart can also be useful for decision makers to illustrate a project from beginning to end. Figure 4-7 illustrates a Gantt chart.

DOS AND DON'TS OF DECISION MAKING

A foundation for good decision making comes with experience and learning from those experiences. Table 4-4 gives the student some additional tips to consider when making decisions.

GROUP DECISION MAKING

Certain situations may call for group decision making. A group may offer innovative alternatives and decisions and afford some protection from mistakes because it uses the combined knowledge of all its members. Today's leadership and management styles include people in the decision-making process who will be most affected by the decision. The effectiveness of groups depends greatly on the group's members. The size of the group and the personalities of group members are important considerations when choosing participants. More ideas can be generated with

The vice president for nursing plans to change all units to include case managers. She believes that this can be accomplished within a year and one half. In order for this to be achieved, the following activities and events have to occur:

Activity Symbol	Activity Descriptions	Immediate Predecessor
A.	Form a multidisciplinary advisory group	None
B.	Agree upon definitions	A
C.	Notify members of subcommittees	B
D.	Write job descriptions	C
E.	Advertise for candidates for case manager	D
F.	Review qualifications of candidates	E
G.	Select candidates for case manager	F
H.	Review patient charts	None
I.	Write patient care maps	H
J.	Meet with case managers	None
K.	Orient case managers	J
L.	Orient unit and hospital staff	K
M.	Utilize case management process	L

	Events
1.	Project begins
2.	Meeting of multidisciplinary committee
3.	Formation of subcommittees
4.	Subcommittee for description meets
5.	Subcommittee for patient care maps meets
6.	Candidates for case managers are interviewed
7.	Candidates are hired
8.	Subcommittee for patient care maps meets to finalize maps
9.	Orientation begins
10.	Implementation begins
11.	Project is evaluated

Expected	Time Calculations
Activity	*Duration*
A	0.5 month
B	1 month
C	0.5 month
D	1 month
E	1 month
F	2 month
G	1 month
H	1 month
I	2 month
J	1 month
K&L	1 month
M	3 month

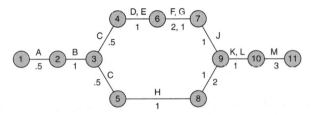

Figure 4-6 PERT diagram with critical path for implementation of case management. (Delmar/Cengage Learning).

A nurse manager has agreed to have her unit pilot a new care delivery system within six months. The Gantt chart can be used to plan the progression of the project.

Activities	Sept	Oct	Nov	Dec	Jan	Feb	Mar	Apr	May
Discuss project with staff	------ X								
Form an ad hoc planning committee	------	X							
Receive report from committee			------ X						
Discuss report with staff			------	X					
Educate all staff about the plan				------ —— X				
Implement new system						------ ———— X			
Evaluate system and make changes							------ ——	X	

Key
------ Proposed Time
—— Actual Time
  X   Complete

Figure 4-7 Gantt chart: implementation of care delivery system. (Delmar/Cengage Learning).

groups, thus allowing for more communication and more choices. This increases the likelihood of higher-quality outcomes.

A major disadvantage of group decision making is the time involved. Without effective leadership, groups can waste time and be nonproductive. Group decision making can be more costly and can also lead to conflict. Groups can be dominated by one person or become the battleground for a power struggle among assertive members.

Group decision making may, however, increase the acceptance of the decision by all members. Vroom and Yetton (1973) identified elements individuals should consider before making a decision alone or with a group. See Table 4-5.

TECHNIQUES OF GROUP DECISION MAKING

There are various techniques of group decision making. The *nominal group technique, Delphi technique,* and *consensus building* are different methods to facilitate group decision making.

NOMINAL GROUP TECHNIQUE

The nominal group technique was developed by Delbecq, Van de Ven, and Gustafson in 1971. The word *nominal* refers to the nonverbal aspect of this approach. In the first step, there is no discussion; group members write out their ideas or responses to the identified issue or question posed by the group leader. The second step involves

TABLE 4-4	DOS AND DON'TS OF DECISION MAKING

Do	**Don't**
Get good information before making a decision.	Make snap decisions.
Make notes and keep ideas visible about decisions to utilize all relevant information.	Waste your time making decisions that do not have to be made.
Write down pros and cons of an issue to help clarify your thinking.	Distort your memories of chosen and rejected options to make the chosen options seem relatively more attractive.
Make necessary decisions as you go along rather than letting them accumulate.	Prolong deliberation about decisions.
Consider those affected by your decision.	Be unduly influenced by initial information that shapes your view of subsequent information.
Trust yourself. Delay or revise a decision as needed.	Always base decisions on the "way things have always been done."

Source: Adapted from *The Small Business Knowledge Base* (1999). Retrieved January 19, 2002, from www.bizmove.com

TABLE 4-5	INDIVIDUAL VS. GROUP DECISION MAKING

1. Does the individual have all the information and resources needed to make the best decision?
2. Does the group have supplementary information needed to make the best decision?
3. Will individual personalities within the group work well together?
4. Is it absolutely critical that the group be involved in the decision and accept the decision prior to implementation?
5. Will the group accept a decision made by an individual? By the group?
6. Is there time for a group decision?
7. Will the course of action chosen make a difference to the organization?
8. Do the group and individual have the best interest of the organization foremost in mind when considering the decision?
9. Will the decision cause undue conflict among the group?

Source: Adapted from Vroom, V. & Yetton, P. (1973). *Leadership and Decision-Making* (pp. 21–30). Pittsburgh, PA: University of Pittsburgh Press.

presentation of the ideas to the group members, along with the advantages and disadvantages of each. These ideas are presented on a flip board or chart. The third phase offers an opportunity for discussion to clarify and evaluate the ideas. The fourth phase includes private voting on the ideas. The ideas receiving the highest number of votes are the solutions implemented.

DELPHI GROUP TECHNIQUE

The Delphi technique differs from the nominal technique in that group members are not meeting face to face. Questionnaires are distributed to group members for their opinions, and the responses are then summarized and disseminated to the group members. This process continues for as many times as necessary for the group members to reach consensus. An advantage of this technique is that it can involve a large number of participants and thus a greater number of ideas.

CONSENSUS BUILDING

Consensus is defined by the Merriam-Webster's Collegiate Dictionary (2003) as "a general agreement; the judgment arrived at by most of those concerned; group solidarity in sentiment and belief" (p. 265). A common misconception is that consensus means everyone agrees with the decision 100%. Contrary to this misunderstanding,

consensus means that all group members can live with and fully support the decision regardless of whether they totally agree. Building consensus is useful with groups because all group members participate and can realize the contributions each member makes to the decision. A disadvantage to the consensus strategy is that decision making requires more time.

USE OF TECHNOLOGY IN DECISION MAKING

The best source of clinical decision making and judgment is the professional practitioner. However, computer technology offers many ways to support evidence-based information needs of nurses.

These include:

- Electronic Health Records
- Patient decision support tools, clinical- and business-related
- Laboratory and x-ray results reporting and viewing systems
- Computerized prescribing and order entry, including barcoding
- Community and population health management and information
- Communication, patient classification staffing systems, and administrative systems
- Evidence-based knowledge and information retrieval systems
- Quality improvement data collection/data summary systems
- Documentation and care planning
- Patient monitoring and problem alerts
- Inventory control

Many nurses today are using PDAs (see Figure 4-8) to improve patient care. PDAs are used for obtaining information about medications and pathophysiology, and for developing nursing care plans and nursing diagnoses. NCLEX questions are also available on PDAs.

CASE STUDY 4-1

You have been working on a medical-surgical unit. As you complete your nursing program, you begin to interview at several hospitals. Set up a decision-making grid to help you analyze your choices. What factors are most important to you as you begin to consider your decision? Use Figure 4-5.

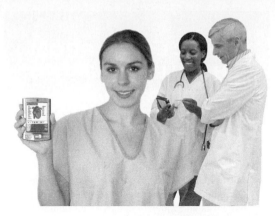

Figure 4-8 Nurse with a PDA. (*Source:* Courtesy PEPID, Heather Hautman).

JOINT COMMISSION NATIONAL PATIENT SAFETY GOALS

Several other forces have highlighted the need for increased patient technology. The Joint Commission (JC), formerly the Joint Commission on Accreditation of Healthcare Organizations (JCAHO), has set the following National Patient Safety Goals for 2006, many of which require the use of technology:

- Improve the accuracy of patient identification
- Improve the effectiveness of communication among caregivers
- Improve the safety of medication use
- Eliminate wrong site, wrong patient, wrong procedure surgery
- Improve the effectiveness of patient-specific clinical alarm systems that alert staff to patient emergencies
- Reduce the risk of health care-associated infections
- Accurately and completely reconcile medications across the continuum of care
- Reduce the risk of patient harm from falls
- Reduce the risk of influenza and pneumococcal disease in older adults
- Reduce the risk of surgical fires
- Encourage active involvement of patients and families in patients' own care as a patient safety strategy
- Prevent health care-associated pressure ulcers

For 2007 and 2008, the changes and additions to these goals include:

- Provide a complete list of medications to the patient when discharged
- Encourage patient's active involvement in his own care as a patient safety strategy
- Tell patients and their families how they can report concerns about safety and encourage them to do so
- Offer the influenza vaccine to all staff
- Identify safety risks in the patient population
- Improve recognition of and response to changes in a patient's condition
- Psychiatric hospitals should identify patients at risk for suicide
- General hospitals should identify those patients being treated for emotional or behavioral disorders who are at risk for suicide (www.jointcommission.org/~Click on *National Patient Safety Goals*).

Attainment of many of these Goals requires the judicious use of technology.

LEAPFROG GROUP

The Leapfrog Group is another force advocating for technology. Leapfrog is a voluntary program aimed at using employer purchasing power to alert America's health industry that big leaps in health care safety, quality, and customer value will be recognized and rewarded. Among other initiatives, Leapfrog works with its employer members to encourage transparency and easy access to health care information, as well as rewards for hospitals that have a proven record of high quality care. Leapfrog measures how hospitals are doing with respect to the following:

- Computerized practitioner order entry into computers linked to error-prevention software
- ICUs staffed by practitioner intensivists
- Evidence-based hospital performance on five high-risk procedures and care for two high-risk neonatal conditions
- Progress on 13 National Quality Forum Safe Practices (www.leapfroggroup.org). Data support services are offered to Leapfrog by Thomson Medstat (see www.medstat.com).

THE NATIONAL QUALITY FORUM

The National Quality Forum (NQF) is a not-for-profit membership organization created to develop and implement a national strategy for health care quality measurement and reporting (www.qualityforum.org). A shared sense of urgency about the impact of health care quality on patient outcomes, workforce productivity, and health care costs prompted leaders in the public and private sectors to create the NQF as a mechanism to bring about national change.

In 2003, the NQF endorsed a set of 30 safe practices that should be universally utilized in applicable clinical care settings to reduce the risk of harm to patients. NQF has now formally launched the Safe Practices Consensus Standards Maintenance Committee to review the practices and recommend additions or changes for members to consider so that the set remains current and appropriate (see www.qualityforum.org; click on *Safe Practices*).

THE SPECIALTY OF NURSING INFORMATICS

According to the American Nurses' Association (ANA, 2001), nursing informatics (NI) is a discipline-specific practice within the broader perspective of health informatics. NI was recognized as a specialty for RNs in 1992.

EVIDENCE FROM THE LITERATURE

Citation: White, A., Allen, P., Goodwin, L., Breckinridge, D., Dowell, J., & Garvy, R. (2005). Infusing PDA technology into nursing education. *Nurse Educator,* 30(4), 153–154.

Discussion: Article discusses the Nursing Education program at Duke University, where students use PDAs and software to access current drug and infectious disease information, calculations, growth charts, immunization guidelines, and Spanish and English language translations to improve clinical decision making. Information about this can be accessed at www.pepidedu.com.

Implications for Practice: Use of the PDA can improve clinical decision making. Go to www.rnpalm.com.

In 2004, 18 regional nursing informatics groups, representing 2,000 nurses, formed the Alliance for Nursing Informatics (ANI) in collaboration with Healthcare Information and Management Systems Society (HIMSS), the American Nurses Association (ANA), and Capital Area Roundtable on Informatics in Nursing Group (CARING). Several nursing and health informatics scholarly journals, such as *Computers, Informatics, and Nursing* (www.cinjournal.com) and *Journal of the Medical Informatics Association* (www.jamia.org), provide essential nursing informatics education. The American Nurses Credentialing Center (ANCC) offers certification examinations for a variety of specialties in nursing, including informatics (www.nursingworld.org/ancc).

USING THE INTERNET FOR DECISION MAKING

You can use a variety of strategies to search the Internet, including quick and dirty searching, links, and brute force. Keep in mind that you must be persistent: no single search strategy or search engine is

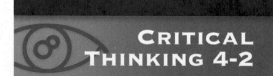

CRITICAL THINKING 4-2

Visit the American Nurses Credentialing Center at www.nursingworld.org. Click on "careers and credentialing/certification." Choose a specialty in which a nurse can be certified and compare it to the certification in informatics. How are they similar? How are they different?

going to work all the time. Here are some strategies and tactics to render Internet searches more efficient and reduce search time (Jones, 2003):

- Use Web sites published by governmental or professional organizations or other reputable organizations. See Table 4-6.
- Use Consumer health sites organized by medical librarians.
- Use precise terms, such as "Diabetes Type I" instead of just "Diabetes," to reduce the number of hits when searching for very specific information.

- Draw on search engines, such as Mayo Clinic (www.mayoclinic.com), WebMD (www.webmd.com), and so forth, that collect information from reliable online health resources rather than relying on the "bots" or robots typically used by search engines to "crawl" the Web, such as Google.
- Refine your Internet searches with filters. Filtering is mechanically blocking Internet content from being retrieved through the identification of key words and phrases. For example, you can narrow your search by the type of medical viewpoint (traditional or

TABLE 4-6	**LIST OF FAVORITE HEALTH CARE WEB SITES**
www.ach.org	www.healthy.net
www.acsh.org	www.intelihealth.com
www.ahrq.gov	www.kidshealth.com
www.allnursingschools.com	www.lungusa.org
www.ama-assn.org	www.mayoclinic.com
www.americanheart.org	www.medlineplus.gov
www.arthritis.org	www.medscape.com
www.cancer.org	www.ncsbn.org
www.cancernet.nci.nih.gov	www.netwellness.org
www.caringinfo.org	www.nhlbi.nih.gov
www.cdc.gov	www.nia.nih.gov
www.cinahl.com	www.ngc.gov
www.clinicaltrials.gov	www.nih.gov
www.cms.hhs.gov	www.noah-health.org
www.cochrane.org	www.nursingworld.org
www.diabetes.org	www.oncolink.com
www.digestive.niddk.nih.gov	www.pain.com
www.eatright.org	www.pdr.net
www.eMD.com	www.personalMD.com
www.epilepsyfoundation.org	www.rarediseases.org
www.fda.gov	www.realage.com
www.familydoctor.org	www.rxlist.com
www.healthAtoZ.com	www.shapeup.org
www.healthcentral.com	www.vh.org
www.healthfinder.gov	www.webMD.com
www.healthgrades.com	www.yourtotalhealth.ivillage.com
www.health.discovery.com	

alternative), reading level (easy, moderate, or complex), and type of site (commercial, non-commercial, government, or nonprofit) that you use in your key words to filter your search (Nicoll, 2003).

The result of your searches after using these strategies will probably be a more focused and helpful list of links matching your specific request. You will then want to evaluate your search data using P-F-A Assessment.

THE P-F-A ASSESSMENT

One strategy to develop your Internet search is to conduct a "purpose-focus-approach" (P-F-A) assessment. To determine your purpose, ask yourself why you are doing the search and why you need the information. Consider questions such as the following:

- Is it for personal interest?
- Do you want to obtain information to share with coworkers or a client?
- Are you verifying information given to you by someone else?
- Are you preparing a report or writing a paper for a class or project?

Based on your purpose, your focus may be as follows:

- Broad and general (basic information for yourself)
- Lay-oriented (to give information to a patient) or professionally-oriented (for colleagues)
- Narrow and technical with a research orientation (Nicoll, 2003)

Purpose combined with focus determines your approach. For example, information that is broad and general can be found using brute force methods or quick and dirty searching.

QUICK AND DIRTY SEARCHING AND LINKS

Quick and dirty searching is a very simple, but surprisingly effective, search strategy. First, start with a search engine, such as AltaVista (*www.altavista.com*) or Google (*www.google.com*). Next, type in the term of interest. At this point, do not worry about being overly broad or general. You may retrieve an enormous number of found references (called "hits"), but you are interested only in the first 10 to 20. Look at the universal resource locators (URLs), that is, the addresses of the sites that are returned by your search, and try to decipher what they mean. Pay attention to the domains: .com is commercial; .edu is an educational institution; .gov is the government. Quickly visit a few sites. Look for the information you need, or useful links. If a site is not relevant, use the back button on your browser to return to your search results and go to the next site. Once you find a site that appears to be useful, begin to explore the site. Many sites will connect you to other sites, using links, or hot buttons. If you click on a link, it will take you to a related site. If the site you are looking at has links (most do), use them to connect to other relevant sites. This process—quick search, quick review, clicking, and linking—can provide a starting point for finding useful information in a relatively short period of time. When you find a site of interest, "bookmark" it and add it to your list of favorites.

A bookmark list, or list of favorites, is like a personal address book. Each time you find a site that is particularly useful, you can add it to your list of favorites, using the appropriate feature in your browser. Eventually, you will have a comprehensive list of sites that are relevant to your work and interests. By having this list, you will be able to quickly return to sites during future Internet sessions.

BRUTE FORCE

Brute force searching is another alternative. To do this, type in an address in the URL box (the address box at the top of the browser window) and see what happens. The worst outcome is an annoying error message, but you may land on a site that is exactly what you want. To be effective, think how URLs work: they usually start with "www" (for "World Wide Web"). Then there is the "thing in the middle" followed by a domain. Perhaps you are trying to find a school of nursing at a certain university. What is the common name for the university? *www.unh.edu* is the very logical URL for the University of New Hampshire. Organizations are also quite logical in their URLs: *www.aorn.org* is the Association of periOperative Registered Nurses

(AORN); *www.aone.org* is the American Organization of Nurse Executives (AONE).

FULL TEXT ARTICLES

The final element of searching for literature online is finding full-text articles. The databases so far discussed (MEDLINE and so on) do not contain full text—they include only literature citations. One option is to use a document delivery service, such as UnCover (www.uta.eou/library/uncover.html). This resource allows you to conduct a search. It identifies which articles can be sent to you, and what the fees will be (including article fees, service charges, and copyright fees). If you elect to order an article, you can identify how you want to have it sent to you (mail, fax, or other).

You can also use a search engine, for example, www.google.com. Search for full text nursing journal articles and see what you get. A final option is to use Google Scholar (scholar.google.com), which allows you to conduct a search, identify the articles needed, and search the publisher's site for delivery costs, including article fees, service charges, and copyright fees. If you elect to order an article, you can identify how you want to have it sent to you, that is, by e-mail, fax or other.

EVALUATION OF INFORMATION FOUND ON THE INTERNET

Traveling through the Internet, one must always evaluate the information that is found. Check the Health on the Net Foundation at www.hon.ch. A simple mnemonic, "Are you PLEASED with the site?" is very helpful (Nicoll, 2003). (Table 4-7).

To determine whether you are PLEASED, consider the following:

- *P—Purpose:* What is the author's purpose in developing the site? Are the author's objectives clear? Many people will develop a Web site as a hobby or way of sharing information they have gathered. It should be immediately evident to you what the true purpose of the site is. At the same time, consider your purpose; that is, think back to your P-F-A assessment. There

should be congruence between the author's purpose and yours.
- *L—Links:* Evaluate the links at the site. Are they working? (Links that do not take you anywhere are called "dead links.") Do they link to reliable sites? It is important to critically evaluate the links at sites hosted by organizations, businesses, or institutions because these entities are usually presenting themselves as authorities on the subject at hand. Some pages, such as those created by individuals, are really nothing more than a collection of links. These can be useful as a starting point for a search, but it is still important to evaluate the links that are provided at the site.
- *E—Editorial (site content):* Is the information contained in the site accurate, comprehensive, and current? Is there a particular bias, or is the information presented in an objective way? Who

TABLE 4-7

WEB SITE EVALUATION: ASK YOURSELF, "AM I PLEASED WITH THE SITE?"

Purpose

Links

Editorial (site content)

Author

Site navigation

Ethical disclosure

Date site last updated

Source: Compiled with information from Health on the Net Foundation. HONcode Site Evaluation form. (2009). Available at www.hon.ch/cgi-bin/HONcode/Inscription/site_evaluation.pl?language=en&userCategory=individuals. (accessed 4-16-09)

is the consumer of the site: is it designed for health professionals, patients, consumers, or other audiences? Is the information presented in an appropriate format for the intended audience? Look at details, too. Are there misspellings and grammatical errors? "Under construction" banners that have been there forever? These types of errors can be very telling about the overall quality of the site.

- *A—Author:* Who is the author of the site? Does that person or group of people have the appropriate credentials? Is the author clearly identified by name, and is contact information provided? One suggestion is to double-check an author's credentials by doing a literature search in MEDLINE. When people advertise themselves as "the leading worldwide authority" on such and such a topic, they should have numerous publications to their credit that establish their reputations. It is surprising how many times this search brings up nothing.

Be wary of how a person presents her credentials, too. Consider a site where "Dr. X" is touted as an expert. Upon further exploration, you may find that, in fact, Dr. X does have a PhD (or MD or EdD), but the discipline in which this degree was obtained has nothing to do with the subject matter of the site. Remember that there is no universal process of peer review on the WWW and anyone can present herself in any way that she wants. Be suspicious.

Keep in mind that the webmaster and the author may be two (or more) different people. The webmaster is the person who designed the site and is responsible for its upkeep. The author is the person who is responsible for the content and is the expert in the subject matter provided. In your evaluation, make sure you determine who these people are.

- *S—Site navigation:* Is the site easy to navigate? Is it attractive? Does it download quickly or have too many graphics and other features that make it inefficient? A site that is pleasing to the eye will invite you to return. Sites that cause your computer to crash should be viewed with skepticism.

- *E—Ethical disclosure:* Is there contact information for the site developer and author? Is there full disclosure of who the author is and the purpose of the site? Is this information easy to find or is it buried deep in the Web site? There are many commercial services, particularly pharmaceutical companies, that have excellent Web sites with very useful information. But some of them exist only to sell their product, although this is not immediately evident on evaluation.

- *D—Date site last updated:* When was the site last updated? Is it current? Does the information need to be updated regularly? Generally, with health and nursing information, the answer to that last question is yes. You should be concerned about sites that have not been updated within 12 to 18 months. The date the site was last updated should be prominently displayed on the site. Keep in mind that different pages within the site may be updated at different times. Be sure to check the date on each of the pages that you visit.

As you become more proficient at evaluating Web sites, you may have additional criteria that you would add to this list or criteria that are important to you for a specific purpose, but, in general, this simple group of seven is surprisingly comprehensive. Test them for yourself. Do a quick search on a topic of interest, visit a number of sites, and determine just how PLEASED you are with what you find (Nicoll, 2003).

KEY CONCEPTS

- In the decision-making process, there are five levels.

- Critical thinking involves examining problems or situations from every viewpoint. Use of the universal intellectual standards will improve a nurse's critical thinking.

- Practicing reflective thinking, intuitive thinking, and problem solving helps individuals become better critical thinkers.

- Decision-making tools are helpful when the nurse needs to separate multiple factors surrounding a situation during the decision-making process.

- Effective searching for information on the Internet requires that you target your search. One technique is to conduct a P-F-A: a purpose-focus-approach assessment to determine what you are looking for and the best way to find it.

- PubMed is a search engine developed by the National Library of Medicine that allows you to search MEDLINE. It is free to anyone with an Internet connection.

- It is important to evaluate information found on the Internet. Ask yourself, "Am I PLEASED with the site?"

  P-Purpose
  L-Links
  E-Editorial (site content)
  A-Author
  S-Site navigation
  E-Ethical disclosure
  D-Date site last updated

- There are situations in which the nurse makes an individual decision. Other situations call for group decision making.

KEY TERMS

consensus

critical thinking

decision making

intuitive thinking

problem solving

reflective thinking

REVIEW QUESTIONS

1. A new nurse is trying to set her goals for the next five years. She plans to eventually become an acute care nurse practitioner in the ICU setting. She knows she needs to become more experienced, obtain appropriate certification, go back to school, and take the practitioner exam. She would like to see a visual of the time it will take her to realistically accomplish those goals. She should use which of the following?
   A. Decision tree
   B. Gantt chart
   C. Decision grid
   D. Problem-solving process

2. A task force designed to examine solutions for low patient satisfaction in an emergency department has decided to write their ideas down, present their ideas to the task force, discuss the ideas, and then, privately vote on the ideas. This is an example of which group process?
   A. Consensus building
   B. Delphi technique
   C. Problem-solving process
   D. Nominal group technique

3. A nurse manager decides to form a task force to identify reasons and solutions for patient dissatisfaction on your unit. What are the advantages of forming this task force? Select all that apply.

    ____A. The decisions will be made more quickly.

    ____B. High quality decision making is possible due to more solutions being generated.

    ____C. Acceptance of decisions is more likely.

    ____D. There is access to a larger resource base.

    ____E. Conflict during the decision-making process is less likely.

    ____F. Ownership of the solution will be promoted.

4. A nurse needs to assist a patient in walking down the hall twice daily as part of the patient's postoperative activities. It is the middle of the afternoon, and the patient is asleep. The nurse would like to allow the patient to sleep because the patient was awake a majority of the night. However, if the nurse does not ambulate the patient now, it is possible that the rest of the nurse's afternoon activities will prevent her from returning to the patient to ambulate before the end of her shift. The nurse must decide whether to ambulate the patient now. What is the next step of the decision-making process?

    A. Determine the outcome or goal that is desired.

    B. Identify alternatives and determine benefits and consequences of each.

    C. Make the decision.

    D. Evaluate the decision.

REVIEW ACTIVITIES

1. You are taking the NCLEX in 10 weeks and need to prepare. Draw a PERT diagram to depict the sequence of tasks necessary for the successful completion of the NCLEX.

2. The education forms are not being filled out correctly for new admissions in your medical-surgical unit. Decide on your own the best action to take in this situation. Then, get into a group and decide on the best action to take. Compare the differences between individual and group decision making. What did you learn?

3. Identify a problem that you have been considering. Using the decision-making grid below, rate the alternative solutions to the problem on a scale of 1 to 3 on the elements of cost, quality, importance, location, and any other elements that are important to you. Did this exercise help you to clarify your thinking?

	Cost	Quality	Importance	Location	Other
Alternative A					
Alternative B					
Alternative C					

EXPLORING THE WEB

- Review these sites for extra information on intuitive thinking:

  www.typelogic.com

  www.intuitivethinking.com

- Search for *Books*, then *PDA* at:

  www.barnesandnoble.com

- The Unified Medical Language System is developed to compensate for differences in

concepts in several biomedical terminologies:
www.umlsks.nlm.nih.gov

■ Note the universal intellectual standards
at the Foundation for Critical Thinking:
www.criticalthinking.org

■ Visit these critical thinking sites:
www.insightassessment.com

■ Review this site on applying artificial intelligence
to clinical situations:
www.medg.lcs.mit.edu

REFERENCES

Alfaro-LeFevre, R. (2003). *Critical thinking and clinical judgment: A practical approach* (3rd ed.). Philadelphia, PA: W. B. Saunders.

American Nurses Association (ANA). (2001). Scope and standards of practice for nursing informatics.

DeLaune, S., & Ladner, P. (2006). *Fundamentals of nursing, standards and practice* (3rd ed.). Clifton Park, NY: Delmar Cengage Learning.

Delbecq , A. L. & Van de Ven, A. H., "A Group Process Model for Problem Identification and Program Planning," *Journal of Applied Behavioral Science* VII (July/August, 1971), 466–91 and Delbecq, A. L., Van de Ven, A. H., & D. H. Gustafson, *Group Techniques for Program Planners* (Glenview, Illinois: Scott Foresman and Company, 1975).

Gardner, P. (2003). *Nursing process in action.* Clifton Park, NY: Delmar Cengage Learning.

Health on the Net Foundation. HONcode Site Evaluation form. (2009). Available at www.hon.ch/cgi-bin/HONcode/Inscription/site_evaluation.pl?language=en&userCategory=individuals. (accessed 4-16-09)

Horrigan, J., & Rainie, L. (2006). When facing a tough decision, 60 million Americans now seek the Internet's help. Observation Deck: Analysis of public opinion, demographic and policy trends. Retrieved May 3, 2006, from pewresearch.org/obdeck/?ObDeckID=19.

Joint Commission (JC). (2008). Hospital/Critical Access Hospital National Patient Safety Goals. Retrieved June 10, 2008 from www.jointcommission.org/. Click on Patient Safety National Patient Safety Goals.

Jones, J. (2003). Patient education and the WWW. *Clinical Nurse Specialist, 17*(6), 281–283.

Jones, R. A. P., & Beck, S. E. (1996). *Decision making in nursing.* Clifton Park, NY: Delmar Cengage Learning.

Merriam-Webster. (2006). *Merriam-Webster's Collegiate® Dictionary* (11th ed.). Springfield, MA.

Nicoll, L. H. (2003). Nursing and health care informatics. In P. L. Kelly-Heidenthal (Ed.), *Nursing leadership & management.* Clifton Park, NY: Delmar Cengage Learning.

Paul, R, (1992). *Critical thinking: What every person needs to survive in a rapidly changing world.* Santa Rosa, CA: Foundation for Critical Thinking.

Paul, R. and Elder, L. (1996, June). Foundation For Critical Thinking, online at website: www.criticalthinking.org.

Pesut, D. J., & Herman, J. (1999). *Clinical reasoning: The art & science of critical & creative thinking.* Clifton Park, NY: Delmar Cengage Learning.

Ruth-Sahd, L., & Hendy, H. (2005). Predictors of novice nurses' use of intuition to guide patient care decisions. *Journal of Nursing Education, 44*(10), 450–458.

The Small Business Knowledge Base. (1999). Retrieved January 19, 2002, from www.bizmove.com.

Vroom, V. H., & Yetton, P. (1973). *Leadership and Decision-Making.* Pittsburgh, PA: University of Pittsburgh Press.

White, A., Allen, P., Goodwin, L., Breckinridge, D., Dowell, J., & Garvy, R. (2005). Infusing PDA technology into nursing education. *Nurse Educator, 30*(4), 153–154.

SUGGESTED READINGS

Bowles, K. H., & Baugh, A. C. (2007, Jan.–Feb.). Applying research evidence to optimize tele-homecare. *Journal of Cardiovascular Nursing, 22*(1), 5–15.

Evans, C. (2005). Clinical decision-making theories: Patient assessment in autonomy and extended roles. *Emergency Nurse, 13*(5), 16–20.

Hao, A. T., Chang, H. K., & Chong, P. P. (2006). *Mobile learning for nursing education.* American Medical Informatics Association Annual Symposium Proceedings, 943.

Manias, E. (2004). Decision-making models used by "graduate nurses" managing patients' medications. *Journal of Advanced Nursing, 47*(3), 270–278.

Murphy, J. (2004). Using focused reflection and articulation to promote clinical reasoning: An evidence-based teaching strategy. *Nursing Education Perspectives, 25*(5), 226–231.

O'Callaghan, N. (2005). The use of expert practice to explore reflection. *Nursing Standard, 19*(39), 41–47.

Poon, E. G., Keohane, C., Featherstone, E., Hays, B., Dervan, A., Woolf, S., et al. (2006). *Impact of bar-code medication administration technology on how nurses spend their time on clinical care.* American Medical Informatics Association Annual Symposium Proceedings, 1065.

Shortell, S., & Kaluzny, A. (2006). *Health Care Management* (5th ed.). Clifton Park, NY: Delmar Cengage Learning.

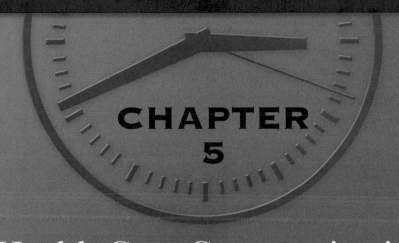

CHAPTER 5

Health Care Communication

Teamwork is the ability to work together toward a common vision, the ability to direct individual accomplishment toward organizational objectives. It is the fuel that allows common people to attain uncommon results.

(Andrew Carnegie, 1984)

OBJECTIVES

Upon completion of this chapter, the reader should be able to:

1. Discuss the purpose of a health care team.
2. Review the process of communication.
3. Review the Health Insurance Portability and Accountability Act of 1996 (HIPAA).
4. Discuss the stages of group process and common team member roles.
5. Identify elements of the Myers-Briggs Type Indicator.
6. Explore crew resource management.
7. Discuss organizational communication.
8. Discuss how to overcome communication barriers.
9. Discuss groupthink.

As a new nurse, you are making the day's assignments for a 34-bed medical–surgical unit. Working with you today will be another two registered nurses, two licensed practical nurses, and one nursing assistant. You graduated only a year ago and you were recently promoted to the role of charge nurse. Today, one of the licensed practical nurses and the nursing assistant are challenging your patient care assignments, saying you do not have enough experience to make a fair assignment. They are trying to get the two registered nurses to side with them. It appears that the two registered nurses often work together, as do the two licensed practical nurses. You know you made the best assignment given the staff available, yet you are wondering if there is a better solution.

What would be the best way to address their concerns?

How can you work with your team to ensure fair patient assignments?

I n today's health care environment, great demands are placed on each health care professional to provide the best quality of care efficiently, safely, and cost-effectively to optimize patient care outcomes. Many administrators and nurse managers recognize that effective interprofessional communication and collaboration through teamwork is needed to create a safe patient care environment. Collaboration and teamwork among staff nurses and other disciplines in the health care setting is so critical to optimizing patient care safety and outcomes that it is a priority for most health care administrators, directors, and managers (Amos, Hu, & Herrick, 2005). This chapter discusses the key factors that build a successful nursing team. It also discusses the group process and ways in which a nurse can communicate on effective teams. Finally, it discusses organizational communication.

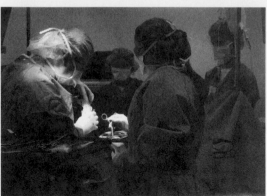

Courtesy of Advocate Good Shepherd Hospital, Barrington, Illinois*

TEAMS AND COMMUNICATION

Katzenbach and Smith (1993) define a **team** as "a small number of people with complementary skills who are committed to a common purpose, performance goals, and approach for which they hold themselves accountable (p. 45)." On health care teams, the purpose is to meet patient care needs. On some teams, such as a nursing policy and procedure team, all members may have similar backgrounds and abilities. Other teams may be developed with interdisciplinary members who have a variety of skills and talents, to provide different perspectives and ideas on how to solve problems.

Everyone on an interdisciplinary team is trained in his or her specialty and looks at care delivery with a different focus, e.g., as nurses, physicians, social workers, dieticians, or case managers. Sometimes having so many viewpoints can be difficult, though, especially if a single decision is needed and everyone has varying opinions.

To get the work of an organization completed, multiple formal and informal teams or groups may develop. Formal teams or groups may include a temporary ad hoc group that meets to accomplish a specific purpose, such as preparing for accreditation by the Joint Commission. Another formal team may be a permanent standing group or committee that meets regularly to accomplish organizational objectives, such as the Intensive Care Committee.

Informal teams may also evolve in organizations. Shortell and Kaluzny (2006) state that the importance of informal workgroup structure and group processes has been recognized for many years. The Hawthorne experiments firmly established the proposition that an individual's performance is determined in large part by informal relationship patterns that emerge within workgroups (Roethlisberger & Dickson, 1939). The workgroup has an impact on individual behaviors and attitudes because it controls so many of the stimuli to which the individual is exposed in performing organizational tasks (Hasenfeld, 1983).

Informal groups are not directly established or sanctioned by the organization but often form naturally by individuals in the organization to fill a personal or social interest or need. Shortell and Kaluzny (2006) identify a number of circumstances under which informal groups can have a negative impact on an organization. Groups may become overly exclusionary and lead to interpersonal conflict. In other cases, informal groups can become so powerful that they undermine the formal authority structure of the organization.

Informal groups can assume a change agent role. Informal groups are often responsible for facilitating improvements in working conditions. Such informal groups sometimes evolve into formal groups. Informal groups may also emerge to deal with a particular organizational problem or to work toward changes in organizational policies and procedures. In sum, informal groups play a unique role in organizations. These roles may be positive or negative.

A team may be advisory, such as a committee that meets to discuss concerns of the professional nursing staff and then reports back to the chief nurse executive for decision making, or the team may be self-directed and make decisions on its own.

Whatever the type, formal or informal, all teams must communicate to achieve their objectives.

COMMUNICATION PROCESS

Communication is an interactive process that occurs when a person (the sender) sends a verbal or nonverbal message to another person (the receiver) and receives feedback. The communication process is influenced by emotions, needs, perceptions, values, education, culture, goals, literacy, cognitive ability, the communication mode, and noise (Figure 5-1).

Communication in health care is used to coordinate patient care. Several studies of ICUs indicate that effective communication and coordination among clinical staff results in more efficient and better quality of care (Baggs, Ryan, Phelps, Richeson, & Johnson, 1992; Knaus, Draper, Wagner, & Zimmerman, 1986; Shortell et al., 1994; Gittell et al., 2000; Young et al., 1997; Young et al., 1998). Additionally, research suggests that ineffective coordination and communication among hospital staff contributes substantially to adverse events. For example, one study of the care of 1,047 patients in a large tertiary care hospital found that approximately 15% of the 480 adverse events identified, for example, failure to order indicated tests and misplaced test results, had causes related to the interaction of staff, such as the failure of a consultant team to communicate adequately with the requesting team (Andrews et al., 1997).

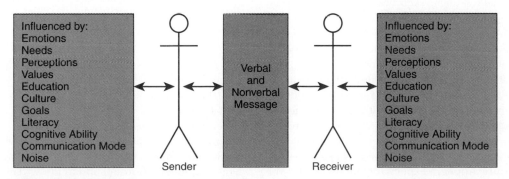

Figure 5-1 Communication process. (Delmar/Cengage Learning).

For many types of health care organizations, staff communication and coordination is also relevant to their ability to comply with the requirements of accrediting bodies. In particular, both the Joint Commission (JC) (www.jointcommission.org), and the National Committee on Quality Assurance (web.ncqa.org), two leading accrediting bodies in the health care industry, have adopted standards that address coordination among professional groups, patient care units, and service components within health care organizations.

Note that communication is affected by following the rules of civility, e.g., do not demean others, show consideration, keep your voice low in public places, give praise, admit you are wrong, smile, etc. (Forni, 2003).

ELECTRONIC COMMUNICATION

Communication is shifting to an electronic mode, with computer technology playing an increasingly dominant role. Health care providers are using a variety of technologies, including telephones, voice mail, personal data assistants, BlackBerry, fax, e-mail, and video conferencing. These methods require careful communication. For example, e-mail now allows almost instantaneous communication around the world, but it also accommodates individual preferences with respect to the timing of the response. This allows a person to send a message early in the day and allows the team members the opportunity to respond as their schedules permit. Using e-mail may save a patient and caregiver from travel or loss of work. However, using e-mail requires that nurses acting in such a caregiver role have keen writing skills. The speed with which exchanges can now be made using technology has reduced the acceptable response time. Therefore, the first tip when communicating using technology is that it is important that both parties have an understanding about the circumstances under which different modes of communication will be used. Although one practitioner who is "connected" may be comfortable receiving urgent patient information such as an elevated potassium level electronically, perhaps by e-mail, most practitioners expect a telephone call if the data being shared is potentially life-threatening.

Practitioners may be satisfied to receive a fax if the data are not urgent. Often, organizations have policies that guide under what circumstances a particular mode of communication is used, so be sure to understand your institution's policy for communicating urgent information.

Another tip is to respond in a timely manner. Timeliness is defined by what information is being shared and the route being used. A fax delivered to a practitioner's office over the weekend will likely not generate a reply before Monday. E-mail, in general, provides greater immediacy, but the telephone remains the primary tool for communicating urgent information. Other tips for communicating on e-mail include the following:

- NO CAPITAL LETTERS—this looks like you are shouting.
- Be brief and reply sparingly, as appropriate.
- Use clear subject lines.
- Cool off before responding to an angry message. Answer tomorrow.
- Forward e-mail messages from others only with their permission.
- Forward jokes selectively, if ever.
- Use good judgment; e-mail may not be private.

Keep in mind that accurate spelling, correct grammar, and organization of thought assume greater importance in the absence of verbal and nonverbal cues that are given in face-to-face encounters. Always proofread correspondences prior to sending them. Imagine yourself as the recipient of the document. Look for complete sentences, logical development of thought and reasoning, accuracy, and appropriate use of grammar, punctuation, and capitalization.

Electronic record keeping is increasingly being adopted by health care systems, particularly acute care settings. However, these systems are expensive to implement, so there is a lag between what's available to improve record keeping and what is actually being used. The types and features of the systems adopted are almost as numerous as the institutions using them, so specific details will not be elaborated here. Orientation to each institution likely includes an introduction to the system(s) in use. In general, as with all patient records, issues of

| TABLE 5-1 | ELEMENTS THAT ARE CONSIDERED PATIENT IDENTIFIERS UNDER HIPAA |

- Names
- All geographic subdivisions smaller than a state, including street address, city, county, precinct, ZIP code
- All elements of dates (except year) for dates directly related to an individual, including birth date, admission date, discharge date, date of death; all ages over 89
- Telephone numbers
- Fax numbers
- E-mail addresses
- Social security numbers
- Medical record numbers
- Health plan beneficiary numbers

- Account numbers
- Certificate/license numbers
- Vehicle identifiers and serial numbers
- Device identifiers and serial numbers
- Web universal resource locators (URLs)
- Internet Protocol (IP) address numbers
- Biometric identifiers, including fingerprints and voiceprints
- Full-face photographic images and any comparable images
- Any other unique identifying number, characteristic, or code unless otherwise permitted

Source: Compiled with information from U.S. Department of Health and Human Services. (2003). *Protecting personal health information in research: Understanding the HIPAA privacy rule.* NIH Publication Number 03–5388.

confidentiality are of utmost importance, so nurses must be mindful of their important role in maintaining privacy and accessing and granting access to the system appropriately.

HEALTH INSURANCE PORTABILITY AND ACCOUNTABILITY ACT (HIPAA) OF 1996

As nurses communicate today, they must increasingly be aware of patient privacy. The Department of Health and Human Services (HHS) has issued regulations known as the Privacy Rule that protect all individually identifiable health information held or transmitted by a covered entity or its business associate, in any form or media, whether electronic, paper, or oral. It applies to all health care plans, health care clearinghouses, and to any health care provider who transmits health information. The

law introduced new standards for protecting the privacy of individuals' identifiable health information. There are 18 personal health identifiers. This law also may apply to health information that is shared for research purposes (www.hhs.gov/ocr/privacy/index.html.); see Table 5-1.

STAGES OF GROUP PROCESS

All teams go through predictable phases of group development as they evolve from an immature stage to a mature stage. It is critical to note that not all teams reach maturity, for a variety of reasons: perhaps there is ineffective leadership, problematic members, unclear goals and communication, or lack of focus or energy. Some teams may become fully functional and mature quickly, bypassing a stage or two along the way. It is typical for high-functioning teams whose members are trusting of one another to be able to make decisions quickly and accurately; it may take longer for other teams, whose members need to get to know and trust one another, before the actual work can take place.

Tuckman and Jensen (1977) identified five stages that a group normally progresses through as it develops. These stages are known as **group process** and consist of: Forming, Storming, Norming, Performing, and Adjourning (Table 5-2).

The first stage of the team process is the Forming stage. This stage occurs when the group is created and meets as a team for the first time. The team members come to the meeting with zest and a sense of curiosity, adventure, and even apprehension as they orient themselves to each other and get to know each other through personal interaction and perhaps team-building activities. With the help of the team leader or facilitator, they will explore the purpose and goals of the team, what contribution they can bring to the table, and set boundaries for the teamwork.

The second stage of the team process is the Storming stage. As the group relaxes and becomes more comfortable, interpersonal issues or opposing opinions may arise that may cause conflict between members of the team and with the team leader. This may cause feelings of uneasiness in the group. It is important at this stage to understand that conflict is a healthy and natural process of team development. When members of the team come from various disciplines and specialties, they are likely to approach an issue from several completely different standpoints. These differences need to be openly confronted and addressed so that effective resolution of the issue may occur in a timely manner. Real teams don't emerge unless individuals on them take risks involving conflict, trust, interdependence, and hard work (Katzenbach & Smith, 2003).

The third stage is called Norming. After resistance is overcome in the Storming stage, a feeling of group cohesion develops. Team members master the ability to resolve conflict. Although complete resolution and agreement may not be attained at all times, team members learn to respect differences

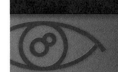

CRITICAL THINKING 5-1

You are having a coffee break with another nurse who mentions a problem she is having with care delivery. The nurse is not sure how to solve it. You want to be helpful and supportive and yet avoid giving advice. Ask the nurse if she can describe the problem fully for you. Do not interrupt. Then, ask the nurse some questions about the problem, and seek clarification until you are clear on the problem and the nurse has fully described it. Do not give advice. Use your communication skills, such as attending, clarifying, and responding, and ask the nurse such things as, tell me more about that, what did you think about it, and so forth, until you are both clear on the issue. At the end of this process, you can just finish by relaxing for the rest of your break or you can ask the nurse, "Do you want advice about your problem?"

Many times, this process will help the nurse solve the problem by himself or herself. If the nurse does want advice, you can give some suggestions if you are comfortable doing so. Do you think this process can strengthen people's ability to find answers to their problems? Do you think this process would be helpful to you in working with others on the unit? Do you think this approach honors people's integrity and ability to solve their own problems?

Source: Adapted from M. Parsons (personal communication, 2003).

	TUCKMAN AND JENSEN'S STAGES OF TEAM PROCESS
TABLE 5-2	

Stages	Description
Forming	*Relationship development:* Team orientation, identification of role expectations, beginning team interactions, explorations, and boundary setting occurs.
Storming	*Interpersonal interaction and reaction:* Dealing with tension and conflict or confrontation may occur.
Norming	*Effective cooperation and collaboration:* Personal opinions are expressed and resolution of conflict with formation of solidified goals and increased group cohesiveness occurs.
Performing	*Group maturity and stable relationships:* Team roles become more functional and flexible, structural issues are resolved leading to supportive task performance through group-directed collaboration and resources sharing.
Adjourning	*Termination and consolidation:* Team goals and activities are met leading to closure, evaluation, and outcomes review. This may also lead to reforming when the need for improvement or further goal development is identified.

Source: Compiled with information from Tuckman, B. W., & Jensen, M. A. C., (1977) Stages of Small Group Development Revisited. *Group and Organizational Studies, 2*(4), 419–427; Hall, P., & Weaver, L. (2001). Interdisciplinary Education and Teamwork: A Long and Winding Road. *Medical Education, 35,* 867-875; Polifko-Harris, K. (2003). Effective Team Building. In P. L. Kelly, *Nursing Leadership & Management.* (2nd ed.). Clifton Park, NY: Delmar Cengage Learning.

of opinion and may work together through these obstacles to achieve team goals. Communication of ideas, opinions, and information occurs through effective cooperation among the team members. Overcoming barriers to performance is how groups become teams (Katzenbach & Smith, 2003).

The fourth stage of the team development process is the Performing stage. In this stage, group cohesion, collaboration, and solidarity are evident. Personal opinions are set aside to achieve group goals. Team members openly communicate, know each other's roles and responsibilities, take risks, and trust or rely on each other to complete assigned tasks. The group reaches maturity at this stage. One of the biggest strengths of this stage is the emphasis on maintaining and improving interpersonal relationships within the team as each member functions

as a whole. Kenneth Blanchard, one of the authors of *The One Minute Manager,* sums it up with his comment, "None of us is as smart as all of us."

The fifth and final stage of team process development is the Adjourning stage. Termination and consolidation occur in this stage. When the team has achieved its goals and assigned tasks, the team closure process begins. The team reviews its activities and evaluates its progress and outcomes by answering the questions: Were the team goals sufficiently met? Was there anything that could have been done differently? The team leader summarizes the group's accomplishments and the role played by each member in achieving its goals. It is important to provide closure or feedback regarding the team process to leave each team member with a sense of accomplishment.

COMMON TEAM MEMBER ROLES

In any team, there are bound to be both participants who are helpful and those who are not helpful in their behaviors. Sometimes the behaviors are unconsciously acted out. At other times, a team member is quite clear and focused about the role he or she is playing, such as the aggressor. In any case, it is imperative that the astute team leader be aware of everyone's roles and use excellent communication skills to facilitate the group process.

Common member roles in groups fit into three categories: group task roles, group maintenance roles, and self-oriented roles. Note that successful teams include both group leader roles and group follower roles.

Group task roles help a group develop and accomplish its goals. Among these roles are the following:

- Initiator-contributor: Proposes goals, suggests ways of approaching tasks, and recommends procedures for approaching a problem or task
- Information seeker: Asks for information, viewpoints, and suggestions about the problem or task
- Information giver: Offers information, viewpoints, and suggestions about the problem or task
- Coordinator: Clarifies and synthesizes various ideas in an effort to tie together the work of the members
- Orienter: Summarizes, points to departures from goals, and raises questions about discussion direction
- Energizer: Stimulates the group to higher levels and better quality of work

Group maintenance roles do not directly address a task itself, but instead help foster group unity, positive interpersonal relations among group members, and development of the ability of members to work effectively together. Group maintenance roles include the following:

- Encourager: Expresses warmth and friendliness toward group members, encourages them, and acknowledges their contributions
- Harmonizer: Mediates disagreements between members and attempts to help reconcile differences
- Gatekeeper: Tries to keep lines of communication open and promotes the participation of all members
- Standard setter: Suggests standards for ways in which the group will operate and checks whether members are satisfied with the functioning of the group
- Group observer: Watches the internal operations of the group and provides feedback about how participants are doing and how they might be able to function better
- Follower: Goes along with the group and is friendly but relatively passive

Self-oriented roles are related to the personal needs of group members and often negatively influence the effectiveness of a group. These roles include the following:

- Aggressor: Deflates the contributions of others by attacking their ideas, ridiculing their feelings, and displaying excessive competitiveness
- Blocker: Tends to be negative, stubborn, and resistive of new ideas—sometimes in order to force the group to readdress a viewpoint that it has already dealt with
- Recognition seeker: Seeks attention, boasts about accomplishments and capabilities, and works to prevent being placed in an inferior position in the group
- Dominator: Tries to assert control and manipulates the group or certain group members by using methods such as flattering, giving orders, or interrupting others (Bartol & Martin, 1998)

MYERS-BRIGGS TYPE INDICATOR

If a team is to succeed, it is critical to get the right blend of personalities, experience, and temperaments in the group to work toward a common goal.

Personality theories emphasize how personality differences affect communication. Traits such as introversion or extroversion and preference for rational objectivity or instinctive "gut feeling" affect an individual's communication. An example is a theory

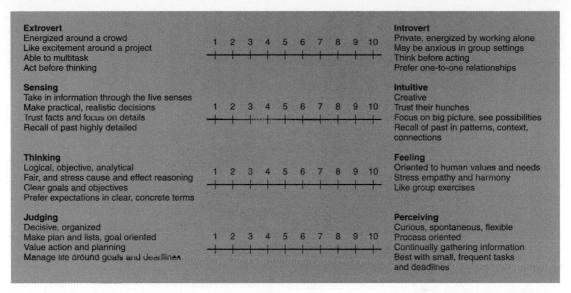

Extrovert
Energized around a crowd
Like excitement around a project
Able to multitask
Act before thinking

1 2 3 4 5 6 7 8 9 10

Introvert
Private, energized by working alone
May be anxious in group settings
Think before acting
Prefer one-to-one relationships

Sensing
Take in information through the five senses
Make practical, realistic decisions
Trust facts and focus on details
Recall of past highly detailed

1 2 3 4 5 6 7 8 9 10

Intuitive
Creative
Trust their hunches
Focus on big picture, see possibilities
Recall of past in patterns, context, connections

Thinking
Logical, objective, analytical
Fair, and stress cause and effect reasoning
Clear goals and objectives
Prefer expectations in clear, concrete terms

1 2 3 4 5 6 7 8 9 10

Feeling
Oriented to human values and needs
Stress empathy and harmony
Like group exercises

Judging
Decisive, organized
Make plan and lists, goal oriented
Value action and planning
Manage life around goals and deadlines

1 2 3 4 5 6 7 8 9 10

Perceiving
Curious, spontaneous, flexible
Process oriented
Continually gathering information
Best with small, frequent tasks and deadlines

Figure 5-2 Myers-Briggs personality dichotomies. (*Source:* Compiled from Briggs Myers, I., & Myers, P.B. [1995]. *Gifts Differing.* Palo Alto, CA: Davies–Black; and *Patient Teaching* by P. Heidenthal, et al, in Kelly, P.L. [2008]. *Nursing Leadership & Management* [2nd ed.]. Clifton Park, NY: Delmar Cengage Learning).

based on the Myers-Briggs Personality Dichotomies (Figure 5-2), which in turn is based on personality theories of Carl Jung (Briggs Myers & Myers, 1995).

This theory suggests that personality is made up of four complementary sets of traits: extroversion-introversion, sensing-intuition, thinking-feeling, and judging-perceiving. Within each of these sets, there is a sliding scale, so to speak. For example, on the extroversion-introversion scale, 1 might be completely extroverted, 10 completely introverted, and 5 equally both. In most cases, one or the other usually dominates. Through testing, an individual can be identified as one of 16 possible types, based on the person's score in each of the four areas. The personality type is identified by a four-letter indicator. For example, an INTJ would be an introverted-intuitive-thinking-judging personality. An ESFP would be an extroverted-sensory-feeling-perceiving personality. In the theories of Jung and Myers-Briggs, each personality type has specific characteristics that affect the individual's approach to life experiences, including learning. Extroverts prefer to interact with people; introverts prefer to be alone. Thinking personalities prefer an objective, unwavering approach; feeling personalities are more likely to bend the rules if they think it makes people happy. Sensing people rely on their senses and prefer facts and structure to make decisions, whereas intuitive people are creative and see possibilities. Judging people like to be organized and decisive, whereas perceiving people work well in a spontaneous, flexible atmosphere.

Such personality differences can affect the way individuals approach and engage in communication. Staff who are the extroverted and judging type may have difficulty understanding and working with staff who are the introverted and perceiving type. It is important to remember when working with all staff that not everyone sees the world and approaches goals in the same fashion. As one works with various personality types, it is crucial to work toward clarification and common understanding of team goals.

GREAT TEAM GUIDELINES

Great teams don't just happen; there is behind-the-scenes planning, preparation, and forward thinking before anyone works together. Theories of effective teams have been discussed in the literature for several decades by Lewin (1951), McGregor (1960), Argyris (1964), Burns (1978), Bennis (1989), and Senge (1990). What are the guidelines for encouraging great teams? A great team accomplishes what it sets out to do, with everyone on the team participating to achieve the desired outcomes. Effective teamwork is achieved when there is synergy. Mark Twain defines synergy as "the bonus that is achieved when things work together harmoniously." Steven Covey maintains that synergy means that the whole is greater than the sum of its parts (1989). The American Association of Critical Care Nurses has a Synergy Model of Professional Caring & Ethical Practice that guides the nurse and results in synergy, where the needs and

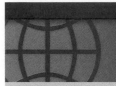

REAL WORLD INTERVIEW

An elderly nonverbal patient with a history of schizophrenia was admitted to our surgical unit for dehydration. She was in need of total care, especially with respect to hygiene, which had been neglected. She was dependent on staff to turn and position her. Her level of awareness suggested she was unable to use a call light for help.

This patient challenged staff for a variety of reasons. First, due to multiple other health problems, she was not a candidate for surgery. This placed her among the patients who don't really "fit" the surgical unit where she was admitted. Nonetheless, my goal was to advocate for comfort care with her physician while also encouraging subordinates to provide quality care even though the goal was not for cure with this particular patient. The patient's inability to communicate verbally added to the challenge. It was unclear how aware the patient was of the care she was receiving. Her nonverbal status blocked her ability to dialogue. This caused us to rely on nonverbal cues. Respect for patients with or without their verbal feedback is essential. The CNA and I tackled the needed bed bath together. Teamwork kept the focus on the goal for the patient, which was to optimize comfort and maintain skin integrity. It allowed me to complete a thorough assessment and to model desired communication with the patient, whom I addressed by name. I inquired whether she was in pain, to which she responded with twisting motions. I continued the one-way conversation, attempting to clarify what her nonverbal responses meant. She pointed to her shoulder, so we repositioned her and she settled down, resting quietly. As is often the case, the CNA willingly returned to reposition the patient with confidence the remainder of the shift. The patient's inability to verbalize needs was perceived as less of a barrier once we were successful in overcoming it together.

I find that CNAs will often volunteer to complete entire tasks they feel capable of performing independently. They also need to be assured that they will not be expected to handle clinical situations for which they do not feel qualified. This mutual respect for each other is essential to an ongoing working relationship. They honor my standard of care and will often complete tasks, going above and beyond what I ask. For example, later in the afternoon, the CNA returned to the patient and washed and braided her hair. Since this same patient would not likely use the call light, I also explained our goal to the high school student volunteer and I asked her to check the patient's position whenever she went by the room. I instructed her to let me know if the patient appeared uncomfortable, assuring her that I would reposition the patient as needed. The student expressed that she thought it was cool how nurses communicate with patients who can't talk. I believe through effective communication our team achieved the goal of optimizing this patient's comfort in spite of many potential barriers.

Lari Summa, RN, BSN
Team leader
Peorla, Illinois

characteristics of a patient, clinical unit, or system are matched with a nurse's competencies (Hardin & Kaplan, 2005). Effective nurses and teams achieve synergy. They develop the ingredients for creating a winning team where people with different ideas, backgrounds, and beliefs work together synergistically and harmoniously.

First and foremost, the team must have a clearly stated purpose: what are the goals? What are the objectives? What does the leader see the team accomplishing? Are any budget requirements, decision-making ability, and lines of authority for the team spelled out? An effective team keeps the larger organization's goals in mind as it progresses; otherwise, its goals will be inconsistent with those of the parent organization.

Second is an assessment of the team's composition: what are the team members' personal strengths and weaknesses? How do the team members see themselves as individuals? Do they see themselves as part of a cohesive team? Are the contributions of all team members valued? Are all team members' opinions respected? Does the team have a plan to avoid groupthink? Are any additional members with special expertise needed? What are the roles of each team member?

Third is the communication link. Are effective communication patterns in place? Is there a need to improve communication, either in written or verbal format? Does the team work well together and is communication open, with minimal hidden agendas of the members? Can the truth be told in a compassionate and sympathetic manner in order to reach a difficult decision?

Active participation by all team members is a critical fourth item. Does everyone have a designated responsibility? Do people listen to one another? Is "we versus they" thinking discouraged? Are all team members involved in shaping plans and decisions? Are they all carrying their weight on the team, or are some members not doing their part? What are the relationships of the team members? Is there mutual trust and respect for members and their decisions, however unpopular? Are there political turf issues that must be resolved before proceeding? The climate of the team should be relaxed but supportive.

Is there a clear plan as to how to proceed? Is there a way to acknowledge team accomplishments and positive change? This fifth element leads to an action plan that everyone agrees with early on, and one that is revisited at certain designated times. Feedback by team members and others affected by the team's decisions is necessary to keep focus.

The sixth guideline is actually ongoing, in that assessment and evaluation are continuous throughout the team's history. Outcomes have to be consistent and related to the expectations of the organization. Creativity is also encouraged at the team level; perhaps a member has an idea to solve a problem that no one has ever tried. In a supportive environment, pros and cons of all reasonable ideas should be freely discussed. A team needs to periodically evaluate its progress. See Table 5-3.

TEAMWORK ON A PATIENT CARE UNIT

The role of the nurse is multifaceted. Depending on the scenario, a nurse may work directly or indirectly with a wide variety of staff on the health care team. A registered nurse (RN) is directly responsible for the care of the patient, but that care encompasses ensuring that the nursing and medical practitioner's orders are carried out and that nursing assistive personnel document the intakes and outputs accurately for the shift. The RN ensures that the licensed practical nurse completes the ordered treatments; that discharge planning is coordinated with the social worker, the case manager, the pharmacist, and the administration; that the family understands how to dress the patient's wound; and, finally, that the patient understands the discharge instructions. The role of the RN team leader incorporates the entire spectrum of care provided to the family by a wide variety of people. The effective nurse will possess excellent communication skills, both written and verbal; be sensitive of others' cultural and value differences; be aware

TABLE 5-3	TEAM EVALUATION CHECKLIST		
		Yes	**No**
1.	Is the environment/climate conducive to team building?	_____	_____
2.	Do the team members have mutual respect for and trust in one another?	_____	_____
3.	Are the team members honest with one another?	_____	_____
4.	Does everyone actively participate in the team's decision making and problem solving?	_____	_____
5.	Are the purpose, goals, and objectives of the team obvious to all participants?	_____	_____
6.	Are the goals met?	_____	_____
7.	Are creativity and mutual support of new ideas encouraged by all team members?	_____	_____
8.	Does the team work to avoid groupthink?	_____	_____
9.	Is the team productive, and does it see actual progress toward goal attainment?	_____	_____
10.	Does the team begin and end its meetings on time?	_____	_____
11.	Does the team leader provide vision and energy to the team?	_____	_____
12.	Do any persons on the team serve in the common team member roles of group task role, group maintenance role, or self-oriented role, as identified earlier in this chapter?	_____	_____

Source: Compiled with information from Polifko-Harris, K. (2003). Effective team building. In P. L. Kelly, *Nursing Leadership & Management.* (2nd ed.). Clifton Park, NY: Delmar Cengage Learning.

of others' abilities; and show genuine interest in the team members.

STATUS DIFFERENCES

Status is the measure of worth conferred on an individual by a group. Status differences are seen throughout organizations and serve some useful purposes (Shortell & Kaluzny, 2006). Differences in status motivate people, provide them with a means of identification, and may be a force for stability in the organization (Scott, 1967).

Status differences have a profound effect on the functioning of teams. Research findings are fairly consistent in showing that high-status members initiate communication more often, are provided more opportunities to participate, and have more influence over the decision-making process (Owens, Mannic, & Neale, 1998). Thus, an individual from a lower-status professional group may be intimidated or ignored by higher-status team members. The group, as a result, may not benefit from this person's expertise. This situation is very likely in health care, where status differences among the professions are well entrenched (Topping, Norton, & Scafidi, 2003). Often, multidisciplinary teams are idealistically expected to operate as a company of equals, yet the reality of the situation makes this difficult (Shortell & Kaluzny, 2006). In a study of end-stage renal disease teams in which the equal participation ideology was accepted by most team participants, it was clear that the medical practitioners, who were perceived as having higher professional status than other groups, had greater involvement in the actual decision-making process (Deber & Leatt, 1986). The mismatch between expectations and reality made many team members, particularly staff nurses, feel a sense of role deprivation, with accompanying implications for morale and job satisfaction. This problem is exacerbated in teams characterized by gender diversity. In one study, men were more likely to want to exit teams that were female-dominated for those that were male-dominated or homogenous. Men have historically been perceived as having higher status in managerial roles in organizations, thereby affecting the men's satisfaction with the team (Chatman & O'Reilly, 2004).

Status differences may significantly impact patient outcomes. According to the recent report, *Keeping Patients Safe: Transforming the Work Environment of Nurses,* "counterproductive hierarchical communication patterns that derive from status differences" are partly responsible for many medical errors (Institute of Medicine, 2003, p. 361). Further, a review of medical malpractice cases from across the country found that medical practitioners, perceived by some as the higher-status members of the team, often ignored important information communicated by nurses, perceived by some as the lower-status members of the team. Nurses in turn were found to withhold relevant information for diagnosis and treatment from medical practitioners (Schmitt, 2001). In this status-conscious environment, opportunities for learning and improvement can be missed because of unwillingness to engage in quality-improving communication.

CREW RESOURCE MANAGEMENT

Patient care, like other technically complex and high-risk fields, is an interdependent process carried out by teams of individuals with advanced technical training who have varying roles and decision-making responsibilities. While technical training assures proficiency in specific tasks, it does not address the potential for errors created by communication and decision making in dynamic environments. Experts in aviation have developed safety training focused on effective team management, known as Crew Resource Management (CRM). Improvements in the safety record of commercial aviation may be due, in part, to this training (Helmreich et al., 1999). Over the past 20 years, lessons from aviation's approach to team training have been applied to medicine (Pizzi, et al., 2000) notably in the Intensive Care Unit (ICU) (Shortell et al., 1994), and anesthesia training (Howard et al., 1992). CRM training encompasses a wide range of knowledge, skills, and attitudes including communication, assertiveness, situational awareness, problem solving, decision making, and teamwork.

Assertiveness is the willingness to actively participate, state, and maintain a position until convinced by the facts that other options are better. It requires initiative and the courage to act. Assertiveness differs from passive behavior which is often submissive to avoid conflict, and demonstrates a lack of initiative. Assertiveness also differs from aggressive behavior which can be dominating, hostile, belligerent, and argumentative. Situational awareness refers to the degree of accuracy by which one's perception of his or her current environment mirrors reality. Factors that reduce situational awareness include insufficient communication, fatigue/stress, task overload, task underload, group mindset, "press on regardless" philosophy, and degraded operating conditions.

CRM fosters a climate or culture where the freedom to respectfully question authority is encouraged. However, the primary goal of CRM is not enhanced communication, but enhanced situational awareness. It recognizes that a discrepancy between what is happening and what should be happening is often the first indicator that an error is occurring. This is a delicate area for many organizations, especially ones with traditional hierarchies like health care. Appropriate communication techniques must be taught to all nursing and medical practitioners so they understand that the questioning of authority need not be threatening, and so that all understand the correct way to question orders.

Todd Bishop, a CRM expert, developed a five-step assertive statement process that encompasses inquiry and advocacy steps. The five steps are:

- Opening or attention getter—Address the individual as, for example, "Dr. Karen" or "Michelle", or whatever name or title will get the person's attention.
- State your concern—State what you see in a direct manner. "Mr. Jones has a pulse of 160."
- State the problem as you see it—"Mr. Jones is going into ventricular tachycardia."
- State a solution—"Mr. Jones needs an antiarrhythmic medication."
- Obtain agreement (or buy-in)—"Do you want to order an antiarrhythmic medication?"

The five steps are difficult but important skills to master, and they require a change in interpersonal dynamics and organizational culture.

COMMUNICATING WITH SUPERVISORS

Communicating with a supervisor about team problems can be intimidating, especially for a new nurse. It is important to communicate with your boss in order to develop a good working relationship (Gabarro & Kotter, 1993). See Table 5-4. Note that observing professional courtesy is an important first step. Alert your supervisor to any problems immediately, follow the policy and procedure of your agency, and, if it is not an emergency, request an appointment to discuss a problem further. This demonstrates respect and allows for the conversation to occur at an appropriate time and place. Be prepared to state the concern clearly and accurately. Provide supporting evidence. State a willingness to cooperate in finding a solution and then match behaviors to words. Persist in the pursuit of a solution.

COMMUNICATING WITH COWORKERS

Nurses depend on their coworkers in many ways to collectively provide quality patient care. Nowhere is this more important than in the acute care setting

TABLE 5-4	HOW TO IMPROVE YOUR ABILITY TO WORK WITH YOUR BOSS
Know your boss's: ■ Goals and objectives ■ Pressures ■ Strengths, weaknesses, and blind spots ■ Working style *Understand your own:* ■ Objectives ■ Pressures ■ Strengths, weaknesses, and blind spots	■ Working style ■ Predisposition toward dependence on authority figures *Develop a relationship that:* ■ Meets both your objectives and styles ■ Keeps your boss informed ■ Is based on dependability and honesty ■ Selectively uses your boss's time and resources

Source: Adapted from Gabarro, J. & Kotter, J. P. (1993, May–June). Managing your boss. *Harvard Business Review,* 150–157.

where nursing services are nonstop around the clock. Transfer of patient care from nurse to nurse is one of the most important and frequent communications between coworkers. Fluid communication is crucial to achieving quality nursing care.

THE GOLDEN RULE

An excellent guide for communicating with coworkers is the golden rule: "Do unto others as you would have them do unto you." As a nurse who will be responsible for overseeing others' work, a valuable perspective for you to maintain is that all members of the team are important to successfully realize quality patient care. Offering positive feedback such as, "I appreciate the way you interacted with Mr. T. to get him to ambulate twice this shift," goes a long way toward team building, and it improves coworkers' sense of worth. Nurses also have an opportunity to act as teachers to coworkers. Often in a hospital setting, nurses teach by example. Demonstrating the desired behavior allows the coworker to copy the behavior. It is important to allow time for return demonstrations to evaluate whether the coworker has learned the intended skill. For example, as the nurse, you may demonstrate how to position a patient with special needs, encouraging the coworker to assist and ask questions. The next time repositioning is indicated, accompany the coworker and observe

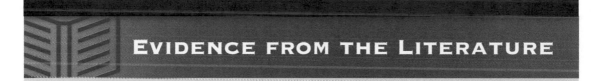

EVIDENCE FROM THE LITERATURE

Citation: Sirota, T. (2008). Nurse/Physician Relationships: Survey Report. July, 28–31.

Discussion: More than half of respondents (57%) to this survey of nurses say they're generally satisfied with their professional relations with physicians; a significant minority, 43%, reports dissatisfaction. Although relationships have improved some since an earlier survey in 1991, respondents' comments indicate that they perceive several factors to be at play here:

■ male physicians' perceptions of traditional gender and cultural roles

■ physicians' arrogance and feelings of superiority

■ nurses' feelings of inferiority

■ hospital culture or policy reinforcing a subordinate role for nurses

Important ways to improve nurse/physician overall collaboration identified in the article includes workplace empowerment for nurses, nurse/physician rounds, team meetings, collaborative educational programs, and collaborative membership on hospital committees.

The article states that the bottom line is that nurses aren't expendable. In the current nursing shortage, the climate is ripe for nurses to speak up as a group and let facility administrators know that they need to pay attention to nurses' legitimate concerns about nurse/physician collaboration, and then correct deficiencies.

Perhaps most important, improving relationships between nurses and physicians will benefit both professional groups by improving job satisfaction and productivity, and will benefit patients by enhancing their overall safety, welfare, and clinical progress. This can be accomplished by promoting greater nurse/physician professional respect, improving communication and collaboration, educating physicians about nursing roles and skills, and addressing physician misconduct (Rosenstein, 2002).

Implications for Nursing: Nursing and medical practitioner communication has improved since the 1991 survey. Good communication by all members of the health care team affects patient safety and must be facilitated by nursing, medical, and hospital team members to build an environment for patient safety.

his or her ability to successfully complete the task. Offer constructive feedback. Be patient. Remember your own learning curve when mastering new skills and behaviors and allow those you supervise the opportunity to grow. Be open to the possibility that coworkers, particularly those with experience, may have a few pearls of wisdom to share with you as well.

COMMUNICATING WITH OTHER NURSING AND MEDICAL PRACTITIONERS

Sometimes new graduates are intimidated by other nursing and medical practitioners they work with. Cardillo (2001) gives several tips on working with other practitioners. She suggests that it is useful to establish rapport and introduce yourself to the other practitioners you work with. Do not be intimidated. You and the other practitioners are

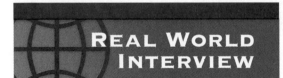

REAL WORLD INTERVIEW

As an emergency medicine physician, I am frequently interfacing with nurses during life-threatening medical scenarios. Whether it is an acute myocardial infarction or respiratory failure or even a very sick child, the dialogue is standard. There is a set tone of urgency on both our parts, and we get straight to work with little discussion. I think when we work as a team, we are like a well-oiled machine. The nurse anticipates my needs and I hers or his, and we follow our protocols. The absolute focus is on the patient and getting him or her out of immediate danger. That is what the emergency department does best. We "stabilize" the patient's acute life-threatening event. The rapport between MD and RN is built from an understanding of mutual competency. I know my nurses in the ED and they know me. I could not save lives day in and day out without the team work mentality.

Dr. Elizabeth Horvath, D.O.
Crystal Lake, Illinois

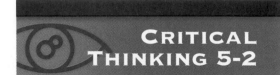

CRITICAL THINKING 5-2

Teamwork on a patient care unit—Day Shift routine

Throughout the day shift, nursing and unit staff communicate and work together to deliver quality patient care.

7:00 am	Day shift takes hand-off shift report from night shift
7:15 am	Charge nurse reviews patient care assignments with all nurses and unit staff, goals and priorities are set
7:20 am	Patient assessment, vital sign assessment, lab work, IV assessment, etc.
7:30 am	Breakfast served
7:45 am	A.M. care begins
8:00 am	Medications given, practitioners make rounds, patient sent for diagnostic tests, nursing care standards followed, documentation begun, hourly regular patient rounds and planning care with other disciplines, etc.
11:30 am	Vital sign assessment
12:00 pm	Lunch served
2:00 pm	Intake and output reports completed; documentation completed
3:00 pm	Hand-off shift report from day shift to evening shift

How does teamwork get patient care completed? Does patient care on your clinical unit follow a similar time sequence as this routine above?

all on the health care team to meet the patient's goals. At least one study has indicated that when nurses and physicians work together, patient death rates or readmission rates decrease (Baggs & Ryan, 1990). Both you and the other practitioners are important to your patient's welfare. Use the SBARR method in Table 5-5 to organize your calls to other practitioners.

Cardillo (2001) also suggests that nurses be assertive. Do not call another practitioner or doctor and say, "I'm sorry to bother you." You are not bothering her. That is her job and you are doing your job by calling her. If you do not understand something, ask questions. Many practitioners and physicians love to teach. Be honest and up front. Tell the practitioner if something is new to you.

TABLE 5-5	SBARR TOOL TO ORGANIZE INFORMATION FOR CALLING ANOTHER NURSING OR MEDICAL PRACTITIONER FOR ASSISTANCE

Situation:

Identify date and time of call

Identify nurse name and unit.

Identify patient name, room number, admitting diagnosis, and date of admission.

State the problem: What it is, when it started, and the severity of it.

Background:

Review pertinent history related to the situation. Postop day, current treatments, medications, allergies, IV fluids and sites, vital signs, level of consciousness, urine output, status of airway, breathing, circulation, pain level, pulse oximeter, cardiac rhythm, mobility, lab results, patient code status, falls, suicide risk, seizure, restraint, isolation precautions, wounds, dressings, other clinical information, and family/significant other involvement.

Assessment:

What is your assessment of the patient? Is the patient's problem severe? Is his or her condition deteriorating? Does the patient need medication?

Recommendation:

What is needed from the practitioner? Know what you want from the practitioner before you call. Don't hang up without communicating this to the practitioner and ensuring that your patient's needs are met, for example, the patient needs to be admitted, needs to be seen, needs medication, and so on.

Response:

Document response of practitioner. Document all calls to practitioner and messages left. Notify supervisor when needed for follow-up. Continue response until patient safety assured.

Source: Adapted from Haig, K.M., Sutton, S., & Whittington, J. (2006). *The SBARR Technique: Improves Communication, Enhances Patient Safety.* Joint Commission's Perspectives on Patient Safety, 5(2), 1–2.

Show respect and consideration for the practitioner you work with, but do not be a doormat. Give due respect and expect the same from him or her. Present information in a straightforward manner, clearly delineating the problem and supporting it with pertinent evidence. This is especially important when reporting changes in patient conditions. Nurses are responsible for knowing classic symptoms of conditions, orally apprising the physician of changes, and recording all observations in the chart (Sanchez-Sweatman, 1996). If the other practitioner is out of line, you might say, "I don't appreciate being spoken to in that way," or "I would appreciate being spoken to in a civil tone of voice and I promise to do the same with you," or something similar.

Calfee (1998) offers suggestions for handling telephone miscommunications. For example, if a physician hangs up, document that the call was terminated and fill out an incident report. If, for example, the physician gives an inappropriate answer or gives no orders for a patient complaint of pain, document the call, the information relayed, and the fact that no orders were given. In addition, document any other steps, such as notifying the supervisor, that were taken to resolve the problem.

Cardillo (2001) suggests that nurses seek clarification from the practitioner if an order is unclear. If an order is inappropriate or incorrect, rather than saying, "This order does not seem appropriate for this patient," which would likely put the practitioner on the defensive, try, "Teach me something, Dr. Jones; I've never seen a dose of Lopressor that high. Can you explain the therapeutic dynamics to me?" or "Dr. Smith, I can't figure out why you ordered a brain scan on this patient. Can you help me out here?" This approach often results in the practitioner either reevaluating an order or changing it. If the practitioner does not change an order that you think is inappropriate or you can't reach the practioner, let your supervisor know and follow the chain of command guidelines of the agency where you work.

COMMUNICATING WITH PATIENTS AND FAMILIES

Communication with patients and families is optimized by many skills, including touch. Nurses routinely use touch as a way to communicate caring and concern. Occasionally, language barriers will limit communication to the nonverbal mode. For instance, a stroke patient who cannot process words can still interpret a gentle hand on his or her shoulder.

Communication requires an openness and honesty with concurrent respect for patients and families. In addition, it is important to honor and protect patients' privacy with the nurse's actions and words.

MENTOR AND PRODIGY

The final pattern of communication that occurs in the workplace that will be discussed is between mentor and prodigy. Mentoring may be an informal process that occurs between an expert nurse and a novice nurse, but it may also be an assigned role. This one-on-one relationship focuses on professional aspects and is mutually beneficial. The optimal novice is hardworking, willing to learn, and anxious to succeed. Communication entails using the skills previously described in this chapter to help the novice develop expert status and career direction. The novice accomplishes this by gleaning the mentor's wisdom. This wisdom is typically shared through listening, affirming, counseling, encouraging, and seeking input from the novice. A strategy that facilitates mentoring is to share the same work schedule so that the novice is exposed to the mentor. This allows for sharing and shadowing opportunities. The mentor can also anticipate added challenges that will likely occur with increasing responsibility. Outlining these challenges with suggestions for how to manage them prepares the novice for his or her expanding responsibilities (Ihlenfeld, 2005). Role-playing, in which the expert preceptor nurse describes a theoretical situation and allows the novice to practice his or her response to new and sometimes challenging situations, is another strategy that can be used.

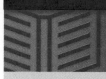

EVIDENCE FROM THE LITERATURE

Citation: Longo, J. and Sherman, R.O. (2007). Leveling horizontal violence. *Nursing Management*, March 2007, 34–37.

Discussion: Horizontal violence has been described as an expression of oppressed group behavior evolving from feelings of low self-esteem and lack of respect from others. Despite recent research that indicates a significant improvement in RNs' perceptions of satisfaction with their careers and work environments, the majority of nurses still disagree when asked if nursing is a good career for people who want respect in their jobs. Nurses have been described as an oppressed group because the nursing profession is primarily female and has existed under a historically patriarchal system headed by male physicians, administrators, and marginalized nurse managers.

Horizontal violence between nurses is an act of aggression perpetrated by one colleague toward another colleague. Although horizontal violence usually consists of verbal or emotional abuse, it can also include physical abuse and may be subtle or overt. Acts of horizontal violence can include talking behind one's back, belittling or criticizing a colleague in front of others, blocking information or a chance for promotion, and isolating or freezing a colleague out of group activities. Repeated acts of horizontal violence against another are often referred to as bullying.

Common behaviors characterized as horizontal violence include:

- nonverbal behaviors such as the raising of eyebrows or making faces in response to comments from the victim
- verbal remarks that could be characterized as being snide, or abrupt responses to questions raised by the victim
- activities that undermine the victim's ability to perform professionally, including either refusing or not being available to give assistance
- the withholding of information about a practice or patient that will undermine a victim's ability to perform professionally
- acts of sabotage that deliberately set victims up for negative situations in their work environment
- group infighting and establishing of cliques designed to exclude some staff members
- scapegoating or attributing all that goes wrong in a situation to one individual
- failure to resolve conflicts directly with the individual involved, choosing instead to complain to others about an individual's behavior
- failure to respect the privacy of others
- broken confidences

Implications for Nursing: Nurses can work to recognize horizontal violence in the profession. As these behaviors are recognized, they can be eliminated.

ORGANIZATIONAL COMMUNICATION

Avenues of communication are often defined by an organization's formal structure. The formal structure establishes who is in charge and identifies how different levels of personnel and various departments relate within the organization. When the chief executive officer of an organization announces that the company will adopt a new policy that all employees will follow, that is downward communication. The message starts at the top and is usually disseminated by levels through the chain of communication (Figure 5-3).

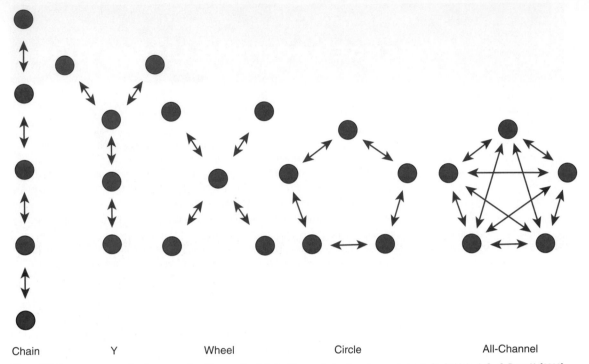

| Chain | Y | Wheel | Circle | All-Channel |

Figure 5-3 Common communication networks. (*Source:* Reprinted with permission from Longest, Jr., B. B., Rakich, J. S., & Darr, K. [2000]. *Managing Health Services Organizations and Systems* [4th ed.]. Baltimore, MD: Health Professional Press).

Upward communication is the opposite of downward communication. The idea originates at some level below the top of the structure and moves upward. For example, when a nurse recommends a more efficient approach to organizing care to his nurse manager, who takes the recommendation to her superior, who uses the recommendation to develop a new policy, that is upward communication. The Y pattern of communication shows two people reporting to another person who reports to others. An example is two staff nurses who report to the nursing unit director, who reports to the vice president for nursing, who reports to the president. The wheel pattern shows a situation in which four nurses report to one nurse manager. There is no interaction among the four nurses, and all communications are channeled through the nurse manager at the center of the wheel. This pattern is rare in health care organizations. Even though this network pattern is not used routinely, it may

be used in circumstances in which urgency or secrecy is required. For example, the president of an organization who has an emergency might communicate with the vice presidents in a wheel pattern because time does not permit using other modes.

The circle pattern allows communicators in the network to communicate directly only with two others, but since each communicates with another communicator in the network, the effect is that everyone communicates with someone, and there is no central authority or leader. The all-channel network is a circle pattern except that each communicator may interact with every other communicator in the network.

Communication networks vary along several dimensions. The most appropriate pattern depends upon the situation in which it is used. The wheel and all-channel networks tend to be fast and accurate compared with the chain or Y-pattern networks. The chain or Y patterns promote clear-cut lines of authority and responsibility. The circle and all-channel networks enhance morale among those in the networks better than other patterns, but these patterns result in relatively slow communication. This is a serious problem if an immediate decision or response is needed. Nurses must construct communication networks to fit the various communication situations they face (Shortell & Kaluzny, 2006). Note that e-mail has had the effect of flattening some organizational communications to sometimes allow more direct access between levels that were formerly controlled through middle managers.

A final avenue worth mentioning, which is not a formal avenue, is the grapevine. The **grapevine** is an informal avenue in which rumors circulate. It ignores the formal chain of command. The major benefit of the grapevine is the speed with which information is spread, but its major drawback is that it often lacks accuracy. For example, nurses who inform an oncoming shift about a rumor that layoffs or mandatory overtime is imminent in the absence of any information from the hospital's administration are participating in grapevine communication.

OVERCOMING COMMUNICATION BARRIERS

DuBrin (2000) has identified nine strategies and tactics for overcoming communication barriers. See Table 5-6.

In addition to these strategies, it is helpful to use stress management techniques to avoid communication barriers.

AVOIDING GROUPTHINK

Effective leaders work to avoid groupthink. The concept of groupthink emerged from Janis's studies of high-level policy decisions by government

CRITICAL THINKING 5-3

The Luck Factor, published in 2004, authored by R. Wiseman, discusses research that illustrates luck as something that can be learned if one pays attention to four principles:

■ Lucky people create, notice, and act on the chance opportunities in their life.

■ Lucky people make successful decisions by using their intuition and gut feeling.

■ Lucky people's expectations about the future help them fulfill their dreams and ambitions.

■ Lucky people are able to transform their bad luck into good fortune.

Do you agree with Wiseman's findings? Can you use "luck" as well as careful planning to improve your nursing career? Your life? Discuss.

leaders, including decisions about Vietnam, the Bay of Pigs, and the Korean War. Groupthink occurs when maintaining the pleasant atmosphere of the team becomes more important to members than reaching a good decision (Shortell & Kaluzny, 2006). There is a reduced willingness to disagree and challenge other's views in groupthink. Some or all of the following symptoms may indicate the presence of groupthink (Janis, 1972):

■ *The illusion of invulnerability:* Team members may reassure themselves about obvious dangers and become overly optimistic and willing to take extraordinary risks.

■ *Collective rationalization:* Teams may overlook blind spots in their plans. When confronted with conflicting information, the team may spend considerable time and energy refuting the information and rationalizing a decision.

■ *Belief in the inherent morality of the team:* Highly cohesive teams may develop a sense of self-righteousness about their role that makes them insensitive to the consequences of decisions.

TABLE 5-6	OVERCOMING COMMUNICATION BARRIERS

Concept	Application
Understand the receiver	Ask yourself, What's in it for the other person?
	Work to develop an understanding of the other person's needs.
Communicate assertively	Be direct. Use "I" statements; e.g., "I want you to . . ."
	Explain ideas clearly and with feeling.
	Repeat important messages.
	Use various communication channels; e.g., written, e-mail, and verbal.
Use two-way communication	Ask questions.
	Communicate face to face.
Unite with a common vocabulary	Define the meaning of important terms, such as high quality, so all understand their meaning.
Elicit verbal and nonverbal feedback	Request and offer verbal feedback often.
	Document important agreements.
	Observe nonverbal feedback.
Enhance listening skills	Pay attention to what is said, what is not said, and nonverbal signals.
	Continue listening carefully even when you don't like the message.
	Give summary reflections to ensure understanding; e.g., "You say you were late giving medication because the pharmacy did not deliver meds on time"
	Engage in concluding discussions; e.g., "Has your unit been late with medications due to problems with pharmacy deliveries before?"
	Ask questions to explore problems.
	Paraphrase the speaker's words to decrease miscommunication, rather than blurting out questions as soon as the other person finishes speaking.
Be sensitive to cultural differences	Know that cultural communication barriers exist.
	Show respect for all workers.
	Minimize use of jargon specific to your culture.
	Be sensitive to cultural etiquette; e.g., use of first names, eye contact, hand gestures, personal appearance.

(continues)

TABLE 5-6	OVERCOMING COMMUNICATION BARRIERS (CONTINUED)

Concept	Application
Be sensitive to gender differences	Be aware that men and women may have some differences in communication style; e.g., men may call attention to their accomplishments and women tend to be more conciliatory when facing differences.
	Know that male-female stereotypes often don't fit the person you are working with.
	Avoid barriers by knowing differences exist, and don't take things personally.
	Males can improve communication by showing more empathy, and females by becoming more direct.
Engage in metacommunication	Communicate about your communication to resolve a problem; e.g., "I'm trying to get through to you, but either you don't react to me or you get angry. What can I do to improve our communication?"

Source: Compiled with information from DuBrin, A.J. (2000). *The active manager.* London: South-Western College Publishing.

- *Stereotyping others:* Victims of groupthink hold biased, highly negative views of competing teams. They assume that they are unable to negotiate with other teams, and rule out compromise.
- *Pressures to conform:* Group members face severe pressures to conform to team norms and to team decisions. Dissent is considered abnormal and may lead to formal or informal punishment.
- *The use of mindguards:* Mindguards are used by members who withhold or discount dissonant information that interferes with the team's current view of a problem.
- *Self-censorship:* Teams subject to groupthink pressure members to remain silent about possible misgivings and to minimize self-doubts about a decision.

- *Illusion of unanimity:* A sense of unanimity emerges when members assume that silence and lack of protest signify agreement and consensus.

Shortell and Kaluzny (2006) state that the consequences of groupthink are that teams may limit themselves, often prematurely, to one possible solution and fail to conduct a comprehensive analysis of a problem. When groupthink is well entrenched, members may fail to review their decisions in light of new information or changing events. Teams may also fail to consult adequately with experts within or outside the organization, and fail to develop contingency plans in the event that the decision turns out to be wrong.

Team leaders can help avoid groupthink. First, leaders can encourage members to critically

CASE STUDY 5-1

Your nurse manager has assigned you as the new member of the task force on patient falls. This task force has been meeting for almost a year without making much progress. In coming to your first meeting, you note that there are several challenging personalities on the team and wonder if they will ever be able to work together effectively.

Jamie is a new graduate nurse and volunteers for everything. Angela likes details, often asking members to repeat what they said so that she can get more information on the topic. Samantha is the passive one and seems annoyed at having to be there. You noticed she was doing some of her patient charting while in the meeting. Anabelle attempts to keep the team on track, but with her soft-spoken voice, she is not well heard. Finally, no matter what anyone says, Beth is critical and comes up with a reason why something will not work.

Would the Myers-Briggs Type (MBTI) Indicator give you any more information about the members of this team?

Use the MBTI and have every member of the team identify his or her personal MBTI type. See the online test in the Web Exercises.

evaluate proposals and solutions. When a leader is particularly powerful and influential, yet still wants to get unbiased views from team members, the leader may refrain from stating his or her own position until later in the decision-making process. Another strategy is to assign the same problem to two separate work teams. Most importantly, groupthink can be avoided by proactively engaging in a process of critical appraisal of ideas and solutions, and by understanding the warning signs of groupthink (Shortell & Kaluzny, 2006).

KEY CONCEPTS

- Teams consist of people who come together for a common purpose and who need each other's contributions to achieve the overall goal.
- Crew Resource Management (CRM) is a method for improving team communication.
- Team members perform various roles, which may ultimately enhance or hinder the team's progress toward goal attainment.

- The MBTI helps identify personality types.
- Great teams have clearly stated purposes, goals, effective communication, an action plan, and continuously evaluate their progress toward outcomes.
- Clear communication is essential to achieving organizational goals.
- Groupthink must be avoided to ensure effective team functioning.

KEY TERMS

communication

grapevine

group process

team

REVIEW QUESTIONS

1. Based on the Tuckman and Jensen Team Process, what stage of team development consists of team members working harmoniously together, engaging in open communication, taking risks, and trusting each other to complete assigned tasks?
   A. Forming
   B. Storming
   C. Norming
   D. Performing

2. Which of the following is not a characteristic of groupthink?
   A. Use of mindguards
   B. Illusion of unanimity
   C. Free discussion of ideas
   D. Pressure to conform

3. Which of the following showed that an individual's performance is often determined in large part by the work group?
   A. Kaluzny study
   B. Dickson research
   C. Carnegie study
   D. Hawthorne experiments

4. All but which of the following are steps to improve communication using the SBARR technique?
   A. Share the situation.
   B. Provide background information.
   C. Ensure patient safety.
   D. Ask for a recommendation from the practitioner.

REVIEW ACTIVITIES

1. You are a nurse on a 38-bed medical surgical unit. In light of some vacancies, the nurse manager has hired a licensed practical nurse to fill a position in which only registered nurses had worked before.

   ■ What are some things you can do to assist the new person in becoming a member of your team?

   ■ Would nursing assignments change with the addition of the new practical nurse?

2. On the unit on which you work as a registered nurse, the team is quite interdisciplinary in nature: you directly work with licensed practical nurses, nursing assistive personnel, a secretary, one housekeeper, one respiratory therapist, one case manager, and one clinical nurse specialist.

   ■ What are some of the advantages of working with interdisciplinary teams?

   ■ What are some of the challenges of working with interdisciplinary teams?

   ■ How does one best communicate with an interdisciplinary team?

EXPLORING THE WEB

■ Search for additional information on effective team building:
www.accel-team.com

■ Check the type descriptions and online test based on Jung Myers-Briggs typology or the updated version of the Jung Typology Test:
www.humanmetrics.com

REFERENCES

Amos, M., Hu, J., & Herrick, C. A. (2005). The impact of team building on communication and job satisfaction of nursing staff. *Journal for Nurses in Staff Development, 21*(1), 10–16.

Andrews, L. B., Stocking, C. T., Krizek, T., Gottlieb, L., Krizek, C., Vargish, T., et al. (1997, Feb.). An alternative strategy for studying adverse events in medical care. *Lancet, 349,* 309–313.

Argyris, C. (1964). *Integrating the individual and the organization*. New York: Wiley.

Baggs, I. G., & Ryan, S. A. (1990). ICU nurse physician collaboration and nursing satisfaction. *Nursing Economics, 8*(6), 386–392.

Baggs, J. G., Ryan, S. A., Phelps, C. E., Richeson, J. F., & Johnson, J. E. (1992). The association between interdisciplinary collaboration and patient outcomes in a medical intensive care unit. *Heart and Lung, 21*(1), 18–24.

Bartol, K. M., & Martin, D. C. (1998). *Management* (3rd ed.). Boston: McGraw-Hill.

Bennis, W. (1989). *Why leaders can't lead*. San Francisco: Jossey-Bass.

Blanchard, K. H., & Johnson, S. (1981). The one minute manager. New York: Partnership and Candle Communications Corporation.

Briggs Myers, I., & Myers, P. B. (1995). *Gifts differing*. Palo Alto, CA: Davies-Black.

Burns, J. M. (1978). *Leadership*. New York: Harper & Row.

Calfee, B. E. (1998). Making calls to the physician. *Nursing, 98,* 10, 17.

Cardillo, D. W. (2001). *Your first year as a nurse*. Roseville, CA: Prima.

Chatman, J., & O'Reilly, C. (2004). Asymmetric effects of work group demographics on men's and women's responses to work group composition. *Academy of Management Journal, 47*(2), 193–208.

Covey, S. (1989). *The 7 habits of highly effective people*. New York: Fireside.

Deber, R. B., & Leatt, P. (1986). The multidisciplinary renal team: Who makes the decisions? *Health Matrix, 4*(3), 3–9.

DuBrin, A. J. (2000). *The active manager*. London: South-Western College Publishing.

Forni, P. (2003). *Choosing civility*. Parade Magazine. New York: St. Martin's Press.

Gabarro, J., & Kotter, J. P. (1993, May–June). Managing your boss. *Harvard Business Review*, 150–157.

Gittell, J. H., Fairfield, K. M., Bierbaum, G., Head, W., Jackson, R., Kelly, M., et al. (2000). Impact of relational coordination of quality of care, postoperative pain and functioning, and length of stay: A nine-hospital study of surgical patients. *Medical Care, 38*(8), 807–819.

Haig, K. M., Sutton, S., & Whittington, J. (2006). The SBARR Technique: Improves Communication, Enhances Patient Safety. *Joint Commission's Perspectives on Patient Safety, 5*(2), 1–2.

Hall, P., & Weaver, L. (2001). Interdisciplinary education and teamwork: A long and winding road. *Medical Education, 35,* 867–875.

Hardin, S. R., & Kaplan, R. (2005). *Synergy for Clinical Excellence, American Association of Critical Care Nurses*. Boston: Jones & Bartlett.

Hasenfeld, Y. (1983). *Human service organizations*. Englewood Cliffs, NJ: Prentice-Hall.

Heidenthal, P. (2004). Patient teaching. In P. Kelly-Heidenthal, *Essentials of Nursing Leadership & Management* (pp. 300–325). Clifton Park, NY: Delmar Cengage Learning.

Helmreich, R.L., Merritt, A.C., & Wilhelm, J.A. (1999). The evolution of Crew resource management training in commercial aviation. *The International Journal of aviation psychology. 9*(1), 19–32.

Howard, S. K., Gaba, D. M., Fish, K. J., Yang, G., & Sarnquist, F. H. (1992) Anesthesia crisis resource management training: teaching anesthesiologists to handle critical incidents. *Aviation, Space, and Environmental Medicine, 63,* 763–70.

Ihlenfeld, J. T. (2005). Hiring and mentoring graduate nurses in the intensive care unit. *Dimensions of Critical Care Nursing, 24*(4), 175–187.

Institute of Medicine (IOM). (2003). *Keeping patients safe: Transforming the work environment of nurses*. Washington, DC: The National Academies Press.

Janis, L. (1972). *Victims of groupthink*. Boston: Houghton-Mifflin.

Katzenbach, J. R., & Smith, D. K. (1993). *The wisdom of teams: Creating the high-performance organization.* New York: Harper Business.

Katzenbach, J. R., & Smith, D. K. (2003). *The wisdom of teams: Creating the high-performance organization.* New York: HarperCollins Publishers, Inc.

Knaus, W. A., Draper, E. A., Wagner, D. P., & Zimmerman, J. E. (1986). An evaluation of outcome from intensive care in major medical centers. *Annals of Internal Medicine, 104*(3), 410–418.

Lewin, K. (1951). *Field theory in social sciences.* New York: Harper & Row.

Longest, Jr., B. B., Rakich, J. S., & Darr, K. (2000). *Managing Health Services Organizations and Systems* (4th ed.). Baltimore, MD: Health Professional Press.

Longo, J. & Sherman, R.O. (2007). Leveling horizontal violence. *Nursing Management,* 2007 March ,*38*(3) 34-7, 50–1.

McGregor, D. (1960). *The human side of enterprise.* New York: McGraw-Hill.

Owens, D. A., Mannic, E. A., & Neale, M. A. (1998). Strategic formation of groups: Issues in task performance and team member selection. In D. H. Gruenfeld (Ed.), *Research on managing groups and teams* (pp. 149–165). Stamford, CT: MAI Press.

Parsons, M. (2003). From personal communication.

Pizzi, L., Goldfarb, N.I., &. Nash, D.B. (2000). Crew Resource Management and its Applications in Medicine. Available at www.ahrq.gov/clinic/ptsafety/chap44.htm.

Polifko-Harris, K. (2003). Effective team building. In P. L. Kelly, *Nursing Leadership & Management.* (2nd ed.). Clifton Park, NY: Delmar Cengage Learning.

Protecting personal health information in Research: Understanding the HIPPA Privacy Rule. NIH 03-5388. (2003). Available at privacyruleandresearch.nih.gov/pdf/HIPAA_Privacy_Rule_Booklet.pdf

Roethlisberger, F. J., & Dickson, W. J. (1939). *Management and the worker.* Cambridge, MA: Harvard University Press.

Rosenstein, A. H., Russell, H., & Lauve, R. (2002, Nov.–Dec.). Disruptive physician behavior contributes to nursing shortage. Study links bad behavior by doctors to nurses leaving the profession. *Physician Exec. 28*(6), 8–11.

Sanchez-Sweatman, L. (1996, Sept.). Communicating with physicians. *The Canadian Nurse, 92*(8), 49–50.

Senge, P. M. (1990). *The fifth discipline.* New York: Doubleday Books.

Schmitt, M. H. (2001). Collaboration improves the quality of care: Methodological challenges and evidence from health care research. *Journal of Interprofessional Care, 15,* 47–66.

Scott, W. G. (1967). *Organization theory.* Homewood, IL: Irwin.

Shortell, S. M., & Kaluzny, A. D. (2006). *Health Care Management* (5th ed.). Clifton Park, NY: Delmar Cengage Learning.

Shortell, S. M., Zimmerman, J. E., Rousseau, D. M., Gillies, R. R., Wagner, D. P., Draper, E. A., et al. (1994). The performance of intensive care units: Does good management make a difference? *Medical Care, 32*(5), 508–525.

Sirota T. (2008, July). Nursing2008 nurse/physician relationships survey report. *Nursing. 38*(7), 28–31.

Topping, S., Norton, T., & Scafidi, B. (2003). Coordination of services: The use of multidisciplinary, interagency teams. In S. Dopson & A. L. Mark (Eds.), *Leading Health Care Organizations* (pp. 100–112). New York: Palgrave Macmillan.

Tuckman, B. W., & Jensen, M. A. C. (1977). Stages of small group development revisited. *Group and Organizational Studies, 2*(4), 419–427.

Wiseman, R. (2004). The Luck Factor.

Young, G. J., Charns, M. P., Daley, J., Forbes, M. G., Henderson, W., & Khuri, S. F. (1997). Best practices for managing surgical services: The role of coordination. *Health Care Management Review, 22*(4), 72–81.

Young, G. J., Charns, M. P., Desai, K., Khuri, S. F., Forbes, M. G., Henderson, W., et al. (1998). Patterns of coordination and surgical outcomes: A study of surgical services. *Health Services Research, 33*(5).

SUGGESTED READINGS

Joint Commission. (2005). The SBARR technique: Improves communication, enhances patient safety. *Joint Commission's Perspectives on Patient Safety, 5*(2), 1–2.

Leonard, M., Graham, S., & Bonacum, D. (2004). The human factor: The critical importance of effective teamwork and communication in providing safe care. *Quality and Safety in Health Care 2004, 13,* 85–90.

Murray, T., & Kleinpell, R. (2006). Implementing a rapid response team: Factors influencing success. *Critical Care Nursing Clinics of North America, 18*(4), 493–501.

Smith, M. K. (2005). Bruce W. Tuckman—forming, storming, norming and performing in groups. *Encyclopedia of Informal Education.* Retrieved April 23, 2006, from www.infed.org/thinkers/tuckman.htm.

Williamson, S. (2006). Training the team: Talk is cheap—but vital in keeping patients safe. *Inside: Duke University Medical Center & Health System Newsletter, 15*(5).

CHAPTER
6

Change, Innovation, and Conflict

*Never doubt that a small
group of thoughtful,
committed citizens can
change the world; indeed, it's
the only thing that ever has.*

(Margaret Mead)

OBJECTIVES

Upon completion of this chapter, the reader should be able to:

1. Discuss traditional theories of change.
2. Discuss chaos theory and the concept of the learning organization.
3. Review the concept of innovation.
4. Discuss the concept of conflict.
5. Review conflict management.

Lakeisha is a new graduate. She is in her fifth week of orientation with her preceptor, Denise, and has been doing fairly well. Recently, Lakeisha disagreed privately with Denise about how to do a patient care procedure. While Lakeisha was careful to disagree in a professional manner, Denise has been acting irritated with her ever since the discussion. How can Lakeisha deal with this conflict with Denise? Is conflict ever useful?

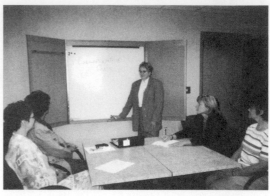

This chapter is designed to introduce the concepts of change, innovation, and conflict. The ability to change and be innovative is useful both in life and in health care situations. The ability to manage any conflict that may ensue from change and innovation requires that the nurse gain understanding of these concepts.

CHANGE

Change can be defined as "making something different from what it was" (Sullivan & Decker, 2005, p. 217). The outcome may be the same, but the actions performed to get to the outcome may be different.

There are many types of change—personal, professional, and organizational. For example, a change to new patient admission forms may necessitate a different method of assessing the patient or change the number of people involved in the admission process. Rather than one registered nurse conducting the entire admission process, the process may be broken down so that individuals with different skill levels conduct parts

of the process. The goal of the change is still the admission of the patient to a unit; how it is done may be different. Adoption of the new admission form may involve personal, professional, and organizational changes. See Table 6-1.

Individual persons, professionals, and organizations that adapt successfully to change are more likely to survive in a competitive health care environment.

TRADITIONAL CHANGE THEORIES

The change theories illustrated here are Lewin's Force-Field Model (1951), Lippitt's Phases of Change (1958), Havelock's Six-Step Change Model (1973), and Rogers' Diffusion of Innovations Theory (1995). These are classic change theories. See Table 6-2.

Lewin's model has three simple steps: unfreezing, moving to a new level, and refreezing. Unfreezing means that the current or old way of doing is thawed. People begin to be aware of the need for

TABLE 6-1	TYPES OF VOLUNTARY AND INVOLUNTARY CHANGE
Personal	A change made in one's life, often for self-improvement.
Professional	A change in one's career, such as obtaining additional academic credentials or being promoted to a new work position.
Organizational	A change in an organization to achieve organizational goals.

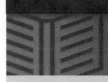

EVIDENCE FROM THE LITERATURE

Citation: Haase-Herrick, K. (2005). The Opportunities of Stewardship. *Nursing Administration Quarterly, 28*(2), 115–118.

Discussion: This article discusses goals for improving the current health care system, which were first recommended by the Institute of Medicine. These were published in *Crossing the Quality Chasm: A New Health System for the 21st Century* in 2002. The recommendations were that health care should be safe, effective, patient-centered, efficient, and equitable. Haase-Herrick challenges nurses to strive to change the status quo and health care delivery system as it currently exists. She recommends that nurses do this by increasing their knowledge level of health care economics, health care financing, and statistical and financial analysis.

Nurses are applying these strategies and are, in fact, changing the way that health care is delivered. Through the establishment of new nurse-run centers, care is being provided that is cost-effective and patient-centered. These centers are meeting the needs of many underserved populations in their respective communities. (www.nncc.us)

The author also advocates for nurses to become more actively involved in the political process in order to ensure that the most current standards of practice are applied to professional organizations, licensing, and accrediting agencies. The profession of nursing can impact the quality of care through continuous involvement in these processes.

Implications for Practice: Nurses must ask themselves, in what ways can I as a nurse become involved in the political processes that are unfreezing, moving, and re-freezing health care? Change is inevitable. Increasing one's knowledge level continuously is imperative.

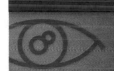

CRITICAL THINKING 6-1

LaTonya works the night shift on her unit. She is concerned that the medication carts stock high dosages of intravenous potassium chloride. LaTonya knows that high dosages of this medication are lethal. She believes that this medication should be made up by the pharmacy only on an "as needed" basis in response to a specific patient's needs. How can LaTonya work as a change agent, unfreeze the current situation, and move to a new way of preparing this medication? How can she then refreeze this needed change?

doing things differently, that change is needed for a specific reason. This change can be easy for some people and difficult for others. In the next step, moving to a new level, change is implemented. In the third step, refreezing occurs. This means that the new way of doing things is incorporated into the routines or habits of the affected people. Although these steps sound simple, the process of change is, of course, more complicated. See Figure 6-1.

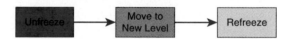

Figure 6-1 Lewin's force field model of change. (*Source:* Lewin, K. [1951] *Field theory in social science.* New York: Harper Row).

The theories described in Table 6-2 are linear in nature, meaning they more or less proceed in an orderly manner from one step to the next for example, from unfreezing to moving to a new level

TABLE 6-2	TRADITIONAL CHANGE THEORIES			
Theorist and Year	Lewin (1951)	Lippitt (1958)	Havelock (1973)	Rogers (1995)
Title of Model	Force-Field Model	Seven Phases of Change	Six-Step Change Model	Diffusion of Innovations Theory
Steps in Model	1. Unfreeze. 2. Move. 3. Refreeze.	1. Diagnose problem. 2. Assess motivation and capacity for change. 3. Assess change agent's motivation and resources. 4. Select progressive change objective. 5. Choose appropriate role of change agent. 6. Maintain change. 7. Terminate helping relationship.	1. Build relationship. 2. Diagnose problem. 3. Acquire resources. 4. Choose solution. 5. Gain acceptance. 6. Stabilize and self-renew.	1. Awareness 2. Interest 3. Evaluation 4. Trial 5. Adoption

Sources: Compiled with information from Lewin, K. (1951). *Field history in social science.* New York: Harper & Row; Lippitt, R., et al. (1958). *The dynamics of planned change.* New York: Harcourt Brace; Havelock, R. G. (1973). *The change agent's guide to innovation in education.* Englewood Cliffs, NJ: Educational Technology; Rogers, E. M. (1995). *Diffusion of Innovations* (4th ed.). New York: Free Press.

to refreezing. Unfortunately, change is not often this simple and often requires more personal, professional, and organizational change.

EMERGING CHANGE THEORIES

Two other emerging theories of change are also useful in understanding health care organizations. These theories are *Chaos theory* and *Learning Organization theory.*

CHAOS THEORY

Chaos theory hypothesizes that chaos actually has an order. That is, although the potential for chaos appears to be random at first glance, further

investigation reveals some order to the chaos. Health care organizations have repeatedly experienced chaos during the past twenty years. Chaos theory would say that this is normal. Most organizations go through periods of rapid change and innovation and then stabilize before chaos erupts again. Even though each chaotic occurrence is similar to the one that occurred before, each is different. The political, scientific, and behavioral components of the organization are different from before, so the chaos looks different. Order emerges through fluctuation and chaos. Thus, the potential for chaos means that nurses and the organization must be able to organize and implement change quickly and forcefully. There is little time for orderly linear change.

LEARNING ORGANIZATION THEORY

Peter Senge (1990) first described **learning organization theory**. Learning organizations are based on five learning disciplines and demonstrate responsiveness and flexibility. Senge believes that because organizations are open systems, they could best respond to unpredictable changes in the environment by using a learning approach in their interactions and interdisciplinary workings with one another. The whole cannot function well without a part, regardless of how small that part may seem. An example in health care is that the billing department cannot submit an accurate bill to the insurance company without the cooperation of the nursing staff. If the patient is not charged appropriately by nursing for items used in his or her care, then the billing department cannot prepare an accurate inventory. Then, the organization cannot be paid for the actual services and supplies used. The learning organization understands these interrelationships and responds quickly to improve relationships. This may be through dialogue and team problem-solving. All parties must understand what is at stake for cooperation and working together to occur. Senge, Kleiner, Roberts, Ross, and Smith (1994) emphasize that the core of the learning organization is based on five "learning disciplines"—lifelong programs of study and practice.

- Personal Mastery. Learning to expand our personal capacity to create the results we most desire, creating an organizational environment that encourages all members of the team to develop themselves toward the goals and purposes they choose.
- Mental Models. Reflecting on, continually clarifying, and improving our internal pictures of the world, and seeing how this vision shapes our actions and decisions.
- Shared Vision. Building a sense of commitment in a group by developing shared images of the future we seek to create, and developing the principles and guiding practices by which we hope to get there.
- Team Learning. Encouraging conversational and collective thinking skills, so groups of people can reliably develop intelligence and ability greater than the sum of individual members' talents.
- Systems Thinking. A way of thinking about and understanding the forces and interrelationships that shape the behavior of systems. *Systems thinking* highlights the fact that change in one area will affect other areas of the system. This discipline helps us to see how we can act more in tune with the larger processes of the natural and economic world.

In organizations, Senge believes the individuals who contribute most to the enterprise are the ones who are committed to the practice of these five learning disciplines. They are expanding their own capacity to improve and master their environment; clarify and share their vision of the world and the future they hope to create; build team learning; and understand the behavior of the systems they are helping to develop.

CHANGE PROMOTION

Bennis, Benne, and Chin (1969) identified three strategies to promote change in groups or organizations. Different strategies work in different situations. The power or authority of the change agent has an impact on the strategy selected. See Table 6-3. The **change agent** is one who is responsible for implementation of a change project. This person may be from within or outside an organization. Most change agents use a variety of approaches to promote successful change. See Table 6-4.

RESPONSE TO CHANGE

Lewin (1951) identified forces that were supportive of, as well as barriers to, change. He called these *driving* and *restraining* forces. If the restraining forces outweigh the driving forces, then the change must be abandoned because it cannot succeed. Driving and restraining forces include political issues, technology issues, cost and structural issues, and people issues. The political issues include the power groups in favor of or against the proposed change. This may include practitioners, administrators, civic and

TABLE 6-3	STRATEGIES FOR CHANGE

Strategy	Description	Example
Power-coercive approach	Used when resistance is expected but change acceptance is not important to the power group. Uses power, control, authority, and threat of job loss to gain compliance with change—"Do it or get out."	Student must achieve a passing grade in a class project to complete the course requirements satisfactorily.
Normative-reeducative approach	Uses the individual's need to have satisfactory relationships in the workplace as a method of inducing support for change. Focuses on the relationship needs of workers and stresses "going along with the majority."	A new RN who is working eight-hour shifts is encouraged by the other unit staff to embrace a new unit plan for twelve-hour staffing.
Rational-empirical approach	Uses knowledge to encourage change. Once workers understand the merits of change for the organization or understand the meaning of the change to them as individuals and the organization as a whole, they will change. Stresses training and communication. Used when little resistance is anticipated.	Staff are educated regarding the scientific merits of a needed change.

community groups, or state or federal regulators. The technology issues include whether to update old equipment, computer systems, or methods for accounting for supply use. Structural issues include the costs, desirability, and feasibility of remodeling or building new construction for the change project. People issues include the commitment of the staff, their level of education and training, and their interest in the project. The most common people issue is fear of job loss or fear of not being valued. It bears repeating that if the restraining forces outweigh the driving forces, then the change will not succeed, and it should be abandoned or rethought. See Figure 6-2.

Several factors affect staff response to change. The first is trust. Staff must trust that each member is doing the right thing and that each is capable of producing successful change. In addition to capability, predictability is important. Another factor is the individual's ability to cope with change.

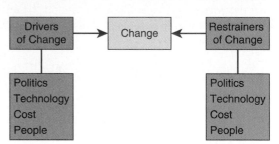

Figure 6-2 Forces driving and restraining change. (Delmar/Cengage Learning).

Silber (1993) points out four factors that affect an individual's ability to cope with change:

1. Flexibility for change; that is, the ability to adapt to change.
2. Evaluation of the immediate situation; that is, if the current situation is unacceptable, then change will be more welcome.

TABLE 6-4	CHANGE AGENT APPROACHES

1. Begin by articulating the vision clearly and concisely. Use the same words over and over. Constantly remind people of the vision.

2. Map out a tentative time line and the steps of the project. Have a good idea of how the project should go.

3. Plant seeds or mention some ideas or thoughts to key individuals from the first step through the evaluation step so that some notion of what is expected is always under consideration.

4. Make sure the committee is heavily loaded with those who will be affected by the change, and other experts as needed. Select a variety of people. For example, an innovator, someone from the late majority group, a laggard, and a rejector (Table 6-5) are probably good to include. These people provide insight into what others are thinking.

5. Set up consistent meeting dates and keep them. Have an agenda and constantly check the time line for target activities.

6. Give regular updates and progress reports, both verbally and in writing, to the executives of the organization and those affected by the change. If the change agent does not do this, someone on the project team will, and the change agent wants to control the messages.

7. Check out rumors of conflict and confront conflict head-on. Do not back away from conflict or ignore it.

8. Maintain a positive attitude and do not get discouraged.

9. Stay alert to political forces, both for and against the project. Get consensus on important issues as the project goes along, especially if policy, financial, or philosophical issues are involved. Obtain consensus quickly from both executives and staff on major issues or potential barriers to the project.

10. Know the formal and informal leaders. Create a relationship with them. Consult them often.

11. Have self-confidence and trust in oneself and one's team. This will overcome a lot of obstacles.

Source: Compiled with information from Lancaster, J. (1999). *Nursing issues in leading and managing change.* St. Louis, MO: Mosby.

3. Anticipated consequences of change; that is, the impact change will have on one's current job.

4. Individual's stake, or what the individual has to win or lose, in the change; that is, the more individuals perceive they have to lose, the more resistance they will offer.

Bushy (1992) has identified six behavioral responses to planned change. See Table 6-5.

Regardless of the importance and necessity of change, the human response is very important and cannot be dismissed. So often, in one's zeal to respond to a need, the change agent forgets that the human side of change must be dealt with. People have a right to their feelings and a right to express them. The important point is that the change agent works with people's responses and helps them move on to the goal of implementing the change.

INNOVATION

Innovation can be defined as the process of creating new services or products. Shortell & Kaluzny (2006) state that *change* and *innovation* are different. *Change* is a generic concept that refers to any modification. *Innovation* is more restricted to new modifications in

TABLE 6-5	**RESPONSES TO CHANGE**

1. Innovators: Change embracers. Enjoy the challenge of change and often lead change.

2. Early adopters: Open and receptive to change, but not obsessed with it.

3. Early majority: Enjoy and prefer the status quo, but do not want to be left behind. They adopt change before the average person.

4. Late majority: Often known as the followers. They adopt change after expressing negative feelings and are often skeptics.

5. Laggards: Last group to adopt a change. They prefer tradition and stability to innovation. They are somewhat suspicious of change.

6. Rejectors: Openly oppose and reject change. May be surreptitious or covert in their opposition. They may hinder the change process to the point of sabotage.

ideas or practices. Tom Kelly, author of *The Ten Faces of Innovation* (2005), stresses that the innovative process is now recognized as a pivotal management tool in all industries including health care. Kelly emphasizes that innovation is a team event that is made up of individuals who possess different strengths and points of view. This team approach results in new innovative ways to effectively solve problems.

An example of innovation in health care has been applied to the problem of medication errors. Injuries and death from medication errors have been identified by internal and external groups, creating pressure for change in performance. Once the medication performance gap was recognized and identified by interdisciplinary health care groups, nursing and medical practitioners, working in collaboration with pharmacists and other team members, analyzed why medication errors were occurring. Rather than blaming the person who administered the medication, an innovative "systems" approach revealed why the errors were occurring. Systems errors included illegible handwriting, unfamiliar medications, dosage calculation errors, food/drug interactions, and lack of documentation of patient allergic reactions.

By applying an innovative systems approach to problem solving, new safety structures and

health care processes were implemented and institutionalized. Health care structures and processes were developed to include a computerized medication order entry system and education of all personnel in the system. This system changed the process of how health care orders were written. Handwritten orders that were prone to interpretation errors were replaced by clear, concise, computer-generated orders. Multiple checks and balances were incorporated into the computer system that documents allergies, health care conditions, and current height and weight to assist in appropriate medication ordering and dosing. Nurses and dietitians reviewed the computerized patient information profiles for possible food/drug allergies and interactions. Pharmacists reviewed orders using this computer system before dispensing medications to analyze whether the medication dosage was indeed correct based on the patient's height and weight. Nurses review computer-generated medication administration records (MARS). Barcoding systems are now used to ensure that the right drug is being administered to the right patient at the right time. Centralized computerized charting for nurses and other health care providers now aids in the accurate and timely flow of information. Patient histories and current lab results can be assessed quickly. Nurses access a database from their portable laptop computers. This use of technology speeds the flow of information to the medical or nursing practitioner and back to the nurse caring for the patient. By improving the flow of essential information, patient safety is enhanced. Hopefully, ongoing evaluation of these innovative measures will indicate that medication errors are occurring less frequently and that patient outcomes are improving.

CONFLICT

An important part of the change process is the ability to resolve conflict. **Conflict** is a disagreement about something of importance to the people involved. Conflict resolution skills are leadership and management tools that all registered nurses should have in their repertoire. Conflict itself is not bad. Conflict can be healthy. It, like change, allows for creativity, innovation, new ideas, and new ways of doing things. It allows for the healthy discussion of different views and values and adds an important dimension to the provision of quality patient care. Without some conflict, groups or work teams tend to become stagnant and routinized. Nothing new is allowed to penetrate the "way we have always done it" mentality. Conflict can be stimulated by such things as scarce resources, invasion of personal space, safety or security issues, cultural differences, scarce nursing resources, increased workload, group competition, and various nursing demands and responsibilities.

THE CONFLICT PROCESS

In 1975, Filley suggested a process for conflict resolution that is widely accepted. In this process, there are five stages of conflict:

1. antecedent conditions,
2. perceived and/or felt conflict,
3. manifest behavior,
4. conflict resolution or suppression, and
5. resolution aftermath.

In Filley's model, conflict and conflict resolution follow a specific course. The process begins with specific preexisting conditions called *antecedent conditions*. As the situation develops, conflict is perceived or felt by the involved parties. This triggers a response or manifest behavior. The conflict is either resolved or suppressed, leading to the development of new feelings and attitudes, and may create new conflicts. Conflict resolution is vital in change. The antecedent conditions that Filley suggests may or may not be the cause of the conflict, but they certainly move the disagreement to the conflict level. The sources of these conditions include disagreement in goals, values, or resource utilization. Other issues may also serve as antecedent conditions such as the dependency of one group on another. For instance, the nursing department is dependent on the pharmacy department to provide drugs for the nursing unit in a timely fashion. The goals and priorities of pharmacy and nursing may be different

REAL WORLD INTERVIEW

Change is all about growing and developing, but the change agent or nurse manager has to be honest and truthful. Once he or she lies to us, then trust is destroyed and the change will surely fail. It's okay to not have the answer or not to be able to give the answer, but don't lie about it.

Caron Martin, RN
Staff Nurse
Highland Heights, Kentucky

at the time the nurse requests the drugs, and so a source of disagreement arises. If the circumstances for disagreement continue, a conflict will develop.

METHODS OF CONFLICT MANAGEMENT

There are essentially seven methods of conflict management. These methods dictate the outcomes of the conflict process. Although some methods are more desirable or produce more successful outcomes than others, there may be a place in conflict management

for all the methods, depending on the nature of the conflict and the desired outcomes. Table 6-6 is a summary of these methods, highlighting some of their advantages and disadvantages.

NEGOTIATION IN CONFLICT MANAGEMENT

According to Lewicki, Hiam, and Olander (1996), there are five basic approaches to negotiating in conflict management: collaborative (win-win),

TABLE 6-6	SUMMARY OF CONFLICT MANAGEMENT METHODS	
Conflict Management Method	**Advantages**	**Disadvantages**
Accommodating—smoothing or cooperating; one side gives in to the other side	One side is more concerned with an issue than the other side; stakes not high enough for one side and that side is willing to give in	One side holds more power and can force the other side to give in; the importance of the stakes are not as apparent to one side as the other; can lead to parties feeling "used" if they are always pressured to give in
Avoiding—ignoring the conflict	Does not make a big deal out of nothing; conflict may be minor in comparison to other priorities; allows tempers to cool	Conflict can become bigger than anticipated; source of conflict might be more important to one person or group than others
Collaborating—both sides work together to develop optimal outcomes	Best solution for the conflict and encompasses all important goals to each side	Takes a lot of time; requires commitment to success
Competing—the two or three sides are forced to compete for the goal	Produces a winner; good when time is short and stakes are high	Produces a loser; may leave anger and resentment on losing side
Compromising—each side gives up something and gains something	No one should win or lose, but both should gain something; good for disagreements between individuals	May cause a return to the conflict if what is given up becomes more important than the original goal
Confronting—immediate and obvious movement to stop conflict at the very start	Does not allow conflict to take root; very powerful	May leave impression that conflict is not tolerated; may make something big out of nothing
Negotiating—high-level discussion that seeks agreement, but not necessarily consensus	Stakes are very high and solution is rather permanent; often involves powerful groups	Agreements are permanent, even though each side has gains and losses

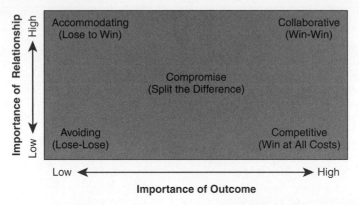

Figure 6-3 Negotiation strategies. (Delmar/Cengage Learning).

competitive (win at all costs), avoiding (lose-lose), accommodating (lose to win), and compromise (split the difference). These five approaches to negotiation are influenced by the importance of maintaining the relationships relative to the importance of achieving one's desired outcomes (Figure 6-3). Note that as the relationship's and the outcome's value increase, the amount of collaboration increases.

STRATEGIES TO FACILITATE CONFLICT MANAGEMENT

Open, honest, clear communication is the key to successful conflict management. The nurse manager/leader and all parties to the conflict must agree to communicate with one another openly and honestly. Courtesy and active listening are encouraged.

The setting for the discussions for conflict management should be private, relaxed, and comfortable. If possible, external interruptions from phones, pagers, overhead speakers, and personnel should be avoided or kept to a minimum. The setting should be on neutral territory so that no one feels overpowered. The ground rules, such as not interrupting, who should go first, time limits, and so on, should be agreed upon in the beginning. Adherence to ground rules should be expected.

In the conflict management process, it is expected that both sides in the conflict will comply with the results. If one party cannot agree to

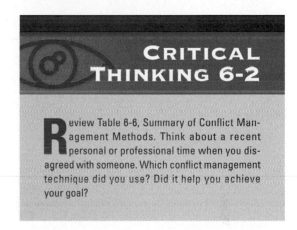

CRITICAL THINKING 6-2

Review Table 6-6, Summary of Conflict Management Methods. Think about a recent personal or professional time when you disagreed with someone. Which conflict management technique did you use? Did it help you achieve your goal?

comply with the decisions or outcomes, there is no point to the process.

CONFLICT MANAGEMENT, CHANGE, AND INNOVATION

Conflict management is an important part of the change and innovation process. Change and innovation can often threaten individuals and groups, making conflict an inevitable part of the process. It is important to keep in mind that some conflicts resolve themselves, so the change agent should not be too quick to jump into an intervention mode.

A guide for assessing conflict is identified in Figure 6-4. Figure 6-5 provides a guide for assess-

Interpersonal or intergroup?

1. **Who?**
   - Who are the primary individuals or groups involved? Characteristics (values; feelings; needs; perceptions; goals; hostility; strengths, past history of constructive conflict management; self-awareness)?
   - Who, if anyone, are the individuals or groups that have an indirect investment in the result of the conflict?
   - Who, if anyone, is assisting the parties to manage the conflict constructively?
   - What is the history of the individuals' or groups' involvement in the conflict?
   - What is the past and present interpersonal relationship between the parties involved in the conflict?
   - How is power distributed among the parties?
   - What are the major sources of power used?
   - Does the potential for coalition exist among the parties?
   - What is the nature of the current leadership affecting the conflicting parties?

2. **What?**
   - What is (are) the issues(s) in the conflict?
   - Are the issues based on facts? Based on values? Based on interests in resources?
   - Are the issues realistic?
   - What is the dominant issue in the conflict?
   - What are the goals of each conflicting party?
   - Is the current conflict functional? Dysfunctional?
   - What conflict management strategies, if any, have been used to manage the conflict to date?
   - What alternatives in managing the conflict exist?
   - What are you doing to keep the conflict going?
   - Is there a lack of stimulating work?

3. **How?**
   - What is the origin of the conflict? Sources? Precipitating events?
   - What are the major events in the evolution of the conflict?
   - How have the issues emerged? Been transformed? Proliferated?
   - What polarizations and coalitions have occurred?
   - How have parties tried to damage each other? What stereotyping exists?

4. **When/Where?**
   - When did the conflict originate?
   - Where is the conflict taking place?
   - What are the characteristics of the setting within which the conflict is occurring?
   - What are the geographic boundaries? Political structures? Decision-making patterns? Communication networks? Subsystem boundaries?
   - What environmental factors exist that influence the development of functional versus dysfunctional conflict?
   - What resource persons are available to assist in constructive conflict management?

Functional or dysfunctional?	YES	NO
Does the conflict support the goals of the organization?	[ ]	[ ]
Does the conflict contribute to the overall goals of the organization?	[ ]	[ ]
Does the conflict stimulate improved job performance?	[ ]	[ ]
Does the conflict increase productivity among work group members?	[ ]	[ ]
Does the conflict stimulate creativity and innovation?	[ ]	[ ]
Does the conflict bring about constructive change?	[ ]	[ ]
Does the conflict contribute to the survival of the organization?	[ ]	[ ]
Does the conflict improve initiative?	[ ]	[ ]
Does job satisfaction remain high?	[ ]	[ ]
Does the conflict improve the morale of the work group?	[ ]	[ ]

A yes response to the majority of the questions indicates that the conflict is probably functional. If the majority of responses are no, then the conflict is most likely a dysfunctional conflict.

Figure 6-4 Guide for the assessment of conflict. (*Source:* From MacFarland, G., Leonard, H., & Morris, M. [1984]. *Nursing Leadership and Management: contemporary strategies.* Clifton Park, NY: Delmar Cengage Learning).

Is conflict too low?	**YES**	**NO**
Is the work group consistently satisfied with the status quo?	[ ]	[ ]
Are no or few opposing views expressed by work-group members?	[ ]	[ ]
Is little concern expressed about doing things better?	[ ]	[ ]
Is little or no concern expressed about improving inadequacies?	[ ]	[ ]
Are the decisions made by the work group generally of low quality?	[ ]	[ ]
Are no or few innovative solutions or ideas expressed?	[ ]	[ ]
Are many work-group members "yes-men"?	[ ]	[ ]
Are work-group members reluctant to express ignorance or uncertainties?	[ ]	[ ]
Does the nurse manager seek to maintain peace and group cooperation regardless of whether this is the correct intervention?	[ ]	[ ]
Do the work-group members demonstrate an extremely high level of resistance to change?	[ ]	[ ]
Does the nurse manager base the distribution of rewards on "popularity" as opposed to competence and high job performance?	[ ]	[ ]
Is the nurse manager excessively concerned about not hurting the feelings of the nursing staff?	[ ]	[ ]
Is the nurse manager excessively concerned with obtaining a consensus of opinion and reaching a compromise when decisions must be made?	[ ]	[ ]

A yes response to the majority of these questions can be indicative of a too-low conflict level in a work group.

Is conflict too high?	**YES**	**NO**
Is there an upward and onward spiraling escalation of the conflict?	[ ]	[ ]
Are the conflicting parties stimulating the escalation of conflict without considering the consequences?	[ ]	[ ]
Is there a shift away from conciliation, minimizing differences, and enhancing goodwill?	[ ]	[ ]
Are the issues involved in the conflict being increasingly elaborated and expanded?	[ ]	[ ]
Are false issues being generated?	[ ]	[ ]
Are the issues vague or unclear?	[ ]	[ ]
Is job dissatisfaction increasing among work-group members?	[ ]	[ ]
Is the work-group productivity being adversely affected?	[ ]	[ ]
Is the energy being directed to activities that do not contribute to the achievement of organizational goals (e.g., destroying opposing party)?	[ ]	[ ]
Is the morale of the nursing staff being adversely affected?	[ ]	[ ]
Are extra parties getting dragged into the conflict?	[ ]	[ ]
Is a great deal of reliance on overt power manipulation noted (threats, coercion, deception)?	[ ]	[ ]
Is there a great deal of imbalance in power noted among the parties?	[ ]	[ ]
Do the individuals or groups involved in the conflict express dissatisfaction about the course of the conflict and feel that they are losing something?	[ ]	[ ]
Is absenteeism increasing among staff?	[ ]	[ ]
Is there a high rate of turnover among personnel?	[ ]	[ ]
Is communication dysfunctional, not open, mistrustful, and/or restrictive?	[ ]	[ ]
Is the focus being placed on nonconflict relevant to sensitive areas of the other party?	[ ]	[ ]

A yes response to the majority of these questions can be indicative of a conflict level in a work group that is too high.

Figure 6-5 Guide for the assessment of level of conflict. (*Source:* From MacFarland, G., Leonard, H., & Morris, M. [1984]. *Nursing Leadership and Management: contemporary strategies.* Clifton Park, NY: Delmar Cengage Learning).

CASE STUDY 6-1

James's staff was about three weeks into the latest change in care delivery when one of the staff nurses, Linda, returned from maternity leave. Linda tends to be negative about change, but she has terrific clinical skills and has often served as a preceptor for new staff. James knew that if Linda could avoid her tendency toward the negative, then not too much would happen to get the change off course. Linda's first words to James were, "Whose brilliant idea is this? I do not want to work with Kathy. She is an idiot." James smiled and said, "Welcome back, Linda. We have missed you. How's the baby? Any pictures?" What do you think James should do to help Linda adjust to the change? Should James explore Linda's feelings about Kathy? Which is more stressful for Linda, the change or working with Kathy? Should James have done something to prepare Linda for this change in her assignment to work with Kathy?

ment of the level of conflict. If the level of conflict is too high, the nurse manager must apply conflict management strategies. Change, innovation, and conflict are all positive processes that promote growth. Leaders, managers, and staff should be encouraged to embrace all three processes and explore them as opportunities for personal and professional growth.

KEY CONCEPTS

- *Change* is defined as making something different from what it was.

- Major change theorists include Lewin, Lippitt, Havelock, and Rogers.

- Senge's model of five disciplines describes the learning organization.

- The change agent is an important part of the change process. The change agent is responsible and accountable for the project.

- *Chaos theory* says that most organizations go through periods of rapid change and innovation and then stabilize before chaos erupts again.

- *Innovation* is the process of creating new services or products.

- Conflict is a normal part of any change project and is often healthy and positive.

- Conflict can move the change process along if it is handled well. Conflict can stop the change process if it is handled poorly or allowed to get out of control.

- The techniques for conflict management include avoiding, accommodating, compromising, competing, negotiating, confronting, and collaborating.

KEY TERMS

change
change agent
conflict

learning organization theory
innovation

REVIEW QUESTIONS

1. What is often the most desirable conflict management technique?
   A. Avoiding
   B. Competing
   C. Negotiating
   D. Collaborating

2. The change agent and the person responsible for conflict management have what characteristic in common?
   A. Secretive and willful
   B. Trustworthy and a good communicator
   C. Ambitious and avoiding
   D. Powerful and dictatorial

3. Select the best reason why change is necessary.
   A. To maintain the status quo
   B. To enhance the quality of health care
   C. To encourage staff turnover
   D. To increase the cost of patient care

4. Identify the theorist who first proposed the original change theory model.
   A. Rogers
   B. Havelock
   C. Lewin
   D. Lippitt

5. Identify an often unreliable form of communication on a nursing unit.
   A. The grapevine
   B. Minutes from a staff meeting
   C. A memo from the unit director
   D. A medical center newsletter

REVIEW ACTIVITIES

1. Select a change project that you have experienced in a clinical situation and discuss with your classmates how the change agent maintained momentum for the project. What approaches did the change agent use?

2. Discuss with a nurse manager how she determines whether a conflict is occurring and what steps she takes to manage it. Share the information with your classmates.

EXPLORING THE WEB

- Look up the *Journal of Conflict Resolution* and describe its purpose. Would this journal be useful to the new nurse manager? A new nurse? Anyone else in health care?
  www.jcr.sagepub.com

- Explore the following Web sites to learn more about change, conflict management, and innovation:

The International Association for Conflict Management
www.iacm-conflict.org

National League for Nursing
www.nln.org
Click on *position statement* and *Innovation in Nursing Education*.

REFERENCES

Bennis, W., Benne, K., & Chin, R. (Eds.). (1969). *The planning of change* (2nd ed.). New York: Holt, Rinehart, Winston.

Bushy, A. (1992). Managing change: Strategies for continuing education. *The Journal of Continuing Education in Nursing, 23,* 197–200.

Filley, A. C. (1975). *Interpersonal conflict resolution.* Glenview, IL: Scott Foresman.

Haase-Herrick, K. (2005). The opportunities of stewardship. *Nursing Administration Quarterly, 28*(2), 115–118.

Havelock, R. G. (1973). *The change agent's guide to innovation in education.* Englewood Cliffs, NJ: Educational Technology.

Kelly, T. (2005). *The ten faces of innovation.* New York: Doubleday.

Lancaster, J. (1999). *Nursing issues in leading and managing change.* St. Louis, MO: Mosby.

Lewicki, R. J., Hiam, A., & Olander, K. W. (1996). *Think before you speak.* New York: John Wiley & Sons.

Lewin, K. (1951). *Field theory in social science.* New York: Harper & Row.

Lippitt, R., Watson, J., & Westley, B. (1958). *The dynamics of planned change.* New York: Harcourt, Brace.

MacFarland, G., Leonard, H., & Morris, M. (1984). *Nursing Leadership and Management: contemporary strategies.* Clifton Park, NY: Delmar Cengage Learning.

Mead, M. Retrieved October 2002 from www.brainyquote.com.

Rogers, E. M. (1995). *Diffusion of Innovations* (4th ed.). New York: Free Press.

Senge, P. M. (1990). *The fifth discipline: The art and practice of the learning organization.* New York: Doubleday.

Senge, P., Kleiner, A., Roberts C., Ross, R. B., & Smith, B. (1994). *The fifth discipline fieldbook.* New York: Doubleday.

Silber, M. B. (1993, Sept.).The "C"s in excellence: Choice and change. *Nursing Management, 24*(9), 60–62.

Shortell, S. M., & Kaluzny, A. D. (2006). *Health Care Management* (5th ed.). Clifton Park, NY: Delmar Cengage Learning.

Sullivan, E. J., & Decker, P. J. (2005). *Effective leadership & management in nursing* (6th ed.). Menlo Park, CA: Addison-Wesley.

SUGGESTED READINGS

Bushy, A., & Kamphius, J. (1993, March). Response to innovation: Behavioral patterns. *Nursing Management, 24*(3), 62–64.

Begun, J., Zimmerman, B., & Dooley, K. (2006). *Health care organizations as complex adaptive systems.* Retrieved September 8, 2006, from www.change-ability.ca/ComplexAdaptive.pdf.

Gleick, J. (1987). *Chaos: Making a new science.* New York: Viking.

Kotter, J. P. (1996). *Leading change.* Boston: Harvard Business School Press.

MacGuire, J. M. (2006, Jan.). Putting nursing research findings into practice: Research utilization as an aspect of the management of change. *Journal of Advanced Nursing, 53*(1), 65–71.

Marquis, B. L., & Huston, C. J. (2006). *Leadership roles and management functions in nursing: Theory applied* (5th ed.). Philadelphia: Lippincott.

McCartney, P. (2006, Nov.–Dec.). The International Council of Nurses innovations database. *American Journal of Maternal Child Nursing, 31*(6), 389.

Position Statement, Innovation in Nursing Education (2003). NLN available at www.NLN.org.

Senge, P., Flowers, B. S., & Scharmer, C. O. (2005). *Presence: An exploration of profound change in people, organizations, and society.* New York: Doubleday.

Shortell, S., & Kaluzny, A. D. (2000). *Health care management-organization design and behavior* (4th ed.). Clifton Park, NY: Delmar Cengage Learning.

Thomas, L. M., Reynolds, T., & O'Brien, L. (2006, Sept.). Innovation and change: Shaping district nursing services to meet the needs of primary health care. *Journal of Nursing Management, 14*(6), 447–454.

Waldrop, M. M. (1992) *Complexity: The emerging science at the edge of order and chaos.* New York: Simon & Schuster.

Whitehead, D. K., Weiss, S. A., & Tappen, R. M., (4th ed.) (2007). *Essentials of Nursing Leadership and Management* (4th ed.). Philadelphia: F. A. Davis.

CHAPTER
7

Power and Politics

OBJECTIVES

Upon completion of this chapter, the reader should be able to:

1. Define the concept of power.
2. Identify various sources of power, i.e., reward and coercion, legitimacy, expertise, reference or charisma, connection, and information.
3. Discuss the role of the American Nurses Association.
4. Discuss workplace advocacy, including collective bargaining.
5. Discuss politics.

Nurse Pat, a new graduate who just finished orientation, is working with a patient for whom a surgical consult has been written. The unit clerk and a long-time nurse on the unit remark that Dr. Killian, the practitioner doing the surgical consultation, should be named Dr. Killjoy because she humiliates new nurses to try to put them in their place. Based on previous reports by other nurses on the unit, Pat knows Dr. Killian has the reputation of being demeaning and inappropriately demanding when interacting with new nurses. Two hours later, Dr. Killian appears on the unit and asks to see the nurse who did the surgical admission sheet.

What type of power does Dr. Killian illustrate?

How could Pat increase his power to improve his approach to Dr. Killian?

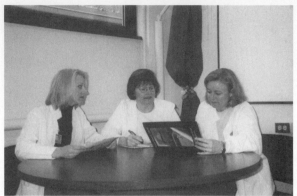

Delmar/Cengage Learning

Effective nurses are powerful. They show objectivity, creativity, and knowledge throughout their practice and regardless of their work setting. They exert power by understanding the concept of power from multiple perspectives and using this understanding to change and improve care.

This chapter discusses power and politics and how they affect patient care.

POWER

Power has been defined in multiple ways, some not so positive. Commonly, **power** is described as the ability to create, get, and use resources to achieve one's goals. If the goals are self-determined, there is an implication of even greater power than if the goals are made by or with others. Power can be seen at various levels: personal, professional, and organizational. Power, regardless of level, comes from the ability to influence others or affect others' thinking or behavior. See Table 7-1.

A person's desire for power takes one of two forms. One form is an orientation toward achieving personal gain and self-glorification. Another form is an orientation toward achieving gain for others or the common good. Orientation to personal gain and power as a bad thing and

therefore something to be avoided is reflected in a quotation from Lord Acton (Seldes, 1985, p. 234): "Power tends to corrupt, and absolute power corrupts absolutely." People having this orientation tend to believe that those wielding or afforded power ultimately should not have power because of their potential to misuse it, that people desiring power should not be trusted because their motivation for acquiring power is inherently wrong—they want power for personal gain at any cost.

The other point of view, that power is a good thing, that is, a force that is used for good purposes, is reflected in Gracian's (1892, p. 172) saying: "The sole advantage of power is that you can do more good." Nurses today are likely to see power as a positive thing and are more inclined to use this positive power to help others.

It would be naive to think that one can necessarily expect easy acceptance, understanding, or even support for one's goals when using power. Machiavelli, an early authority on power, is reported to have said:

There is nothing more difficult to take in hand, more perilous to conduct, than to take a lead in the introduction of a new order of things, because the innovation has for enemies all those who have done well under the old conditions, and lukewarm defenders in those who may do well under the new (Machiavelli & Rebhorn, 2003).

TABLE 7-1	A FRAMEWORK FOR BECOMING EMPOWERED
Personal power	Find and work with a career mentor.
	Find and maintain good sources of evidence-based information.
	Make a plan to develop all sources of personal, professional, and organizational power. Introduce yourself to power holders.
	Identify yourself to others as a professional nurse who gives evidence-based care to assure quality patient outcomes.
Professional power	Collaborate with administrators and other nursing and medical practitioners and health care workers involved in the care of your patients.
	Join your professional nursing organization.
	Monitor and improve patient care quality.
	Continue your education through conferences, certifications, formal higher education.
Organizational power	Get involved beyond direct patient care.
	Volunteer for committee assignments that will challenge you to learn and experience more than what is expected of you in a staff nurse role.
	Think about the following when involved with committees: 1. What is the committee trying to do? 2. What specific information does the committee use to operate and make decisions? 3. How does the committee apply to my practice, to my colleagues, to my patients, to my organizational unit, and to the organization as a whole?
	Readily share appropriate knowledge with others who will value it and use it to a good end.
	Continue to develop all your sources of power.
	Be involved politically with health care at the local, state, and national level.

The entry-level nurse will do well to heed Machiavelli's warning. Machiavelli recognized the fact that power should be employed thoughtfully.

SOURCES OF POWER

Most researchers agree that the sources of power are diverse and vary from one situation to another.

They also agree that these **sources of power** are a combination of conscious and unconscious factors that allow an individual to influence others to do as the individual wants (Fisher & Koch, 1996). Articles and textbooks about nursing administration, educational leadership, and organizational management commonly include references to the work of Hersey, Blanchard, and Natemeyer (1979), an expansion of the power typology originally developed by French and Raven in 1959. The typology helps nurses understand how different people perceive power and subsequently relate to others in the work setting and in attempts to achieve their goals. Power is described as having a basis in expertise, legitimacy, reference (charisma), reward and coercion, or connection. More recently, another power source—information—has been added to the typology (Wells, 1998). Generally speaking, nurses exert influence derived from one or a combination of these power sources. See Table 7-2.

TABLE 7-2	SOURCES AND EXAMPLES OF POWER	
Type	**Source**	**Examples for Nursing**
Expert	Power derived from the knowledge and skills nurses possess. The more proficiency the nurse has, the more the nurse is received as an expert.	Communicating information from current evidence-based journals and bringing expert knowledge to patient care.
Legitimate	Power derived from an academic degree, licensure, certification, experience in the role, and job title in the organization.	Wearing or displaying symbols of professional standing, including license and certification.
Referent	Power based on the trust and respect that people feel for an individual, group, or organization with which one is associated.	Gaining power by affiliating with nurses and others who have power in the organization.
Reward	Power that comes from the ability to reward others to influence them to change their behavior.	Using a hospital award to alter other's behavior.
Coercive	Power that comes from the ability to punish others to influence them to change their behavior.	Using the hospital disciplinary evaluation system to alter another's behavior.
Connection	Power that comes from personal and professional relationships that enhance one's resources and the capacity for learning and information sharing.	Developing good working relationships and mentoring with your boss and other powerful people.
Information	Power based on information that someone can provide to the group.	Sharing useful knowledge gleaned from the Internet and other sources with coworkers.

Source: Developed with information from Hersey, P., Blanchard, K. & Natemeyer, W. (1979). Situational leadership, perception and impact of power. *Group and Organizational Studies, 4*; French, J.P.R, Jr., & Raven, B. (1959). The bases of social power, in D. Cartwright and A. Zander (eds.), *Group Dynamics.* New York: Harper and Row; and Wells, S. (1998). *Choosing the future: The power of strategic thinking.* Boston: Butterworth–Heinemann.

Effective nurses use these sources of power and combine reference (charismatic) power and expert power from a legitimate power base, adding carefully measured portions of reward power and little or preferably no coercive power (Fisher & Koch, 1996). These leaders gather and use information in new and creative ways. They understand that power from all sources should be a means to accomplish a goal instead of a goal in itself.

USE OF POWER

Nursing involvement in power and politics includes using power to improve the position of patients and nurses. Nurses use their power with colleagues, administrators, and subordinates. Nurses can also use power in the legal system, their professional nursing organizations, and the media to work to improve care. Nurses must grow in their ability to work with all of these groups. Many nurses believe that it is helpful to become active participants in some formal part of the nursing profession, such as the American Nurses Association (ANA), the National League for Nursing (NLN), or one of the nursing specialty organizations. See Table 7-3.

Ultimately, health care will be defined and controlled by those wielding the most power. If nurses fail to exert political pressure on health policy makers, they will lose ground to others who are more politically active. It is unrealistic to believe that other stakeholders will take care of nursing while the competition for health care resources increases. It is not useful to complain about other nurses and members of the health care team in order to improve health care.

Nurses strengthen their power by taking ownership of their problems in serving patients. Leddy, Pepper, and Hood (2002) stated, "When nurses blame others such as physicians, administrators, or politicians for the state of the health care delivery system, or constantly look to others for improvement of this system, they weaken their position and power base [p. 331]. . . ." Historically, some stakeholders in health care have never supported nursing as a profession or acknowledged professional

roles for nurses. Nurses, like other health care providers, must stand up and compete, negotiate, and collaborate with others who lobby for health care. See Table 7-4.

POWER AND THE MEDIA

People who work in the media recognize the relationship between power and perception. Those who work in advertising, marketing, and public relations understand how media can be used to create or change perceptions. They have long recognized that the public's perception can be created or changed through advertising and marketing campaigns, damage control, timely press releases, and well-orchestrated media events.

The way the media present nursing to the public will empower or disempower nursing. Nurses must work to consistently use the media as effectively as other, more powerful, occupational groups. To date, the media have failed to recognize nursing as one of the largest and most trusted groups in health care. The media's presentation of the rapidly growing nursing shortage over the next decade can improve the public's perceptions of nursing as a career and human service. The media can show nurses as decision makers, coordinators of care, and primary care providers in health care. Too often, the media has presented a stereotypical, insignificant view of nurses (Kalisch & Kalisch, 1986). According to the Woodhull Study on Nursing and the Media (Sigma Theta Tau International, 1998), nurses are nearly invisible to the media. Sometimes, even nurses fail to view nursing as the honorable profession it is. One strategy for empowering nursing is to employ the media to create a stronger, more powerful image of nursing, for example, by writing opinion editorial (op-ed) pieces and letters to the editor for the local newspaper. Examples on a larger scale include a series of television spots promoting a positive nursing image, such as that recently sponsored by the Johnson and Johnson Corporation as part of its Campaign for Nursing's Future (Johnson & Johnson, 2006). Advocacy for nursing on a national scale requires more nurses to become active participants in some formal part of their profession, that is, the American Nurses

TABLE 7-3   NURSING ORGANIZATIONS

Organization	Web site
Academy of Medical-Surgical Nurses	www.medsurgnurse.org
Air & Surface Transport Nurses Association	www.astna.org
American Academy of Nurse Practitioners	www.aanp.org
American Academy of Ambulatory Care Nursing	www.aaacn.org
American Assembly for Men in Nursing	www.aamn.org
American Association for the History of Nursing	www.aahn.org
American Association of Colleges of Nursing	www.aacn.nche.edu
American Association of Critical-Care Nurses	www.aacn.org
American Association of Legal Nurse Consultants	www.aalnc.org
American Association of Managed Care Nurses	www.aamcn.org
American Association of Neuroscience Nurses	www.aann.org
American Association of Nurse Anesthetists	www.aana.com
American Association of Nurse Life Care Planners	www.aanlcp.org
American Association of Occupational Health Nurses	www.aaohn.org
American Association of Spinal Cord Injury Nurses	www.aascin.org
American College of Nurse-Midwives	www.acnm.org
American Forensic Nurses	www.amrn.com
American Holistic Nurses Association	www.ahna.org
American Nephrology Nurses' Association	www.annanurse.org
American Nurses Association	www.ana.org
American Nursing Informatics Association	www.ania.org
American Organization of Nurse Executives	www.aone.org
American Pediatric Surgical Nurses Association	www.apsna.org
American Psychiatric Nurses Association	www.apna.org
American Radiological Nurses Association	www.arna.net
American Society of Ophthalmic Registered Nurses	webeye.ophth.uiowa.edu
American Society of PeriAnesthesia Nurses	www.aspan.org
American Society of Plastic Surgical Nurses	www.aspsn.org
Association of Camp Nurses	www.campnurse.org
Association of Child Neurology Nurses	www.acnn.org
Association of Nurses in AIDS Care	www.anacnet.org
Association of Pediatric Gastroenterology and Nutrition Nurses	www.apgnn.org
Association of Pediatric Hematology/Oncology Nurses	www.apon.org
Association of PeriOperative Registered Nurses	www.aorn.org
Association of Rehabilitation Nurses	www.rehabnurse.org

(continues)

TABLE 7-3	NURSING ORGANIZATIONS (CONTINUED)

Organization	Web site
Association of Women's Health, Obstetric and Neonatal Nurses	www.awhonn.org
Chi Eta Phi Sorority, Inc.	www.chietaphi.com
Dermatology Nurses' Association	www.dnanurse.org
Developmental Disabilities Nurses Association	www.ddna.org
Emergency Nurses Association	www.ena.org
Family Medicine Residency Nurses Association	www.fmrna.com
Home Healthcare Nurses Association	www.hhna.org
Hospice and Palliative Nurses Association	www.hpna.org
Infusion Nurses Society	www.ins1.org
International Association of Forensic Nurses	www.iafn.org
National Organization of Nurse Practitioner Faculties	www.nonpf.com
National Association of Clinical Nurse Specialists	www.nacns.org
National Association of Hispanic Nurses	www.thehispanicnurses.org
National Association of Nurse Practitioners in Women's Health	www.npwh.org
National Association of Neonatal Nurses	www.nann.org
National Association of Orthopedic Nurses	www.orthonurse.org
National Association of Pediatric Nurse Practitioners	www.napnap.org
National Association of School Nurses	www.nasn.org
National Conference of Gerontological Nurse Practitioners	www.ncgnp.org
National Council of State Boards of Nursing	www.ncsbn.org
National Black Nurses Association	www.nbna.org
National Gerontological Nursing Association	www.ngna.org
National League for Nursing	www.nln.org
National Nursing Staff Development Organization	www.nnsdo.org
Nurses Organization of Veterans Affairs	www.vanurse.org
Oncology Nursing Society	www.ons.org
Nurses for a Healthier Tomorrow	www.nursesource.org
Pediatric Endocrinology Nursing Society	www.pens.org
Preventive Cardiovascular Nurses Association	www.pcna.net
Sigma Theta Tau International	www.nursingsociety.org
Society of Gastroenterology Nurses and Associates, Inc.	www.sgna.org
Society of Otorhinolaryngology and Head-Neck Nurses, Inc.	www.sohnnurse.com
Society of Pediatric Nurses	www.pedsnurses.org
Society of Urologic Nurses and Associates	www.suna.org
Wound, Ostomy and Continence Nurses Society	www.wocn.org

TABLE 7-4	HEALTH CARE LOBBYING GROUPS

AFL-CIO	Chamber of Commerce
America's Health Insurance Plans	Coalition to Advance Health Care Reform
American Association of Retired Persons	Health Care Equipment Companies
American Hospital Association	National Coalition on Benefits
American Medical Association	National Federation of Independent Business
American Nurses Association	Pharmaceutical Companies

Association (ANA), the National League for Nursing (NLN), or one of the nursing specialty organizations, for example, the Emergency Nurses Association.

DIMENSIONS OF NURSING

To build power, nurses must be able to clearly articulate at least four dimensions of nursing to any audience or stakeholder: what nursing is; what distinctive services nurses provide to consumers; how nursing benefits consumers, including improvement in nurse sensitive outcomes; and what nursing services cost in relation to other health care services. Although anecdotal stories and emotional appeals may be effective with certain audiences, it is far more powerful to present research-based evidence to support the political position of the nursing profession. Table 7-5 details responses to four essential dimensions of nursing.

AMERICAN NURSES ASSOCIATION

The American Nurses Association (ANA) is a full-service professional organization representing the nation's entire RN population. The ANA represents the 2.6 million RNs in the United States through its 54 constituent state and territorial associations. The ANA's mission is to work for the improvement of health standards and availability of health care services for all people, foster high standards for nursing, stimulate and promote the professional development of nurses, and advance their economic and general welfare (ANA, 2003). The National Labor Relations Board (NLRB) recognizes the ANA as a collective bargaining agent. The fact that the ANA has a dual role of being a professional organization and a collective bargaining agent causes controversy. Some nurses believe that unionization is not professional and that the ANA cannot truly support nursing as a profession if it is also a collective bargaining agent. Because nurse managers are excluded from union membership, many nurse managers believe they have been left outside the organization that is supposed to represent all of nursing. Other nurse managers do not feel this separation (Fitzpatrick, 2001).

The ANA represents the interests of nurses in collective bargaining and in many other areas as well. The ANA advances the nursing profession by fostering high standards for nursing practice and lobbies Congress and regulatory agencies on health care issues affecting nurses and the general public. The ANA initiates many policies involving health care reform. It also publishes its position on issues ranging from whistle-blowing to patients' rights. The ANA recently launched a major campaign to mobilize nurses to address the staffing crisis, to educate and gain support from the public, and to develop and implement initiatives designed to resolve

TABLE 7-5	FOUR ESSENTIAL DIMENSIONS OF NURSING

1. *Nursing* is the protection, promotion, and optimization of health and abilities, prevention of illness and injury, alleviation of suffering through the diagnosis and treatment of human response and advocacy in the care of individuals, families, communities, and populations (American Nurses Association, 2003).

2. *Distinctive services* that nurses provide focus on the response of the individual and the family to actual or potential health problems. Nurses are educated to be attuned to the whole person, not just the unique presenting health problem. While a medical diagnosis of an illness may be fairly circumscribed, the human response to a health problem may be much more fluid and variable and may have a great effect on the individual's ability to overcome the initial medical problem. It is often said that physicians cure, and nurses care. In what some describe as a blend of physiology and psychology, nurses build on their understanding of the disease and illness process to promote the restoration and maintenance of health in their clients (American Nurses Association, 2008).

3. *Benefits to consumers* include lower rates of nurse-sensitive outcomes (defined in research study as death of a patient with one of the following life-threatening complications: pneumonia, shock, cardiac arrest, urinary tract infection, gastrointestinal bleeding, sepsis, or deep vein thrombosis, and "failure to rescue") (Needleman, Buerhaus, Mattke, Stewart, & Zelevinsky, 2002).

4. *Costs of nursing services* vary according to the care setting and role of the nurse. Primary care delivered by nurse practitioners and services provided by certified nurse midwives cost less than the same care delivered by physicians (Shi & Singh, 2008).

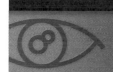

CRITICAL THINKING 7-1

As a beginning nurse, how does your nursing practice identify the four essential dimensions of nursing? How do you define nursing and how do you identify your distinctive services, benefits to consumers, and cost of your services? Does good nursing care prevent nurse-sensitive patient outcomes?

the crisis (United American Nurses, 2006). The American Nurses Credentialing Center, a subsidiary of the ANA, created the Magnet Recognition Program to recognize health care organizations that provide the very best in nursing care. Since 1994, many institutions have received this award.

WORKPLACE ADVOCACY

Workplace advocacy refers to activities nurses undertake to improve work environments and address problems in their everyday workplace settings. The American Nurses Association (ANA), with its partners and through its organizational relationships, is a leader in promoting improved work environments and the value of nurses as professionals, essential providers, and decision makers in all practice settings. The ANA protects, defends, and educates nurses about their rights as employees under the law. The ANA also addresses the growing number of occupational hazards that threaten nurses, such as needle stick injuries, latex sensitivity, back injuries, and violence. Go to: www.nursingworld.org. Click on *health care policy*. Click on *ANA position statements*. Click on *workplace advocacy*.

COLLECTIVE BARGAINING AGENTS

In collective bargaining, the group is bargaining with management for what the group desires. If the group cannot achieve its desires through informal collective bargaining with management, the group may decide to use a collective bargaining agent to form a union. In general, nurses who are content in their workplace do not unionize (Forman & Grimes, 2004). It is when nurses feel powerless that they initiate attempts to unionize. Other motivations to unionize include job stress and physical demands (Budd et al., 2004). Nurses are also motivated to join unions when they feel the need to communicate concerns and complaints to management without fear of losing their jobs. Some nurses believe that they need a collective voice so that management will hear them and changes will be instituted.

Issues that are commonly the subject of collective bargaining include poor wages, unsafe staffing, health and safety issues, mandatory overtime, poor quality of care, job security, and restructuring issues such as cross-training nurses for areas of specialty other than those in which they were hired to practice (United American Nurses, 2006).

Different organizations act as collective bargaining agents for nurses. Some of these are the Teamsters Union, the General Service Employees

REAL WORLD INTERVIEW

I graduated from a diploma nursing program in 1962. I worked for 5 years and then was home for 15 years raising my children. I wanted to return to nursing and took a refresher course. It was very hard. So much had changed. I made it, though. I think that with the shortage of nurses now, hospitals would be smart to try to make it easier for nurses who have left nursing to return by offering reasonable, supportive refresher courses. I stayed at the hospital I went back to and later retired with just short of 19 years of service. When I retired, I was shocked to find out what my pension was going to be. It was $425 a month—this after almost 19 years of service. If it wasn't for my husband's pension, who, with a high school education, gets almost 10 times what I get, I would never be able to retire. My husband worked through a union. I understand that teachers who work through unions often get 75% of their salary when they retire. Some nurses who are single or divorced would like to retire but simply can't afford to do so. You keep hearing about the poor pay for teachers, and while I agree it should be better, at least they can afford to retire. Who thinks about nurses? It seems to me that more and more of the doctors' work is being given to the nurses and yet a survey I read said that the gap between the doctors' and nurses' pay is greater than what it was at the end of World War II. New nurses should start thinking about retirement benefits when they look for their first job. I know my 40 years as a nurse went fast.

Gerri Kane, RN
Retired Staff Nurse
Cedar Lake, Indiana

Union, and the ANA. A large collective bargaining agent for nurses is the United American Nurses AFL-CIO. The United American Nurses (UAN) and its constituent member nurse associations, including state nurses associations, are a division of the ANA that serves as a collective bargaining agent. The UAN represents approximately 100,000 nurses. Another large collective bargaining agent for nurses is the National Union of Hospital and Health Care Employees. It represents 360,000 nurses and health care workers nationally. Another large collective bargaining agent for nurses is the Service Employees International Union. It represents 110,000 combined nurses and health care workers nationally. Other nursing collective bargaining agents are part of the United Autoworkers of America, the United Steelworkers of America, and the AARN (Forman & Davis, 2002). See Table 7-6 for the pros and cons of collective groups.

STRIKING

Many nurses are morally opposed to unions because they believe if they are members of a union, they may be forced to strike. In reality, a collective bargaining agent cannot make the decision to strike. The decision to strike is made only if the majority of union members decide to do so. Most nursing collective bargaining agents insert in the contract a no strike clause, stating that striking is not an option for its members. The union members decide upon the no strike clause. Provisions set forth in the 1974 Taft-Hartley Amendments to the Wagner Act guarantee the continuation of adequate patient care by requiring the union to provide contract expiration notice and advance strike notice, making mediation mandatory, and giving the hospital or agency the option of establishing a board of inquiry prior to work stoppage.

TABLE 7-6	PROS AND CONS OF COLLECTIVE GROUPS

Pros	Cons
The union contract guides standards.	There is reduced allowance for individuality.
Members are able to be a part of the decision-making process.	Other union members may outvote your decisions.
All union members and management must conform to the terms of the contract without exception.	All union members and management must conform to the terms of the contract without exception.
A process can be instituted to question a manager's authority if a member feels something was done unjustly. More people are involved in the process.	Disputes are not handled with an individual and management only; there is less room for personal judgment.
Union dues are required to make the union work for you.	Union dues must be paid even if individuals do not support unionization.
Unions give a collective voice for employees.	Employee may not agree with the collective voice.
Employees are able to voice concerns to management without fear of job security.	Unions may be perceived by some as not professional.

Scheck (2002) reports an instance where a nurses strike has had satisfying outcomes. Nurses in Minnesota had a strike for better working conditions. As a result of the strike, nurses gained the ability to refuse new patients to a unit and "close" the unit until staffing situations are addressed.

In 1995, the California Nurses Association separated from the ANA. In response to the separation of this powerful state organization, a new and quickly growing organization was created in 2000, the American Association of Registered Nurses (AARN). The AARN was created to be a collective bargaining agent for the California Nurses Association and to attract other state nurses associations to become members. Since its creation, many state nurses associations that were originally part of the ANA have switched over to the AARN. The AARN is considered to be aggressive and action oriented (Forman & Davis, 2002).

WHISTLE-BLOWING

As patient advocates, nurses protect patients from known harm. Nurses are often aware of health care fraud in the form of people violating laws or endangering public health or safety. However, some nurses who are aware of health care fraud do nothing because of fear of retribution. Fraud costs the federal government and ultimately costs the taxpayer.

Whistle-blowing is the act in which an individual discloses information regarding a violation of a law, rule, or regulation, or a substantial and specific danger to public health or safety. The government has recouped more than $2 billion since 1995 from whistle-blowers exposing fraud (Weinberg, 2005). Health care fraud can range from filing false claims to performing unnecessary procedures. As patient advocates, nurses have an ethical and moral duty to protect their patients. In 1986, the False Claims Act was modified to encourage whistle-blowers to come forward. Whistle-blowing claims are brought in *qui tam* lawsuits (Weinberg, 2005), which anyone can file on both the government's behalf and their own behalf. If the government believes an individual has a case of fraud, the government will pay all expenses for the lawsuit, and the individual will be entitled to 15% to 25% of the government's recovery. To date, over $199 million has been received by whistle-blowers (Weinberg, 2005). The name of the person filing the suit will not be divulged if the government does not consider the matter to involve health care fraud, thereby protecting the person from any retribution from the employer. The employer will not

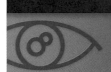

CRITICAL THINKING 7-2

You are caring for Mr. San Filipe, a 65-year-old man who was admitted for congestive heart failure. He is a retired steelworker from an area steel mill. He states, "I worked in that mill for 30 years, and I am thankful for the union. Because of the union, my medical costs are covered for the rest of my life. The union served me well. Do nurses have unions or groups that help them get what they want?"

How will you respond to Mr. San Filipe? Name two collective groups to which you belong. What are these collective groups able to get done as a whole? Are these collective groups more effective and stronger than you are as an individual in these interest areas? What are the downsides of belonging to a collective group?

know who attempted to "blow the whistle." If nurses are aware of fraud in their practice setting, the proper steps for them to take include the following:

- File a *qui tam* lawsuit in secret with the court.
- Do not let the agency or hospital know you filed a lawsuit.
- Serve a copy of the complaint to the Department of Justice with a written disclosure of all the information you have concerning the fraud.
- If the government decides to go forward with the lawsuit, the government will bear responsibility for litigating the lawsuit and will pay for it.

POLITICS

Politics is predominantly a process by which people use a variety of methods to achieve their goals. These methods inherently involve some level of competition, negotiation, and collaboration for the power to achieve desired outcomes, as well as to protect and enhance the interests of groups or individuals. Nurses who can effectively compete, negotiate, and collaborate with others to get what they want or need develop strong political skills. They have the greatest ability to build strong bases of support for themselves, patients, and the nursing profession. Nurses consistently show up as rated number one in consumer opinion polls asking who are considered to be trusted professionals. Nurses can garner consumer support for professional nursing positions to help patients and help the profession of nursing by tapping into this strong support. Nursing is important as a profession only as it meets its societal mandate for professional nursing service. Nurses must garner political support to do this most effectively.

Politics exist because resources are limited, and some people control more resources than others. Resources include people, money, facilities, technology, and rights to properties, services, and technologies. Individuals, groups, or organizations that have the ability to provide or control the distribution of desirable resources are politically empowered. The consumer movement in health care is a political movement about health care resources. It reflects consumer perceptions and values and influences patient care delivery.

CASE STUDY 7-1

You are a nurse working in a cardiac catheterization unit. You notice that a certain practitioner routinely performs cardiac catheterizations on patients who are in their early forties, have no risk factors or cardiac history, and are on Medicaid. The catheterizations are always negative for disease. You love your job, but are troubled by this practice. You are fearful that patients will have complications. You ask the practitioner why these procedures are performed on patients who do not appear to need this testing. The response is, "You don't worry about what I do; these procedures keep us all employed with healthy paychecks." You discuss this with your nursing manager and the chief nursing executive, who both say, "Just do your job and let the practitioner decide what is best for your patients."

You decide that whistle-blowing is your next action. What is your first step? Should you notify management of your whistle-blowing? What policies exist in your agency to guide the nurse when he or she encounters unprofessional activities?

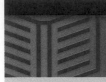

EVIDENCE FROM THE LITERATURE

Citation: McDonald, L. (2006). Florence Nightingale as a social reformer. History Today, 56(1), 9–15.

Discussion: The purpose of this historical research on the work of Florence Nightingale is to illuminate her work as a social reformer of a public health system. She advocated health promotion and disease prevention based on evidence. Ms. Nightingale extended the use of nurses that she had trained in hospitals to the care of the poor in pauper houses. She not only placed nurses in these workhouses for the poor, but she lobbied the powerful for passage of laws for the poor. She persuaded key figures to support her ideas for reform. Due to her hard work, the Metropolitan Poor Bill was passed by Parliament in 1867 and followed by other reforms that improved the lot of the poor and infirmed in Britain. Ms. Nightingale was able to obtain the support of such powerful and influential people due to her meticulous attention to detail and careful, methodical preparation. Florence Nightingale used what is now dubbed "Nightingale Methodology." First, study the best information in print, especially government reports and statistics. Second, interview experts, and if the available information is inadequate, survey others with a questionnaire. When you have a proposed plan, test it at one institution, consult with the practitioners that implemented it, and send out the draft reports for comment before sending the final report out for publication and dissemination to the influential.

Implications for Practice: New nurses often believe that their responsibilities begin and end at the bedside. But historical research demonstrates that from the very beginning of modern nursing, nurses have not only given care but partnered with others to influence public opinion and to change legislation for the benefit of the health care consumer especially the vulnerable—the poor, the mentally ill, the soldier, and children. So, as a new nurse, you may view yourself as a patient advocate who is willing to join with others through professional associations or consumer groups to improve health care and the system within which it is delivered.

STAKEHOLDERS AND HEALTH CARE

Control of health care resources is spread among a number of vested interest groups called stakeholders. Everyone is a stakeholder in health care at some level, but some people are far more politically active about their stake in health care than others. These stakeholder groups include insurance companies; consumer groups; professional organizations, such as the American Nurses Association; health care groups, such as nurses and doctors pharmacists, dieticians, physical therapists, administrators, and educational groups. These stakeholders exert political pressure on health policy makers—local, state, and federal legislative bodies—in an effort to make the health care system work to the economic advantage of the stakeholder.

NURSE AS POLITICAL ACTIVIST

Nurses are the largest health care group, and nurses who are politically active have a definitive voice in their work environments for patient welfare as well as for themselves. Nurses must set their political goals as individual nurses, nurse citizens, nurse activists, and nurse politicians for the future (Table 7-7). Nurses must study the issues, garner political support, and contact policy makers to assure quality care for patients.

TABLE 7-7	POLITICAL GOALS FOR NURSES

Role	Activities
Nurse individual	■ Highlights important role of nurse to prevent nursing-sensitive outcomes, for example, pneumonia, cardiac arrest, and so on. ■ Highlights the essential dimensions of nursing (Table 7-5). ■ Participates as a member in professional and in health care consumer groups, for example, the American Nurses Association, the American Association for Retired Persons, and so on.
Nurse citizen	■ Votes on and writes members of Congress and state legislators regarding issues of interest. ■ Educates patients on how to evaluate Web site sources of health care information.
Nurse activist	■ Lobbies and influences state and federal legislation as active member of nursing professional organization. ■ Notifies hospital Board of Trustees of any quality issues.
Nurse politician	■ Runs for a political office and serves society as a whole. ■ Collaborates with other health care professionals to improve care at the local, state, and national levels.

KEY CONCEPTS

■ Effective nurses are powerful. They show objectivity, creativity, and knowledge throughout their practice and regardless of their work setting.

■ Sources of power are reward and coercion, legitimacy, expertise, reference, information, and connection.

■ The American Nurses Association is a full-service professional organization that represents the nation's entire registered nurse population. The ANA has a dual role of being a professional organization and a collective bargaining agent for nursing. The ANA is politically active and lobbies on issues affecting nursing and the general public.

■ Politics are inherent in any system in which resources are absolutely or relatively scarce and where there are competing interests for those resources.

■ If nursing is defined through politics to be less than critical or professional, nurses will be less empowered and paid less.

KEY TERMS

connection power

expert power

information power

legitimate power

power

referent power

reward power

sources of power

workplace advocacy

REVIEW QUESTIONS

1. Suppose that, as a new nurse, you propose a change in a longstanding unit routine. You can expect:

    A. support from the head nurse.

    B. resistance from your coworkers.

    C. resistance from anyone who is comfortable with the status quo.

    D. support from your coworkers.

2. When a person fears another enough to act or behave differently than he would otherwise, the source of the other person's power is called

    A. coercive power.

    B. reward power.

    C. expert power.

    D. connection power.

3. Politics exist because of which of the following statements?

    A. They are required by law.

    B. Resources cannot be limited by political process.

    C. Some people want to control more resources than others.

    D. Resources must be equally distributed among stakeholders.

4. As a new school nurse, you become aware of some state laws that actually get in the way of providing the best care for your students. What are the best steps in becoming politically active and changing these laws? Choose all that apply.

    ____ A. Join the state school nurse organization, become active, and partner with parent groups.

    ____ B. Vote in the next election, and encourage all your friends to do so.

    ____ C. Study politics, and run for political office.

    ____ D. Write your state legislators, describe your problem, and ask them to initiate laws that will resolve the problem.

REVIEW ACTIVITIES

1. Identify a nursing leader. Observe the leader and note what type of power they use to meet objectives.

2. Sign up for the Freedom Corps at www.freedomcorps .gov. Are there any opportunities at this Web site in which you are interested?

3. Find out who your congress people are. Write or e-mail them and find out what health care legislation they are supporting at www.house.gov or www. senate.gov.

EXPLORING THE WEB

- What site would you access to find out about the history of collective bargaining?
  www.nlrb.gov

- Find two nurses identified on the following site:
  www.distinguishedwomen.com

- Identify some sites for government bodies and health care agencies.
  U.S. Congress:
  www.congress.org
  U.S. Department of Health and Human Services:
  www.hhs.gov

- Go to the site and search for *workplace advocacy*, *collective bargaining*, and your state nursing association:
  www.nursingworld.org

REFERENCES

American Nurses Association. (ANA). (2003). Nursing Social Policy Statement. Available at nursingworld. org/Books/pdescr.cfm?cnum=7#9781558102149.

American Nurses Association. (ANA). (2008). What is Nursing? Silver Spring, MD.

Budd, K., Warino, L., & Patton, M. (2004). *Traditional & nontraditional collective bargaining strategies to improve the patient care environment*. Online Journal of Issues in Nursing, (9). Retrieved from www .nursingworld.org/ojin/topic23/tpc23_5.htm (2/25/07).

Fisher, J. L., & Koch, J. V. (1996). *Presidential leadership: Making a difference*. Phoenix, AZ: American Council on Education and The Oryx Press.

Fitzpatrick, M. (2001). *Collective Bargaining Nursing Management, 32*(2), 40–42.

Forman, H., & Davis, G. (2002). The rising tide of health-care labor unions in nursing. *Journal of Nursing Administration. 32*(7/8), 376-378.

Forman, H. & Grimes, T. C. (2004). *The "new age" of union organizing*. Journal of Nursing Administration, *34*(3), 120–124.

French, J. P. R., Jr., & Raven, B. (1959). The bases of social power. In D. Cartwright and A. Zander (Eds.),

Group Dynamics (pp. 607–623). New York: Harper and Row.

Gracian, B. (1892). *The art of worldly wisdom*. (J. Jacobs, Trans.) Boston: Dover Publications, 2005. (Original work published 1647)

Hersey, P., Blanchard, K., & Natemeyer, W. (1979). Situational leadership, perception and impact of power. *Group and Organizational Studies, 4,* 418–428.

Johnson and Johnson. (2006). Campaign for nursing's future. Retrieved July 3, 2006, from www.jnj. com/our_company/advertising/discover_nursing.

Kalisch, G., & Kalisch, P. (1986). A comparative analysis of nurse and physician characters in the entertainment media. *Journal of Advanced Nursing, 11,* 179–195.

Leddy, S., Pepper, J. M. and Hood, L. (2002). *Conceptual bases of professional nursing* (5th ed.). Philadelphia: Lippincott.

Machiavelli, N., & Rebhorn, W. A. (2003). *The prince and other writings*. New Providence, NJ: Barnes & Noble.

McDonald, L. (2006). Florence Nightingale as a social reformer. *History Today, 56*(1), 9–15.

Needleman, J., Buerhaus, P., Mattke, S., Stewart, M., & Zelevinsky, K. (2002). Nurse staffing levels or the quality of care in hospitals. *New England Journal of Medicine, 346*(22).

Seldes, G. (1985). *The Great Thoughts*. New York: Ballantine Books.

Scheck, T. (2001). *The nurses' strike—one year later*. Minnesota Public radio. Retrieved Feb. 25, 2007, from news.minnesota.publicradio.org/features/20020626_scheckt_nurseupdate.

Shi, L., & Singh, D. A. (2008). *Delivering health care in America* (4th ed.). Gaithersburg, MD: Aspen.

Sigma Theta Tau International. (1998). Woodhull Study on Nursing and the Media. Retrieved September 11,

2003, from www.nursingsociety.org/media/woodhullextract.html.

United American Nurses (2006). *Nurses organize*. Retrieved from www.uannurse.org/organizeindex.html (2/25/07).

Weinberg, N. (2005, March). The dark side of whistle-blowing. *Forbes,* 90-96.

Wells, S. (1998). *Choosing the future: The power of strategic thinking*. Boston: Butterworth-Heinemann.

SUGGESTED READINGS

Armalegos, J., & Berney, J. (2005). 30 years of collective bargaining autonomy, voice in practice. *Michigan Nurse, 78*(2), 6–8.

Buerhaus, P., Donelan, K., Ulrich, B., Norman, L., Williams, M., & Dittus, R. (2005). Hospital RNs' and CNOs' perceptions of the impact of the nursing shortage on the quality of care. *Nursing Economics, 23*(5), 214–221.

Buerhaus, P., Donelan, K., Ulrich, B., Norman, L., & Dittus, R. (2005). Six part series on the state of the registered nurse workforce in the United States. *Nursing Economics, 23*(2), 58–60.

Buresh, B., & Gordon, S. (2005). *From silence to voice: What nurses know and must communicate to the public*. Cornell, NY: ILR Press.

Donelan, K., Buerhaus, P. I., Ulrich, B. T., Norman, L., & Dittus, R. (2005). Awareness and perceptions of the Johnson & Johnson campaign for nursing's future. *Nursing Economics, 23*(4), 150–156, 180.

Wiseman, R. (2003). *The luck factor.* NY: Hyperion Miramax.

CHAPTER 8

Delegation of Patient Care

The authority was delegated to me to care for this patient and, by assuming this responsibility for the patient, I will then be accountable for this patient's care.

(Phyllis Franck and Marjorie Price, 1980)

OBJECTIVES

Upon completion of this chapter, the reader should be able to:

1. Discuss concepts of delegation, authority, responsibility, accountability, supervision, assignment, and competence.
2. Utilize the National Council of State Boards of Nursing Delegation Decision–Making Tree.
3. Describe the five rights of delegation.
4. Identify delegation responsibilities of health team members.
5. Identify organizational responsibility for delegation and the chain of command.
6. Discuss transcultural delegation.

A patient was admitted to 3C with the diagnosis of transient ischemic attack (TIA). She required neurological assessments to be performed at the onset of every shift and whenever necessary as indicated by a change in her condition. The night nurse assessed the patient at the beginning of her shift, noting that the patient's neurologic status was intact. During the night, the nurse periodically checked on the patient every two hours but did not awaken the patient. A sitter was in the room with the patient. The sitter had assured the nurse that the patient was "doing fine." The sitter did not report that when the patient had been assisted to the bathroom initially, she had no difficulty. Upon assisting the patient a second time, the sitter noted that the patient was leaning to one side so badly that she could not stand and required help from two additional nursing assistive personnel. No one reported this to the nurse. When the nurse checked the patient at 6 a.m., she noted that the patient was not able to move her right side.

Should the nurse have checked the patient more carefully during the night?

What are the responsibilities of the nurse and the sitter?

How could delegation have been appropriately performed in this situation?

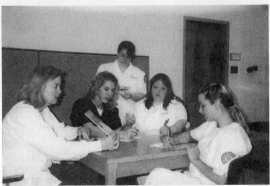

There is more nursing to do than there are nurses to do it. Many nurses are stretched to the limit in the current health care environment, with greater numbers of patients, higher acuity of patient illnesses, more technological advances, and increased complexity of therapies. The topic of nursing delegation has never been more timely. Delegation is a process that, when used appropriately, can result in safe and effective nursing care. Delegation can free the nurse to deal with more complex patient care needs, develop the skills of nursing assistive personnel (NAP), and promote cost containment for the health care organization. The RN determines appropriate nursing practice by using nursing knowledge, professional judgment, and legal authority to practice nursing. RNs must be familiar with their state's Nurse Practice Act, professional nursing standards, and agency policies and procedures related to delegation.

The Patient Safety and Quality Improvement Act of 2005 requires health care institutions to make public specified information on staffing levels, patient mix, and patient outcomes, including the number of RNs providing direct care; the numbers of unlicensed personnel utilized to provide direct patient care; the average number of patients per RN providing direct patient care; the patient mortality rate; the incidence of adverse patient care incidents; and the methods used for determining and adjusting staffing levels and patient care needs.

In addition, health care institutions have to make public their data regarding complaints filed with the state agency, the Health Care Financing Administration, or an accrediting agency related to Medicare Conditions of Participation. The agency would then have to make public the results of any investigations or finding related to the complaint. Recent studies have demonstrated a direct relationship between RN staffing levels and positive patient outcomes. These outcomes are affected by nursing delegation.

This chapter discusses the concepts of delegation, authority, responsibility, accountability, supervision, and assignment of nurses. It also describes the National Council of State Boards of Nursing Delegation Decision–Making Tree, the role of state boards of nursing in delegation, transcultural delegation, the responsibilities of health team members and the heath care organization, the five rights of delegation, and using the chain of command.

DELEGATION

Florence Nightingale is quoted as saying, "But then again to look to all these things yourself does not mean to do them yourself. . . . But can you not insure that it is done when not done by yourself?" (1859, p. 17). Nursing delegation was discussed by Nightingale in the 1800s and has continued to evolve since then. The American Nurses Association defines **delegation** as the transfer of responsibility for the performance of a task from one individual to another while retaining accountability for the outcome. (ANA, Principles for Delegation, 2006, available at www.safestaffingsaveslives.org//WhatisSafeStaffing/SafeStaffingPrinciples/PrinciplesforDelegationhtml.aspx#Definitions). In 2006, both the American Nurses Association and the National Council of State Boards of Nursing adopted papers on delegation and included them as attachments in a Joint Statement on Delegation, 2006, American Nurses Association (ANA) and the National Council of State Boards of Nursing (NCSBN), available at www.ncsbn.org/Joint_statement.pdf. The Joint Statement's two attachments are the ANA Principles of Delegation and the NCSBN Decision Tree-Delegation to Nursing Assistive Personnel.

Note that state nurse practice acts define the legal parameters for nursing practice, available at, www.ncsbn.org. Most states authorize RNs to delegate selected patient care activities. The nursing profession is responsible for determining the scope of nursing practice (Joint Statement, 2006). Competent, appropriately supervised nursing assistive personnel (NAP) are needed in the delivery of affordable, quality health care. The nursing profession defines and supervises the education, training, and utilization of nursing assistants involved in providing direct patient care.

The RN is in charge of patient care and determines the appropriate utilization of any nursing assistant involved in providing direct patient care. All decisions related to delegation are based on the fundamental principles of protection of the health, safety, and welfare of the public. A task delegated to an NAP cannot be redelegated by the NAP. When a nursing task is delegated, the task must be performed in accordance with standards of practice, policies, and procedures established by the nursing profession, the state nurse practice act, the agency, and ethical-legal standards of behavior. Standards are written and used to guide both the provision and evaluation of patient care by RNs and NAP. The nurse who delegates retains accountability for the task delegated (Delegation Concepts and Decision-Making Process, NCSBN Position Paper, 1995).

ANA AND NCSBN

Note that the ANA and NCSBN have different constituencies. The constituency of the ANA is state nursing associations and member RNs. The constituency of NCSBN is state boards of nursing and all licensed nurses. Although for the purpose of collaboration, the 2006 Joint Statement refers to registered nurse practice, NCSBN acknowledges that in many states LPN/LVNs have limited authority to delegate (Joint Statement, 2006).

ACCOUNTABILITY AND RESPONSIBILITY

Accountability is being responsible and answerable for the actions or inactions of self or others in the context of delegation (NCSBN, 1997).

Licensed nurse accountability involves compliance with legal requirements as set forth in the jurisdiction's laws and rules governing nursing. The licensed nurse is also accountable for the quality of the nursing care provided; for recognizing limits, knowledge, and experience; and for planning for situations beyond the nurse's expertise (NCSBN, 2004). Licensed nurse accountability includes the preparedness and obligation to explain or justify to relevant others (including the regulatory authority) the relevant initial and ongoing judgments, intentions, decisions, actions, and omissions . . . and their consequences. RNs are accountable for monitoring changes in a patient's status, noting and implementing treatment for human responses to illness, and assisting in the prevention of complications.

The RN assesses the patient; makes a nursing diagnosis; and develops, implements, and evaluates the patient's plan of care. The RN uses nursing judgment and monitors unstable patients with unpredictable outcomes. The monitoring of other more stable patients cared for by the LPN and NAP may involve the RN's direct continuing presence, or the monitoring may be more intermittent. As stated by the AACN in 2004, the delegation of direct and indirect patient care to other caregivers is reasonable, relevant, and practical. Nursing tasks that do not involve direct patient care can be reassigned more freely and carry fewer legal implications for RNs than delegation of direct nursing practice activities. The assessment, analysis, diagnosis, planning, teaching, and evaluation stages of the nursing process may not be delegated to NAP. Delegated activities usually fall within the implementation phase of the nursing process.

Responsibility involves reliability, dependability, and the obligation to accomplish work when an assignment is accepted. Responsibility also includes each person's obligation to perform at an acceptable level—the level to which the person has been educated. For example, a NAP is expected to provide the patient with a bed bath. She does not administer pain medication or perform invasive or sterile procedures. After the NAP performs the assigned duties, she provides feedback to the nurse about the performance of the duties and the outcome of her actions. This feedback is given to the nurse within a specified time frame. Note that feedback is provided in both directions. It is also the RN's responsibility to follow up with ongoing supervision and evaluation of activities performed by non-nursing personnel. The nurse transfers responsibility and authority for the completion of a delegated task, but the nurse retains accountability for the delegation process.

The decision of whether or not to delegate requires the RN's judgment concerning the condition of the patient; the competence, knowledge, and skill of all members of the nursing team; and the degree of supervision that will be required of the RN if a task is delegated. The RN delegates only those tasks for which she or he believes the NAP has the knowledge and skill to perform, taking into consideration training, culture, experience, and agency policies and procedures. The RN individualizes communication regarding delegation and the patient's situation to the NAP. The communication should be Clear, Concise, Correct, and Complete (Hansten and Jackson, 2008). The RN verifies comprehension with the NAP and assures that the NAP accepts the delegation. NAP are then also answerable for their actions and behavior and the responsibility that accompany them (NCSBN, 2005, Working With Others Position Paper). Communication between the RN and the NAP must be a two-way process. NAP should have the opportunity to ask questions and seek clarification of delegated tasks.

The RN must ensure that all communication is culturally appropriate and that the person receiving the communication is treated respectfully. Note that delegation involves both individual accountability and organizational accountability. It is inappropriate for employers or others to require nurses to delegate when, in the nurse's professional judgment, delegation is unsafe and not in the patient's best interest. In those instances, the nurse should act as the patient's advocate and take appropriate action to ensure provision of safe nursing care. If the nurse determines that delegation may not take place appropriately, but nevertheless delegates as directed, the nurse may be disciplined by the Board of Nursing (Delegation: Concepts and Decision-Making Process, NCSBN Position Paper, 1995). Two types of patient care activities may be delegated: direct and indirect.

CRITICAL THINKING 8-1

A major responsibility of nurses is to keep patients safe. This responsibility is tested on the NCLEX-RN. This responsibility includes not only keeping side rails up on patients who are at risk for falls, but also requires such things as monitoring patients' vital signs and level of consciousness. Maintaining safety also includes implementing safety devices such as a "keep open" IV line on patients who are at risk for poor outcomes. How have you seen nurses monitor patients? Have you noted any strategies nurses use to prevent negative nurse-sensitive patient outcomes?

DIRECT PATIENT CARE ACTIVITIES

Direct patient care activities include following standards for activities such as assisting the patient with feeding, drinking, ambulating, grooming, toileting, dressing, and socializing. Direct patient care activity may also involve following standards for collecting, reporting, and documenting data related to these activities. These data are reported to the RN, who uses the information to make a clinical judgment about patient care. Activities delegated to NAP do not include health counseling or teaching, or require independent, specialized nursing knowledge, skill, or judgment.

INDIRECT PATIENT CARE ACTIVITIES

Indirect patient care activities are necessary to support patients and their environment and only incidentally involve direct patient contact. These activities assist in providing a clean, efficient, and safe patient care milieu. They typically encompass unit routines such as chore services, companion care, and house-keeping, transporting, clerical, stocking, and maintenance tasks (ANA, 1996).

UNDERDELEGATION

Personnel in a new job role, such as new nurse managers or new nursing graduates, often underdelegate. Believing that older, more experienced staff may resent having someone new delegate to them, new nurses may simply avoid delegation. Or they may seek approval from other staff members by demonstrating their capability to complete all assigned duties without assistance. New nurses can become frustrated and overwhelmed if they fail to delegate properly. They may, for example, fail to delegate to those with certain responsibilities the appropriate authority to carry them out. Perfectionism and refusal to allow mistakes also can overwhelm new nurses. More-experienced staff members can help new personnel by intervening early on, assisting in the delegation process, and clarifying responsibilities (Table 8-1).

OVERDELEGATION

Overdelegation of duties can also be a problem. Delegating duties that are inappropriate for personnel to perform because they have been inadequately educated is dangerous and against the state nurse practice act. The reasons for overdelegation are numerous. Personnel may feel uncomfortable performing duties that are unfamiliar to them, and they may depend too much on others. They may be unorganized or inclined to either avoid responsibility or immerse themselves in trivia. Overdelegating duties can overwork some personnel and underwork others. See Table 8-2 for other obstacles to delegation.

TABLE 8-1	DELEGATION CHECKLIST		
Question		**Yes**	**No**
Do you recognize that you retain ultimate responsibility for the outcome of delegated assignments?		——	——
Do you spend most of your time completing tasks that require an RN?		——	——
Do you trust the ability of your staff to complete job assignments successfully?		——	——
Do you allow staff sufficient time to solve their own problems before interceding with advice?		——	——
			(continues)

TABLE 8-1   DELEGATION CHECKLIST (CONTINUED)

Question	Yes	No
Do you clearly outline expected outcomes and hold your staff accountable for achieving these outcomes?	____	____
Do you support your staff with an appropriate level of feedback and followup?	____	____
Do you use delegation as a way to help staff develop new skills and provide challenging work assignments?	____	____
Does your staff know what you expect of them?	____	____
Do you take the time to carefully select the right person for the right job?	____	____
Do you feel comfortable sharing control with your staff as appropriate?	____	____
Do you clearly identify all aspects of an assignment to staff when you delegate?	____	____
Do you assign tasks to the lowest level of staff capable of completing them successfully?	____	____
Do you support your staff, even when they are learning?	____	____
Do you allow your staff reasonable freedom to achieve outcomes?	____	____

Source: Compiled with information from Harvard ManageMentor® Delegating Tools. (2004). *Delegation skills checklist.* Boston: Harvard Business School Publishing.

TABLE 8-2   OBSTACLES TO DELEGATION

Fear of being disliked

Inability to give up any control of the situation

Fear of making a mistake

Inability to determine what to delegate and to whom

Inadequate knowledge of the delegation process

Past experience with delegation that did not turn out well

Poor interpersonal communication skills

Lack of confidence to move beyond being a novice nurse

Lack of administrative support for nurse delegating to LPN and NAP

Tendency to isolate oneself and choosing to complete all tasks alone

Lack of confidence to delegate to staff members who were previously one's peers

Inability to prioritize using Maslow's hierarchy of needs and the nursing process

Thinking of oneself as the only one who can complete a task the way "it is supposed" to be done

Inability to communicate effectively

Inability to develop working relationships with other team members

Lack of knowledge of the capabilities of staff, including their competency, skill, experience, level of education, job description, and so on

AUTHORITY

The right to delegate duties and give direction to nursing assistive personnel (NAP) places the RN in a position of authority. Authority identifies the source of the power to act (NCSBN, 1995). **Authority** occurs when a person who has been given the right to delegate, based on the state nurse practice act, also has the official power from an agency to delegate. Authority given by an agency legitimizes the right of a nurse to give direction to others and expect that they will comply. An understanding of the level of authority at the time the task is delegated and the level of authority that is identified by the state nurse practice act and the agency's job description prevents each party from making inaccurate assumptions about authority for delegated assignments. Note there are four possible levels of authority to be used by the RN when delegating a task to another nurse. See Table 8-3.

An understanding of the level of authority at the time the task is delegated and the level of authority that is mandated by the state nurse practice act prevents each party from making inaccurate assumptions about authority for delegated assignments.

SUPERVISION

NCSBN defines **supervision** as the provision of guidance or direction, oversight, evaluation, and follow-up by the licensed nurse for the accomplishment of a delegated nursing task by assistive personnel. The ANA defines supervision as the active process of directing, guiding, and influencing the outcome of an individual's performance of a task. Both the ANA and NCSBN define supervision as the provision of guidance and oversight of a delegated nursing task (Joint Statement on Delegation, ANA and NCSBN, 2005).

Supervision can be categorized as on-site, in which the nurse is physically present or immediately available while the activity is being performed, or off-site, in which the nurse has the ability to provide direction through various means of written, verbal, and electronic communication (ANA, 1996). On-site supervision generally occurs in the acute care setting where the RN is immediately available. Off-site supervision may occur in community settings.

As a result of the rapidly increasing use of technology in patient care, some operational guidelines for supervision from the ANA are helpful. Ask yourself, who is in control of the activity? If the RN is responsible, the nurse should incorporate measures to determine whether an activity has been completed in a way that meets expectations. Also ask yourself, how should controls be instituted? Controls must be in place that allow the RN delegating an activity to stop the task when inappropriately done, review the measures taken, and take back control of the task (ANA, 1996).

A nurse who is supervising care will provide clear direction to the staff about what tasks are to be performed for specific patients. The supervising nurse must identify when and how the task is to be done and what information must be collected, as well as any patient-specific information. The nurse must also identify what outcomes are expected and the

TABLE 8-3	LEVELS OF AUTHORITY

Level	Authority
One	Delegate to collect data to simply find out the facts or assess the situation and report back.
Two	Delegate to collect data and make a recommendation back to the RN.
Three	Delegate to assess the situation, make a recommendation, report back, and then implement the final RN recommendation.
Four	Delegate to carry out the task, as he or she believes appropriate.

time frame for reporting results. The nurse will monitor staff performance to ensure compliance with established standards of practice, policy, and procedure. The supervising nurse will obtain feedback from staff and patients and intervene, as necessary, to ensure quality nursing care and appropriate documentation.

Hansten and Washburn (2004) identify three levels of supervision based on the task delegated and the education, experience, competency, and working relationship of the people involved:

- An absence of supervision occurs when one RN works with another RN. Both are accountable for their own practice. When an RN is in a management position (for example, charge nurse, nurse manager, and so on) the RN will supervise other RNs.
- Initial direction and periodic inspection occurs when an RN supervises licensed or unlicensed staff, knows the staff's training and competency level, and has a working relationship with the staff. For example, an RN who has worked with NAP for several weeks is now comfortable giving initial directions to ambulate two new postoperative patients. The RN follows up with NAP once and as needed during the shift.
- Continuous supervision occurs when the RN determines that the delegate needs frequent-to-continuous support and assistance. This level is required when the working relationship is new, the task is complex, or the delegate is inexperienced or has not demonstrated competency.

ASSIGNMENT

Assignment is defined by both ANA and NCSBN (2005) as the distribution of work that each staff member is to accomplish on a given shift or work period. The NCSBN uses the verb "assign" to describe those situations when a nurse directs an individual to do something the individual is already authorized to do, e.g., when an RN directs another RN to assess a patient, the second RN is already authorized to assess patients in the RN scope of practice (Joint Statement, 2005). The 2003 survey by the American Organization of Nurse Executives and McCanis & Monsalve Associates, Inc., Healthy Work Environments, Volume 2, Striving for Excellence, states, "Assignments and delegation of activities of care are based on the nurse's assessment of patient needs and are congruent with the caregiver's knowledge and skill." (Available at, www.mcmanis-monsalve. com/assets/publications/healthy_work_environments_full.pdf). During a typical shift, patients range from those needing only occasional care to those requiring frequent care. The charge nurse makes out the assignment sheet taking into consideration the skill, knowledge and judgment of the RNs, LPNs, and NAP. Assignments are given to staff who have the appropriate knowledge and skill to complete the assignment. They must always be within the legal scope of practice. Assignment sheets are used to identify patient care duties for RNs, LPNs, and NAP. See Figure 8-4, later in this chapter.

COMPETENCE

Competence is the ability of the nurse to apply knowledge and interpersonal decision making, and psychomotor skills expected for the practice role of a licensed nurse in the context of public health, safety, and welfare (NCSBN, 1995). Competence is required to practice safely and ethically in a designated role and setting. Licensed nurse competence is built upon the knowledge gained in a nursing education program, orientation to specific settings, and the experiences of implementing nursing care. Nurses must know themselves first, including strengths and challenges; assess the match of their knowledge and experience with the requirements and context of a role; gain additional knowledge as needed; and maintain all skills and abilities needed to provide safe nursing care.

NAP competence is built upon formal training and assessment, orientation to specific settings and groups of patients, interpersonal and communication skills, and the experience of the nurse aide in assisting the nurse to provide safe nursing care.

Health care organizations require employees to demonstrate that they are competent to perform certain technical procedures and apply specific knowledge to safely care for patients. Written documentation of these competencies is maintained in the employee's personnel file. Most

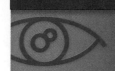

CRITICAL THINKING 8-2

Identify which members of the health care team may do each of the following nursing activities.

Nursing activity	RN	LPN	NAP
Administer blood to a patient			
Assess a patient going to surgery			
Develop a teaching plan for a newly diagnosed patient with diabetes			
Measure a patient's intake and output			
Provide a bath to an immobilized patient			
Give a dressing change to a patient			
Give patient report when transferring a patient from ICU to a step-down unit			
Give insulin			
Evaluate a patient's DNAR status			
Give an oral medication			
Assist a patient with ambulation			
Give an IM pain medication			

health care organizations require employees to undergo annual competency training for elements of care unique to their practice setting. Annual competency testing for RN, LPN, and NAP may include: patient safety, infection control, code blue, medication safety, IV skills, glucose testing, chain of command, HIPAA policies, and restraints.

DELEGATION DECISION-MAKING TREE

The National Council of State Boards of Nursing (NCSBN) has developed a Delegation Decision-Making Tree.

The steps of the Decision-Making Tree are as follows:

- Assessment of the patient, staff, and context of the situation and planning the delegation based on the patient's needs and available resources.

- Communication with the delegate to provide direction and opportunity for interaction during thae completion of the delegated task, including any unique patient requirements and characteristics as well as clear expectations regarding what to do, what to report, and when to ask for assistance.

- Surveillance, supervision, and monitoring of the delegation to ensure compliance with standards of practice, policies, and procedures. This includes the level of supervision needed for the particular situation and the implementation of that supervision, including follow-up for problems or a changing situation.

- Evaluation and feedback to consider the effectiveness of the delegation, including any need to adjust the plan of care to achieve desired patient outcomes (Figure 8-1).

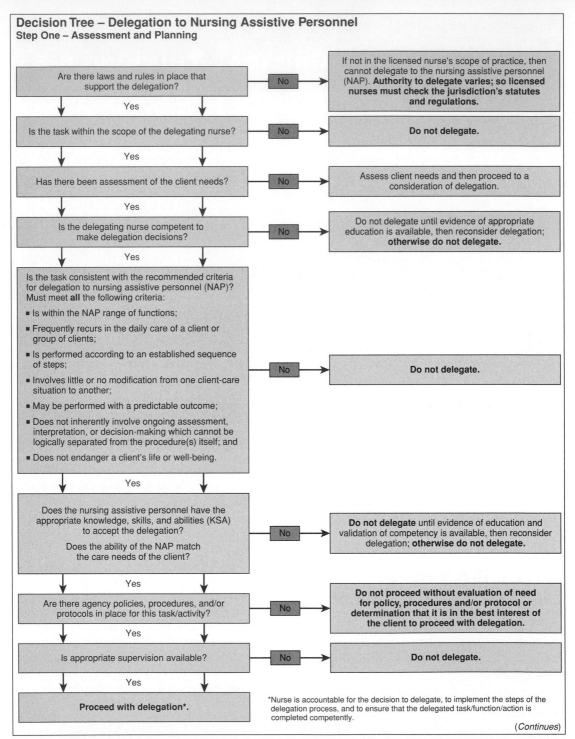

Decision Tree – Delegation to Nursing Assistive Personnel
Step One – Assessment and Planning

Are there laws and rules in place that support the delegation? — No → If not in the licensed nurse's scope of practice, then cannot delegate to the nursing assistive personnel (NAP). **Authority to delegate varies; so licensed nurses must check the jurisdiction's statutes and regulations.**

Yes ↓

Is the task within the scope of the delegating nurse? — No → **Do not delegate.**

Yes ↓

Has there been assessment of the client needs? — No → Assess client needs and then proceed to a consideration of delegation.

Yes ↓

Is the delegating nurse competent to make delegation decisions? — No → Do not delegate until evidence of appropriate education is available, then reconsider delegation; **otherwise do not delegate.**

Yes ↓

Is the task consistent with the recommended criteria for delegation to nursing assistive personnel (NAP)? Must meet **all** the following criteria:

- Is within the NAP range of functions;
- Frequently recurs in the daily care of a client or group of clients;
- Is performed according to an established sequence of steps;
- Involves little or no modification from one client-care situation to another;
- May be performed with a predictable outcome;
- Does not inherently involve ongoing assessment, interpretation, or decision-making which cannot be logically separated from the procedure(s) itself; and
- Does not endanger a client's life or well-being.

— No → **Do not delegate.**

Yes ↓

Does the nursing assistive personnel have the appropriate knowledge, skills, and abilities (KSA) to accept the delegation?

Does the ability of the NAP match the care needs of the client? — No → **Do not delegate** until evidence of education and validation of competency is available, then reconsider delegation; **otherwise do not delegate.**

Yes ↓

Are there agency policies, procedures, and/or protocols in place for this task/activity? — No → **Do not proceed without evaluation of need for policy, procedures and/or protocol or determination that it is in the best interest of the client to proceed with delegation.**

Yes ↓

Is appropriate supervision available? — No → **Do not delegate.**

Yes ↓

Proceed with delegation*.

*Nurse is accountable for the decision to delegate, to implement the steps of the delegation process, and to ensure that the delegated task/function/action is completed competently.

(*Continues*)

Figure 8-1 NCSBN delegation decision-making tree. (*Source:* Joint statement on delegation. ANA and NCSBN. [2005]. Reprinted and used by permission of the National Council of State Boards [1997]).

Decision Tree – Delegation to Nursing Assistive Personnel (Continued)

Step Two – Communication

Communication must be a two-way process.

The nurse:	The nursing assistive personnel:	Documentation:

▪ Assesses the assistant's understanding of:
  ▪ How the task is to be accomplished
  ▪ When and what information is to be reported, including:
    ▪ Expected observations to report and record
    ▪ Specific client concerns that would require prompt reporting.
▪ Individualizes for the nursing assistive personnel and client situation
▪ Addresses any unique client requirements and characteristics, and expectations
▪ Assesses the assistant's understanding of expectations, providing clarification if needed
▪ Communicates his or her willingness and availability to guide and support assistant
▪ Ensures appropriate accountability by verifying that the receiving person accepts the delegation and accompanying responsibility.
	▪ Asks questions regarding the delegation and seeks clarification of expectations if needed
	▪ Informs the nurse if the assistant has not done a task/function/activity before, or has only done it infrequently
	▪ Asks for additional training or supervision
	▪ Affirms understanding of expectations
	▪ Determines the communication method between the nurse and the assistive personnel
	▪ Determines the communication and plan of action in emergency situations.
		Timely, complete, and accurate documentation of provided care
		▪ Facilitates communication with other members of the health care team
		▪ Records the nursing care provided.

Step Three – Surveillance and Supervision

The purpose of surveillance and monitoring is related to the nurse's responsibility for client care within the context of a client population. The nurse supervises the delegation by monitoring the performance of the task or function and ensures compliance with standards of practice, policies, and procedures. Frequency, level, and nature of monitoring vary with needs of client and experience of assistant.

The nurse considers the:	The nurse determines:	The nurse is responsible for:

▪ Client's health care status and stability of condition
▪ Predictability of responses and risks
▪ Setting where care occurs
▪ Availability of resources and support infrastructure
▪ Complexity of the task being performed.
	▪ The frequency of onsite supervision and assessment based on:
	  ▪ Needs of the client
	  ▪ Complexity of the delegated function/task/activity
	  ▪ Proximity of nurse's location.
		▪ Timely intervening and follow-up on problems and concerns. Examples of the need for intervening include:
		  ▪ Alertness to subtle signs and symptoms (which allows nurse and assistant to be proactive, before a client's condition deteriorates significantly)
		  ▪ Awareness of assistant's difficulties in completing delegated activities
		  ▪ Providing adequate follow-up to problems and/or changing situations is a critical aspect of delegation.

Step Four – Evaluation and Feedback

Evaluation is often the forgotten step in delegation.

In considering the effectiveness of delegation, the nurse addresses the following questions:
- Was the delegation successful?
  - Was the task/function/activity performed correctly?
  - Was the client's desired and/or expected outcome achieved?
  - Was the outcome optimal, satisfactory, or unsatisfactory?
  - Was communication timely and effective?
  - What went well; what was challenging?
  - Were there any problems or concerns; if so, how were they addressed?
- Is there a better way to meet the client need?
- Is there a need to adjust the overall plan of care, or should this approach be continued?
- Were there any "learning moments" for the assistant and/or the nurse?
- Was appropriate feedback provided to the assistant regarding the performance of the delegation?
- Was the assistant acknowledged for accomplishing the task/activity/function?

Figure 8-1 NCSBN delegation decision-making tree. (Continued)

THE FIVE RIGHTS OF DELEGATION

The NCSBN has spelled out Five Rights of Delegation (NCSBN, 1997) that nurses may apply to their practice. These five rights are the right task, the right circumstance, the right person, the right direction and communication, and the right supervision

NCSBN, 1997. See the Web site for more information at www.ncsbn.org. See also Table 8-4.

KNOWLEDGE AND SKILL OF DELEGATION

Note that delegation is not a skill that is simply learned in a classroom. Delegation requires discussion of knowledge and concerns related to

TABLE 8-4	THE FIVE RIGHTS OF DELEGATION
Right Task	Does the delegated task confirm to agency established policies, procedures, and standards consistent with the state Nurse Practice Act, federal and state regulations and guidelines for practice, nursing professional standards, and the ANA Code of Ethics? Delegated tasks are often repetitive, require little supervision, and are relatively non-invasive.
Right Circumstance	Does the delegated task require independent nursing management? Do the personnel have the education, experience, resources, equipment, and supervision needed to complete the task safely in the current setting and circumstances?
Right Person	Is a qualified, competent person delegating the right task to a qualified, competent person to be performed on the right patient? Is the patient stable with predictable outcomes? Is it legally acceptable to delegate to this LPN or NAP? Do health care personnel have documented knowledge, skill, and competency to do the task?
Right Direction/Communication	Does the RN communicate the task clearly with standards, directions, specific steps of the tasks, any limitations, and expected outcomes? Are times for reporting back to the RN specified? Is staff understanding of the task clarified? Are staff encouraged to say "I don't know how to do this and I need help," as needed?
Right Supervision	Is there appropriate monitoring, intervention, evaluation, and patient and staff feedback as needed? Are patient and staff outcomes monitored? Does the RN answer staff questions and problem solve as needed? Does the staff report task completion and patient response to the RN? Does the RN provide follow-up teaching and guidance to staff as appropriate? Is there continuous quality improvement of the delegation process and patient care? Are problems, particularly any sentinel events, reported via the chain of command and as needed to the State Board of Nursing and the Joint Commission (JC)?

Source: Adapted from National Council of State Boards of Nursing (NCSBN). (1997). *The Five Rights of Delegation.* Retrieved from www.ncsbn.org/fiverights.pdf.

TABLE 8-5	NURSING PROCESS

Ultimately, some professional activities involving the specialized knowledge, judgment, or skill of the nursing process can never be delegated. These include patient assessment, triage, making a nursing diagnosis, establishing nursing plans of care, extensive teaching or counseling, telephone advice, evaluating outcomes, and discharging patients. Delegated tasks are typically those that occur frequently, are considered technical by nature, are considered standard and unchanging, have predictable results, and have minimal potential for risks. As a professional standard for all nurses in all states, the assessment, analysis, diagnosis, planning, teaching, and evaluation stages of the nursing process may not be delegated. Delegated activities usually fall within the implementation phase of the nursing process.

delegation, clinical mentorship or practice in responsibilities related to delegation, and discussion of how to handle situations where tasks were not accomplished when delegated. See Table 8-5.

RESPONSIBILITIES OF HEALTH TEAM MEMBERS

New graduate nurses may feel overwhelmed with their responsibilities and need to delegate patient care. The consequences and likely effects must be considered when delegating patient care. The AACN (2004) suggests assessment of five factors that must occur before deciding to delegate:

1. *Potential for Harm:* Determine if there is a risk for the patient in the activity delegated.
2. *Complexity of the Task:* Delegate simple tasks. These tasks often require psychomotor skills with little assessment or judgment proficiency.
3. *Amount of Problem Solving and Innovation Required:* Do not delegate tasks that require a creative approach, adaptation, or special attention to complete.
4. *Unpredictability of Outcome:* Avoid delegating tasks in which the outcome is not clear, causing volatility for the patient.
5. *Level of Patient Interaction:* Value time spent with the patient and the patient's family to develop trust, and so on.

Attention to these five factors will improve patient safety associated with delegation.

Other nursing staff can help new graduates begin to develop their role and learn to delegate by making sure that they introduce all the other department staff and explain their roles to the new nurses. See Figure 8-2 and Table 8-6.

NURSE MANAGER RESPONSIBILITY

The nurse manager helps develop staff members' ability to delegate. Guidance in this area is necessary because new graduates, wanting to be regarded favorably, often may try to do everything themselves and not ask for assistance. Orientation will cover staff job descriptions, competency, chain-of-command guidelines, and other delegation resources for the new nurse.

The nurse manager will determine the appropriate mix of personnel on a nursing unit based on the patients' needs, acuity levels, and staff competency. From this personnel mix, the nurse manager will identify who can best perform the direct and indirect nursing duties.

REGISTERED NURSE RESPONSIBILITY

The registered nurse is responsible and accountable for the provision of nursing care. Although nursing assistive personnel may measure vital signs, intake

Elements to Consider

- Federal, state, and local regulations and guidelines for practice, including the State Nurse Practice Act
- Nursing professional standards
- Agency policy, procedure, and standards

- Job description of Registered Nurse, Licensed Practical Nurse/Licensed Vocational Nurse, Nursing Assistive Personnel
- Five rights of delegation
- Ethical-legal standards

- Knowledge and skill of personnel
- Documented personnel competency, strengths, and weaknesses (select the right person for the right job)

RN accountable for application of the Nursing Process
Assessment and Nursing Judgment*
Nursing diagnosis
Planning care
Implementation and teaching
RN delegates as appropriate.
RN retains accountability.
Note that LPNs/LVNs and NAP are also responsible for their actions**

RN assesses, plans, implements, and evaluates care for all patients, especially complex, unstable patients with unpredictable outcomes.

Administer medications, including IV Push and IVPBs.

Start and maintain IVs and blood transfusions.

Perform sterile or specialized procedures, for example, Foley catheter and nasogastric tube insertion, tracheostomy care, and suture removal.

Educate patient and family.

Maintain infection control.

Administer cardiopulmonary resuscitation.

Interpret and report laboratory findings.

Implement patient triage.

Prevent nurse-sensitive patient outcomes, for example, cardiac arrest and pneumonia.

Monitor patient outcomes.

LPN/LVN cares for stable patients with predictable outcomes. They work under the direction of an RN and are responsible for their actions within their scope of practice.

Gather patient data.

Administer medications.

Implement patient care.

Administer CPR.

Maintain infection control.

Perform sterile procedures and respiratory suctioning.

Provide teaching from standard teaching plan.

Insert foley catheters, do colostomy care.

Depending on the state and with documented competency, may do the following:**

- Perform specialized procedures, for example, nasogastric tube insertion, tracheostomy care, and suture removal.
- Start and maintain IV therapy.

NAP assists the RN and the LPN and gives technical care to stable patients with predictable outcomes and minimal potential for risk. NAP work under the direction of an RN and are responsible for their actions within their scope of practice.

Assist with activities of daily living.

Bathe, groom, and dress.

Assist with toileting and bed making.

Perform noninvasive and nonsterile treatments.

Ambulate, position, and transport.

Feed and socialize with patient.

Measure intake and output (I&O).

Document care.

Weigh patient.

Maintain infection control.

Take vital signs.

Depending on the state and with documented competency, may do the following:**

- Perform blood glucose monitoring.
- Administer CPR.
- Perform twelve lead EKGs.
- Perform venipuncture for blood tests.

Evaluation
RN uses judgment and is responsible for evaluation of all patient care.

*Nursing Judgment is the process by which nurses come to understand the problems, issues, and concerns of patients, attend to salient information, and respond to patient problems in concerned and involved ways. Judgment includes both conscious decision making and intuitive response (Benner, Tanner, & Chesla,1996).

**Some variation from state to state and across agencies.

Figure 8-2 Considerations in delegation. (Delmar/Cengage Learning).

TABLE 8-6	**DELEGATION SUGGESTIONS FOR RNs**

- Be clear on the qualifications of the delegate, i.e., education, experience, and competency. Require documentation or demonstration of current competence by the delegate for each task. Clarify patient care concerns or delegation problems. Consult ANA position papers at www. nursingworld.org and your state board of nursing, as necessary.

- Speak to your delegate as you would like to be spoken to. There is no need to apologize for your delegation. Remember, you are carrying out your professional responsibility. Positively reinforce good attitudes and dependability in your staff.

- Communicate the patient's name, room number, and what you want done and when you want it done. Discuss any changes from the usual procedures that might be needed to meet special patient needs and any potential patient abnormalities that should be reported to you. The expectations for personnel before, during, and after duty performance should be stated in a clear, pleasant, direct, and concise manner.

- Identify realistic, attainable standards that you will use to identify completion of the task. Identify the expected patient outcome.

- Identify the authority necessary to complete the task. Include any limits on the delegate's authority also.

- Verify the delegate's understanding of delegated tasks and have him or her repeat instructions, as needed. Be clear, and welcome lots of questions until you are convinced that the delegate understands what you want done. Verify that the delegate accepts responsibility for carrying out the task correctly. Require frequent mini reports about patients from staff, and include any specific reporting guidelines, times for interventions, and deadlines for accomplishing any tasks.

- As needed, explain to the delegate why the task needs to be done, its importance in the overall scheme of things, and any possible complications that may arise during its performance. Invite questions, and don't get defensive if your delegate pushes you for answers. Seek commitment from your delegate to complete the task according to standards and in a timely fashion.

- Avoid changing standards or removing duties once performance has begun. Removing duties should be done only when the duty is above the level of the delegate, such as when the patient's well-being is in jeopardy because his or her status has changed.

- Provide support, and monitor the task completion according to standards. Make frequent walking rounds to assess patient outcomes. Be sure your delegate has the resources, training, and other help to get the task done.

- Accept minor variations in the style in which the duties are performed. Individual styles are acceptable as long as the duty is performed according to standards. Try to provide for continuity of care by the same staff when possible, and consider the geography of the unit and fair, balanced work distribution among staff when assigning care.

- If the delegate doesn't meet the standards, talk with him or her to identify the problem. If this is not successful, inform the delegate that you will be discussing the problem with your supervisor. Document your concerns, as appropriate. Follow up with your supervisor according to your organization's policy.

(continues)

TABLE 8-6	DELEGATION SUGGESTIONS FOR RNs (CONTINUED)

■ Avoid high-risk delegation. The RN may be at risk if the delegated task can be performed only by the RN according to law, organizational policies and procedures, or professional standards of nursing practice; if the delegated task could involve substantial risk or harm to a patient; if the RN knowingly delegates a task to a person who has not had the appropriate training or orientation; or if the RN fails to adequately supervise the delegated activity and does not evaluate the delegated action by reassessing the patient (ANA, 1996).

and output, and other patient status indicators, it is the registered nurse who analyzes these data for comprehensive assessment, planning, nursing diagnosis, implementation and evaluation of the plan of care. Many nurses are reluctant to delegate. This is reflected in NCSBN research findings, a review of the literature, and anecdotal accounts from nursing students and practicing nurses. Many factors contribute to this reluctance, e.g., not having had educational opportunities to learn how to work with others effectively, not knowing the skill levels and abilities of nursing assistive personnel, the fast work pace, and the rapid turnover of patients. At the same time, NCSBN research shows an increase in the complexity of the nursing tasks performed by assistive personnel. With demographic changes and the resultant increase in the need for nursing services, combined with the nursing shortage, nurses need to lean upon the support of nursing assistive personnel (Joint Statement, 2006).

LICENSED PRACTICAL/ VOCATIONAL NURSES RESPONSIBILITY

Licensed practical/vocational nursing (LPN/LVN) caregivers who have undergone a standardized training and competency evaluation are able to perform duties and functions that NAPs are not allowed to do. LPN/LVNs usually care for stable patients with predictable outcomes, though they may help the RN with seriously ill patients in ICU. The LPN does not do initial patient assessment, but after the RN has completed the patient's initial assessment

and the plan of care, the LPN does the ongoing assessment, monitoring vital signs, medication, administration, breath sounds, and so on. In nursing homes in some states, the LPN may assume the charge nurse role with an on-site supervising RN. LPNs report their findings to the RN. The RN is still primarily responsible for overall patient assessment, nursing diagnosis, planning, implementation, and evaluation of the quality of care delegated.

NAP RESPONSIBILITY

According to the ANA (2005), if the RN knows or reasonably believes that the nursing assistant has the appropriate training, orientation, and documented competencies, then the RN can reasonably expect that the NAP will function in a safe and effective manner.

NAP cannot be assigned to assess or evaluate responses to treatment because that is the role of the RN. It may be more cost-effective to have NAP perform non-nursing duties than to have nurses perform them. NAP can deliver supportive care. They cannot practice nursing or provide total patient care.

If the LPN or NAP performs poorly, the RN should tell him or her about the mistakes privately, as much as possible, in a supportive manner with a focus on learning from them. If the LPN or NAP performs in an inappropriate, unsafe, or incompetent manner, the RN must intervene immediately and stop the unsafe activity, counsel the LPN or NAP, document the facts, and report to the nurse manager, as appropriate.

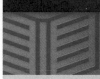

EVIDENCE FROM THE LITERATURE

Citation: Johnson, S. H. (1996). Teaching nursing delegation: Analyzing nurse practice acts. *The Journal of Continuing Education in Nursing, 27*(2), 52–58.

Discussion: This author recommends reviewing your state's nurse practice act. She notes policies common to many state nurse practice acts. These include:

- Only nursing tasks, not nursing practice, can be delegated.
- RNs must perform patient assessment to determine what can be delegated.
- LPNs and NAP do not practice professional nursing.
- RNs can delegate only what is in the scope of nursing practice.
- LPNs work under the direction/supervision of an RN.
- RNs delegate care based on the knowledge and skill of the person selected to perform the task.
- RNs determine competency of those to whom they delegate.
- RNs can't delegate activity that requires RN professional skill and knowledge.
- RNs are accountable and responsible for delegated tasks.
- RNs must evaluate patient outcomes resulting from delegated activity.
- Health care facilities can develop special delegation protocols, provided they meet State Board of Nursing delegation guidelines.
- Delegation requires critical thinking by the RN.

The author recommends looking at the following items in your state's nurse practice act to improve your understanding of delegation:

- Definition of delegation
- Items that cannot be delegated
- Items that cannot be routinely delegated
- Guidelines for RNs on what items can be delegated
- Description of professional nursing practice
- Description of LPN/LVN and unlicensed nursing assistant roles
- Degree of supervision required
- Guidelines for lowering risks of delegation
- Warning about inappropriate delegation
- Restricted use of the word "nurse" to apply only to licensed nurses

Implications for Practice: Reviewing your own state's nurse practice act can increase your knowledge and skill in using delegation appropriately. Note that many State Nursing Board's contact information, as well as information about model nurse practice acts, relisted at www.ncsbn.org.

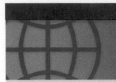

REAL WORLD INTERVIEW

I use delegation now that I have completed school. I began working as a graduate nurse immediately after graduating from nursing school. Prior to graduation, I worked as a nurse technician. I feel that I understand how it feels to be at both ends of patient care delivery. I vowed that when I became a registered nurse, I would delegate appropriately and fairly to others.

As a registered nurse, I make a point to delegate appropriately to certified nursing assistants (CNAs). I delegate duties like taking vital signs, changing beds, bathing patients, feeding patients, and performing an accurate intake and output. I delegate these things after giving my CNA a complete report on my patients.

I work on a medical-surgical floor where our CNAs use an automated DYNAMAP to take blood pressures, pulses, and temperatures. I will take my own manual blood pressure when I am assessing my patient if the readings from the DYNAMAP were high or low. My CNAs bring me the patients' vital signs as soon as they are done taking them so that I can determine what more I need to evaluate.

It is important to mention that I never delegate patient assessments or patient education. These duties are reserved for the registered nurse. I will never delegate to a CNA to watch over a patient while she takes her medication. I never delegate the insertion or removal of Foleys. I believe my CNAs take me seriously as I do not delegate anything that I am not willing to do myself and have not done myself in the past. In essence, I do not give the impression that I am "beyond" or "better" than anyone else.

I get concerned when I see a fellow nurse walk out of a patient's room who has just requested a bedpan and go to find a CNA to get him that bedpan. I would never make my patient wait for a bedpan. Like I said earlier, I have been on both ends of patient care delivery, and I know what it feels like to be unappreciated. So far, I have stuck to my promise to delegate appropriately and fairly. I truly believe my CNAs would agree.

Shelly A. Thompson
New Graduate Nurse
Dyer, Indiana

ORGANIZATIONAL ACCOUNTABILITY FOR DELEGATION

Organizational accountability for delegation includes providing sufficient resources, including sufficient staffing with an appropriate staff mix; documenting competencies for all staff providing direct patient care; ensuring that the RN has access to information regarding all staff competencies; providing opportunities for continuing staff development; creating an environment conducive to teamwork, collaboration, and patient-centered care; and developing organizational policies on delegation with the active participation of all nurses. These policies on delegation must acknowledge that delegation is a professional nursing right and responsibility. Note that Chief Nursing Officers are responsible for establishing systems to assess, monitor, verify, and communicate ongoing competence requirements in areas related to delegation, both for RNs and for other nursing staff. The organization is accountable for delegation through the allocation of resources to ensure sufficient staffing so that the RN can delegate appropriately. The organization must also ensure that the education needs of nursing assistive personnel are met through the implementation of a system that allows for nurse input. See Table 8-7.

TABLE 8-7	ORGANIZATIONAL ELEMENTS NEEDED FOR EFFICIENT DELEGATION

- Follow professional standards for education, licensure, and competency in all hiring decisions, orientation, and ongoing continuing education programs.

- Have clear job descriptions and ongoing licensing and credentialing policies for RNs, MDs, LPN/LVNs, NAP, and other health care staff. The organization must ensure that all staff members are safe, competent practitioners before assigning them to patient care. Orient staff to their duties, chain of command, and the job descriptions of RN, LPN, and NAP.

- Facilitate clinical and educational specialty certification and credentialing of all health care practitioners and staff.

- Provide standards for ongoing supervision and periodic licensure/competency verification and evaluation of all staff.

- Provide access to professional health care standards, policies, procedures, library, Internet, and medication information with unit availability and efficient library and Internet access.

- Facilitate regular evidence-based reviews of critical standards, policies, and procedures.

- Have clear policies and procedures for delegation and chain-of-command reporting lines for all staff from RN to charge nurse to nurse manager to nurse executive and, as appropriate, to risk management, the hospital ethics committee, the hospital administrator, nursing and medical practitioners, the chief of the medical staff, the board of directors, the State Licensing Board for Nursing and Medicine, and the Joint Commission. See Figure 8-3 for an illustration of one such organizational chain of command.

- Provide administrative support for supervisors and staff who delegate, assign, monitor, and evaluate patient care.

- Clarify health care provider accountability; for example, if a medical or nursing practitioner or physician assistant delegates a nursing task to NAP, the health care provider is responsible for monitoring that care delivery. This must be spelled out in hospital policy. If the RN notes

that the NAP is doing something incorrectly, the RN has a duty to intervene and to notify the ordering practitioner of the incident. The RN always has an independent responsibility to protect patient safety. Blindly relying on another nursing or health care provider is not permissible for the RN.

- Provide education and standards for regular RN evaluation of NAP and LPN/LVN, and reinforce the need for NAP and LPN/LVN accountability to the RN. RNs must delegate and supervise. They cannot abdicate this professional responsibility.

- Develop a physical, mental, and verbal "No Abuse" policy to be followed by all professional and nonprofessional health care staff. Follow up on any problems.

- Consider applying for magnet status for your facility. This status is awarded by the American Nurses Credentialing Center to nursing departments that have worked to improve nursing care, including the empowering of nursing decision making and delegation in clinical practice.

- Monitor patient outcomes, including nurse-sensitive outcomes, staffing ratios, and other quality indicators, as well as develop ongoing clinical quality improvement practices. Benchmark with national groups.

- Maintain ongoing monitoring of incident reports, sentinel events, and other elements of risk management and performance improvement of the process and outcome of patient care.

- Develop systematic, error-proof systems for medication administration that ensure the six rights of medication administration, that is, the right patient, right medication, right dose, right time, right route, and right documentation. Develop safe computerized order-entry systems.

- Provide documentation of routine maintenance for all patient care equipment.

- Attain the JC Patient Safety Goals (www. jointcommission.org).

- Develop intrahospital and intra-agency safe transfer policies.

CHAIN OF COMMAND

The RN, including the new graduate nurse, is accountable to the charge nurse and nurse manager of the unit. The nurse manager is accountable to the chief nursing executive, for example, the vice president for nursing. The chief nursing executive is accountable to the chief executive officer of the hospital, who is accountable to the board of directors. The board of directors is accountable to the community it serves and often to another larger hospital corporation, as well as to the state nursing and licensing boards and the accreditation agency. See Figure 8-3.

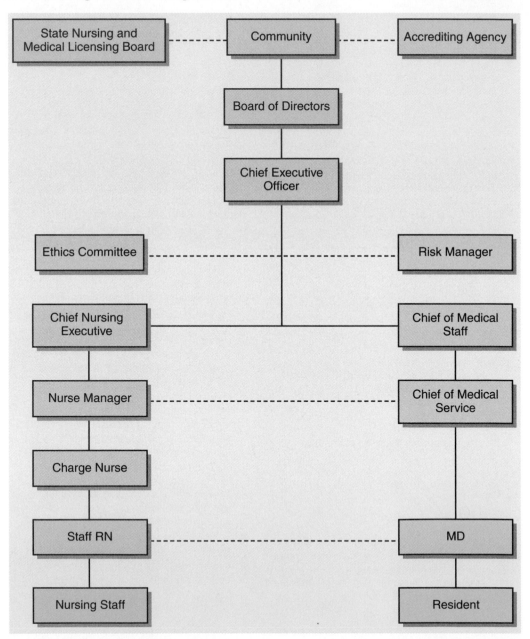

Figure 8-3 Chain of command. (Delmar/Cengage Learning).

CASE STUDY 8-1

You are working with an RN, NAP, an LPN/LVN, and a sitter. Which patient(s) from the list in Figure 8-4 would you give to each of them? Who would you have do the P.M. care for all patients, pass water, answer call lights, and pick up supplies? Who would give the medications and change dressings?

Room/Name	Patient Description	Special Needs
		Report vitals and outcomes to Mary, RN, at 8:30 P.M. Report anything abnormal STAT
2501/Ms. J. D.	68-year-old female, post-op day 1, post-shoulder repair Confused; fall risk; side rails up	Up in chair at 6 P.M. Maintain safety Vitals at 4 P.M. and 8 P.M. check distal pulses Monitor level of consciousness (LOC) Check dressings at 4 P.M. and 8 P.M. Check voiding at 6 P.M. Family at bedside
2502/Mr. D. H.	45-year-old male diabetic, post-op day 1, amputation just below the knee; Insulin sliding scale; Complaining of pain; restlessness; diaphoretic	Vitals and Accucheck STAT and at 4 P.M. and 9 P.M. Up in chair 6 P.M. Pain medication as needed Monitor dressing No pillow under stump
2503/Mr. H. M.	35-year-old male, history of alcohol abuse Complaining of abdominal pain; new hematemesis of coffee-ground fluid; IV of 0.9% normal saline at 125 cc/hour; alert	Vitals Q 15 minutes Monitor LOC, hematemesis, and possible seizures 16 gauge IV, type and crossmatch Possible transfer to ICU
2504/Mr. J. K.	20-year-old male college student, just admitted threatening to commit suicide; alert and oriented	Vitals at 4 P.M. and 8 P.M. Do not leave unattended Maintain safety

Figure 8-4 Assignment form. (Delmar/Cengage Learning).

TRANSCULTURAL DELEGATION

Nurses and patients come from diverse cultural backgrounds. Transcultural delegation requires that personnel perform duties with this cultural diversity taken into consideration. Poole, Davidhizar, and Giger (1995) suggest there are six cultural phenomena to be considered when delegating to a culturally diverse staff: communication, space, social organization, time, environmental control, and biological variations. See Table 8-8.

TABLE 8-8	CULTURAL PHENOMENA

Phenomena	Example
Communication	Consider cultural communication elements such as communication volume, dialect, use of touch, context of speech, and kinesics such as gestures, stance, and eye behavior as you delegate patient care to staff.
Space	Consider physical closeness as you delegate patient care to staff. Some cultures prefer to stand close physically while communicating. Others prefer to maintain more physical distance between themselves and others.
Social Organization	When communicating with patients, consider that cultures vary in the amount of close social supports they maintain with family and others. Note that staff also vary in the amount of social support that they need from other health care staff.
Time	Cultures vary in their past, present, or future orientation. Note that some cultures focus on maintaining past traditions, while other cultures focus on the current activities of today. Still other cultures focus on preparing for the future.
Environmental Control	Note that cultures with an internal locus of control plan and take action. They don't rely on luck or fate. Cultures with an external locus of control wait for fate and luck to determine and guide their actions.
Biological Variations	Note that there are cultural and biological variations in attributes such as physiological strength, stamina, and susceptibility to disease. Consider these as you delegate patient care to staff.

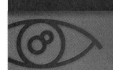

CRITICAL THINKING 8-3

Note the following selected list of values:

Mainstream American Values	Other Cultural Values
Make your own luck.	Fate and luck determine your life.
Change is good.	Like tradition.
Arrive on time.	Frequently arrive late.
Value the individual.	Value the group.
Value competition.	Value cooperation.
Set goals for the future.	Enjoy life and just let it happen.
Value directness.	Value being subtle.
Believe that all have a fairly equal chance to achieve status.	Believe that some people will always have higher status.

Which of these values do you hold? Which do members of your staff hold? How can you work to improve communication around these values and improve your working relationships?

KEY CONCEPTS

- Delegation is the transfer of responsibility for the performance of a task from one individual to another while retaining accountability for the outcome.

- Accountability is being responsible and answerable for the actions or inactions of self or others.

- Responsibility involves reliability, dependability, and the obligation to accomplish work when one accepts an assignment. Responsibility also includes each person's obligation to perform at an acceptable level to which they have been educated.

- Authority occurs when a person who has been given the right to delegate based on the state Nurse Practice Act also has the official power from an agency to delegate.

- The RN is accountable for the delegation and performance of all nursing duties.

- Transcultural delegation is encouraged to provide a patient with optimal care.

- Assignment is the distribution of work that each staff member is to accomplish on a given shift or work period. It is often identified on an assignment sheet.

- Organizations interested in quality patient care provide staff with guidelines on how to use the chain of command, clear standards, and other resources to achieve quality outcomes.

- The NCSBN Delegation Decision-Making Tree is a useful tool when developing skill in delegating patient care.

- All members of the health care team must fulfill their delegated responsibilities.

- Note that the assessment, analysis, diagnosis, planning, teaching, and evaluation stages of the nursing process may not be delegated. Delegated activities usually fall within the implementation phase of the nursing process.

- In a hospital, NAP and LPNs/LVNs are accountable to the RN.

- According to the NCSBN, supervision is the provision of guidance or direction, oversight, evaluation, and follow-up by the licensed nurse for accomplishment of a nursing task delegated to nursing assistive personnel.

- The five rights of delegation are the right task, the right circumstance, the right person, the right direction and communication, and the right supervision.

- Competence is the ability of the nurse to act with and integrate the knowledge skills, values, attitudes, abilities, and professional judgment that underpin effective and quality nursing and is required to practice safely and ethically in a designated role and setting.

KEY TERMS

accountability

assignment

authority

competence

delegation

responsibility

supervision

REVIEW QUESTIONS

1. Which of the following is an inappropriate task for an LPN/LVN?
   A. taking vital signs on a new patient
   B. completing a portable blood glucose monitor and reporting it to the RN
   C. completing a pain assessment that the NAP identified as being changed from an earlier assessment
   D. discharging the patient after teaching has been completed by the RN

2. After a patient's blood transfusion is completed, which health care personnel can obtain the vital signs? Select all that apply.
   A. RN
   B. LPN
   C. NAP
   D. new graduate nurse

3. When a nurse asks another nurse to observe his or her group of patients while the nurse is at lunch and one patient falls out of bed while the nurse is gone, which nurse is responsible?
   A. The nurse who went to lunch is responsible.
   B. The nurse who monitored the patient while the nurse went to lunch is responsible.
   C. Neither nurse is responsible.
   D. The action of both nurses should be reviewed.

4. Which patient will you delegate to the LPN?
   A. the patient who has a fleet enema ordered
   B. the patient who needs to be started on a twenty-four-hour urine collection
   C. the patient who is elderly and needs help with frequent ambulation
   D. the patient who is two days post-op and needs an abdominal wound irrigation and dressing change every shift

REVIEW ACTIVITIES

1. You are caring for a new patient in Room 2510. You are trying to decide whether to delegate his care to NAP Jill or to NAP Penny. Use the Decision Grid below to decide.

   Decision Grid

	Certified	Easy to work with?	Do their fair share?	Other?
Jill				
Penny				

2. Review the job descriptions of NAP and RNs in the institution in which you are doing your clinical rotation. Compare the job descriptions. Do the job descriptions identify what the NAP can do? What the RN can do?

EXPLORING THE WEB

- Log on and search for *Delegation Handbook*. Note what policies consider delegation of care to NAP and LPNs:
www.aacn.org

- The state of California is the first state to require all its licensed hospitals to meet fixed nurse-to-patient ratios. Log on to the California Nurses Association Web site at:
www.calnurse.org.
Click on *ratios, 2008*.

- Visit another resource for delegation information regarding whom to delegate to and what can be delegated. This site also has review questions for NCLEX covering delegation:
nclextestprep.com

REFERENCES

American Association of Critical Care Nurses (AACN). (2004). *AACN Delegation Handbook*. Aliso Viejo, CA: Author.

American Nurses Association (ANA). (1996). *Registered professional nurses and unlicensed assistive personnel*. (2nd ed.). Washington, DC: Author.

American Nurses Association (ANA). (2005). *Principles for Delegation*. Silver Spring, MD: Author.

American Nurses Association (ANA) (2006). Principles for Delegation, 2006, available at www.safestaffingsaveslives.org//WhatisSafeStaffing/SafeStaffingPrinciples/PrinciplesforDelegationhtml.aspx#Definitions).

American Nurses Association (ANA) and the National Council of State Boards of Nursing (NCSBN) (2006). Joint Statement on Delegation, 2006, available at www.ncsbn.org/Joint_statement.pdf.

American Organization of Nurse Executives and McCanis & Monsalve Associates, Inc., *Healthy Work Environments, Volume 2, Striving for Excellence*. Available at www.mcmanis-monsalve.com/assets/publications/healthy_work_environments_full.pdf.

Benner, P., Tanner, C. A., & Chesla, C. A. (1996). *Expertise in nursing practice: Caring clinical judgement and ethics*. New York City, NY: Springer Publishing Company.

Franck, P., & Price, M. (1980). *Nursing Management* (2nd ed.). NCSBN: New York.

Hansten, R. & Jackson, M. (2008). *Clinical delegation skills*. 4th ed. Jones and Bartlett Publishers.

Hansten, R. I., & Washburn, M. J. (2004). *Clinical Delegation Skills*. (3rd ed.). Boston: Jones and Bartlett.

Harvard ManageMentor® Delegating Tools, (2004). *Delegating skills checklist*. Boston: Harvard Business School Publishing.

Johnson, S. H. (1996). Teaching nursing delegation: Analyzing nurse practice acts. *The Journal of Continuing Education in Nursing, 27*(2), 52–58.

Joint statement on delegation. ANA and NCSBN. (2005). National council of state boards of nursing decision tree for delegation to nursing assistive personnel. Available at www.abn.alabama.gov/main/news/Joint_statement.pdf

National Council of State Boards of Nursing (NCSBN). (1995). Delegation Concepts and Decision-Making Process., NCSBN Position Paper. Available at www.ncsbn.org/323.htm#Delegation_Decision-Making_Process

National Council of State Boards of Nursing (NCSBN). (1997). The five rights of delegation. Retrieved from www.ncsbn.org/fiverights.pdf.

National Council of State Boards of Nursing (NCSBN). (2004). Working with others: *NCLEX-RN Test Plan. A Position paper.* Chicago: Author.

National Council of State Boards of Nursing (NCSBN). (2005). *Working with Others: Delegation and Other Health Care Interfaces.* Chicago.

Nightingale, F. (1859). *Notes on nursing: What it is and what it is not.* London: Harrison & Sons.

Poole, V., Davidhizar, R., & Giger, J. (1995). Delegating to a transcultural team. *Nursing-Management, 26*(8), 33–34.

SUGGESTED READINGS

American Nurses Association (ANA). (2004). *Nursing: Scope and standards of practice.* Washington, DC: Author.

Cohen, S. (2004). Delegating vs. dumping: Teach the difference. *Nursing Management, 35*(10), 14–15.

Hanston, R. I. (2005), Relationship and results-oriented health care. *Journal of Nursing Administration, 35*(12), 522–524.

Ireland, A. M., DePalma, J. A., Arneson, L., Stark, L., & Williamson, J. (2004). The oncology nursing society ambulatory office nurse survey. *Oncology Nursing Forum, 31*(6), 147–156.

Kleinman, C. (2004). Leadership strategies in reducing staff nurse role conflict. *Journal of Nursing Administration, 34*(7/8), 322–324.

Mikos, C. A. (2004). Beware the consequences of license relinquishment. *Nursing Management, 35*(10), 16–17.

Nurses Board of South Australia. (2004). *Standards: Delegation by a registered nurse or midwife to an unregulated healthcare worker.* Unpublished manuscript (available at www.ncsbn.org).

O'Keefe, C. (2005, Jan.–Feb.). State laws and regulations for dialysis: An overview. *Nephrology Nursing Journal, 32*(1), 31–37.

CHAPTER 9

Effective Staffing

Best-practice staffing provides timely and effective patient care while providing a safe environment for both patients and staff, as well as promoting an atmosphere of professional nursing satisfaction.

(Carl Ray, et al., 2003)

OBJECTIVES

Upon completion of this chapter, the reader should be able to:

1. Discuss how staffing needs are determined.
2. Calculate full-time equivalents (FTEs) needed to staff a typical inpatient nursing unit.
3. Discuss appropriate units of service used to measure nursing need by unit type.
4. Identify patient classification systems.
5. Review considerations in developing a staffing pattern.
6. Discuss staff scheduling on a patient care unit.
7. Discuss the role of nurse staffing in achieving quality nurse-sensitive outcomes.
8. Compare and contrast models of care delivery and their impact on patient outcomes.
9. Discuss care delivery management tools, such as clinical pathways, case management, and disease management.

You are a new nurse on a 30-bed medical unit that uses primary nursing as the care delivery model. There are 40 employees who work full and part time on this unit with vacancies for 8 additional full-time staff. The current schedule does not accommodate any 12-hour shifts. There are five long-term staff members who are threatening to leave if they are forced to work 12-hour shifts. You have heard there are several new graduates who will come to work on the unit only if there are 12-hour shifts.

How can the needs of both groups of staff be accommodated?

What effect will the 12-hour shifts have on the care delivery model?

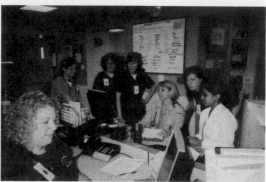

Delmar/Cengage Learning

The ability of a nurse to provide safe and effective care to a patient is dependent on many variables. These variables include the knowledge and experience of the staff, the severity of illness of the patients, patient dependency for daily activities, complexity of care, the amount of nursing time available, the care delivery model, care management tools, and organizational supports in place to facilitate care. This chapter explores these factors, how they affect planning for staffing, scheduling staff, and patient outcomes associated with staffing factors. It also reviews the models of care delivery that can be used with various patient populations.

DETERMINATION OF STAFFING NEEDS

Nurse staffing has varied widely since the inception of nursing as a profession. Nursing staffing ratios have ranged from a ratio of one nurse to many soldiers, as in Florence Nightingale's time, to today when you may see a ratio of one nurse to one patient in a critical care area. Gaining an understanding of the key terms—full-time equivalents (FTEs), productive time, nonproductive time, direct and indirect care, nursing workload, and units of service—is necessary for understanding staffing patterns.

FTEs

A **full-time equivalent (FTE)** is a measure of the work commitment of a full-time employee. A full-time employee has traditionally worked 5 days a week for 40 hours per week for 52 weeks a year. This amounts to 2,080 hours of work time (Figure 9-1). A full-time employee who works 40 hours a week is referred to as a 1.0 FTE. An employee who works 36 hours (three 12-hour shifts) is considered full time for benefit purposes in many agencies, but is assigned 0.9 FTE for budgeting purposes ($36/40 = 0.9$ FTE). A part-time employee who works five days in a two-week period is considered a 0.5 FTE. FTE calculation is used to mathematically describe how much an employee works (Figure 9-2). Understanding FTEs is essential when moving from a staffing plan to the actual number of staff required.

FTE hours are a total of all paid time. This includes worked time as well as nonworked time.

5 days per week	× 8 hours per day	=	40 hours per week
40 hours per week	× 52 weeks per year	=	2,080 hours per year

Figure 9-1 Calculation of full-time equivalent hours. (Delmar/Cengage Learning).

1.0 FTE = 40 hours per week or five 8-hour shifts per week

0.8 FTE = 32 hours per week or four 8-hour shifts per week

0.6 FTE = 24 hours per week or three 8-hour shifts per week

0.4 FTE = 16 hours per week or two 8-hour shifts per week

0.2 FTE = 8 hours per week or one 8-hour shift per week

Figure 9-2 FTE calculation for varying levels of work commitment. (Delmar/Cengage Learning).

Vacation time	15 days	or	120 hours
Sick time	5 days	or	40 hours
Holiday time	6 days	or	48 hours
Education time	3 days	or	24 hours
Total nonproductive time		=	232 hours

2,080 − 232 = 1,848 hours of productive work time available for each staff member with these benefits.

Figure 9-3 Calculation of productive and nonproductive time. (Delmar/Cengage Learning).

Hours worked and available for patient care are designated as productive hours. Benefit time such as vacation, sick time, and education time is considered nonproductive hours. When considering the number of FTEs you need to staff a unit, you must count only the productive hours available for each staff member. Available productive time can be easily calculated by subtracting benefit time from the time a full-time employee would work (Figure 9-3). These figures vary greatly depending on institutional policy and availability of human resource benefits.

In this case, a full-time registered nurse (RN) would have 1,848 hours per year of productive time available to care for patients.

Employees who work with patients can be classified into two categories: those who provide direct care and those who provide indirect care. Direct care is time spent providing hands-on care to patients. Indirect care is time spent on activities that are patient related but are not done directly to the patient. Documentation, time consulting with people in other health care disciplines, and time spent following up on problems are good examples of indirect care. Even though RNs, licensed practical nurses (LPNs), and nursing assistive personnel (NAP) engage in indirect care activities, the majority of their time is spent providing direct care; therefore, they are classified as direct care providers. Nurse managers, clinical specialists, unit secretaries, and other support staff are considered indirect care providers because the majority of their work is indirect in nature and supports the work of the direct care providers.

Units of service include a variety of volume measures that are used to reflect different types of patient encounters as indicators of nursing workload (Figure 9-4). Volume measures are used in budget negotiations to project nursing needs of patients and to ensure adequate resources for safe patient care.

The majority of nurses practice on in-patient units; therefore, further calculations for this chapter's examples will be in Nursing Hours Per Patient Day (NHPPD). **Nursing Hours Per Patient Days (NHPPD)** is the amount of nursing care required per patient in a 24-hour period and is usually based on midnight census and past unit needs, expected unit practice trends, national benchmarks,

Unit Type	Unit of Service
In-patient Unit	Nursing Hours Per Patient Day (NHPPD)
Labor and Delivery	Births
Operating Room	Surgeries/Procedures
Home Care	Patient Visits
Emergency Services	Patient Visits

Figure 9-4 Units of service—volume measures by unit type. (Delmar/Cengage Learning).

20 patients on the unit

5 staff × 3 shifts = 15 staff

15 staff each working 8 hours = 120 hours available in a 24-hour period

120 nursing hours ÷ 20 patients = 6.0 NHPPD

Figure 9-5 Calculation of Nursing Hours Per Patient Day (NHPPD). (Delmar/Cengage Learning).

professional staffing standards, and budget nego-tiations. NHPPD reflects only productive nursing time needed. Calculation of NHPPD is displayed in Figure 9-5.

NURSE INTENSITY

Nurse intensity is "a measure of the amount and complexity of nursing care needed by a patient" (Adomat & Hewison, 2004, p. 304). Nurse inten-sity is dependent on many factors that are difficult to measure: severity of illness, patient dependency for activities of daily living, complexity of care, and amount of time needed for care (Beglinger, 2006). It is vital that nurses measure nurse intensity be-cause staffing needs vary not only with the number of patients being cared for, but also with the type of care provided for each of those patients (Unruh & Fottler, 2006).

Patient turnover affects nurse intensity. Patient turnover is a measure reflecting patient admission, transfer, and discharge, all of which entail RN-intensive procedures. As the health care industry pushes to reduce costs through shorter lengths of stay, these RN-intensive procedures related to

patient turnover consume an increasing propor-tion of the hospital stay. As length of stay shortens, the intensity and need for NHPPD increases. What is not known at this time is the exact nature of this inverse relationship (Unruh & Fottler, 2006).

PATIENT CLASSIFICATION SYSTEMS

A **patient classification system** (PCS) is a measure-ment tool used to articulate the nursing work-load for a specific patient or group of patients over a specific period of time. The measure of nursing workload that is generated for each pa-tient is called the **patient acuity**. PCS data can be used to predict the amount of nursing time needed based on the patient's acuity. As a pa-tient becomes sicker, his acuity level rises, mean-ing the patient requires more nursing care (see Table 9-1). As a patient's acuity level decreases, he requires less nursing care. In most patient classification systems, each patient is classified us-ing weighted criteria that then approximate the nursing care hours needed for the next 24 hours.

TABLE 9-1

COMPARATIVE VALUES OF ACUITY AND CARE HOURS

PCS Acuity	Care Hours
1	3.00
2	3.60
3	6.00
4	9.99
5	15.00

Because patient care is dynamic, it is impossible to capture future patient care needs using a one-time measure (Gran-Moravec & Hughes, 2005). Criteria reflect care needed in assessment, bathing, mobilizing, supervision, monitoring, evaluation, and so on. In most cases, patients are classified once a day. The ideal PCS produces a valid and reliable rating of individual patient care requirements, which are matched to the latest clinical technology and caregiver skill variables. These systems are generally applied to all inpatients in an organization. Other PCS systems exist to measure the workload associated with patient visits in the Emergency Department (ED) or in clinic environments based on relative weights for visit lengths as well as complexity of care. There are two different types of classification systems: factor and prototype. A factor system assigns a time or weight to reflect the amount of time needed to perform a nursing task. The time or weight factor assigned for different nursing activities can be changed over time to reflect the changing needs of the patients or hospital systems. A *prototype* classification system allocates nursing time to large patient groups based on an average of similar patients. For example, specific **diagnostic-related groups (DRGs)** have been used as groupings of patients to which a nursing acuity

is assigned based on past organizational experience. DRGs are patient groupings established by the federal government for reimbursement purposes. DRGs are sorted by patient disease or condition. This model assumes that, on average, this measure will reflect the nursing care required and provided. The data are then used by hospitals in determining the cost of nursing care and negotiating contracts with payers for specific patient populations. Both classification systems have advantages and disadvantages.

UTILIZATION OF CLASSIFICATION SYSTEM DATA

Patient classification data are valuable sources of information for all levels of an organization. On a day-to-day basis, acuity data can be utilized by staff and managers in planning nurse staffing over the next 24 hours. Acuity data and NHPPD are concrete data parameters that are used to educate staff on how to adjust staffing levels. For example, for an acuity range of 1.0 to 1.10, the RN staffing may be five RNs on day shifts. For an acuity of 1.10 to 1.15, the RN staffing on day shifts might be six RNs. Experienced staff have the knowledge to manage staffing to acuity levels given the information, boundaries, and authority to do so. In many organizations, a central staffing office monitors the census and acuity on all units and deploys nursing resources to the areas in most need using the classification system data and recommended staffing levels. The manager reviews the results of staffing over the past 24 to 48 hours to adjust staffing to patient requirements. At the unit level, acuity data are also essential in preparing month-end justification for variances in staff utilization. If your average acuity has risen, then there is often a rise in NHPPD to accommodate the increased patient needs.

At an organizational level, acuity data have been used to cost out nursing services for specific patient populations and global patient types. This information is also very helpful in negotiating payment rates with third-party payers such as insurance companies to ensure that reimbursement reflects nursing costs. In most organizations, the classification or acuity data are also used in preparation of the nursing staffing budget for the upcoming fiscal year. The data can be benchmarked with other organizations to lend credence to any efforts to change nursing hours. Finally, patient acuity data and NHPPD can be used to develop a staffing pattern. Patient classification and NHPPD data provide an enormous amount of information that serves a multitude of needs.

CONSIDERATIONS IN DEVELOPING A STAFFING PATTERN

Benchmarking is a tool used to compare productivity across facilities to establish performance goals. Note, however, that "being the best performer in a group does not necessarily indicate best practice" (Ray, Jagim, Agnew, Inglass-McKay, & Sheehy, 2003, p. 246). Often, benchmarking data provides only comparable unit-of-service performance and does not reflect quality-of-care indicators that can link quality patient care outcomes to productivity measures. In developing a staffing pattern that leads to a budget, it is important to benchmark your planned NHPPD against other organizations with similar patient populations as part of evidence-based decision-making (EBD-M). Purchased patient classification systems often offer acuity and NHPPD benchmarking data from around the country as part of their system. This kind of data can be helpful in establishing a starting point for a staffing pattern or as part of justification for increasing or reducing nursing hours. Caution must be used, however, because each organization has varying levels of support in place at the unit level for the nurse. For example, a nursing unit that has dietary aides from the dietary department distribute and pick up meal trays would need less nursing time than a unit that had no external support for this activity. Practice differences such as these contribute significantly to differences in hours of care from one organization to another.

REGULATORY REQUIREMENTS

Generally speaking, there are few regulatory requirements related to nurse staffing. This is changing, however, as the nursing shortage heightens. Eight states have mandated nurse staffing plans (White, 2006). Note that staffing plans are different from staffing ratios. In 1999, California became the first state to mandate development of nurse-to-patient ratios. By January 2005, California hospitals were required to meet a 1:5 ratio in all medical-surgical units. Similar legislation is pending in Massachusetts. In both cases, the State Nurses Associations were central to the legislation. There is considerable controversy within the nursing profession over this issue. There are nurses who are adamant that they need to be protected by law with stipulated staffing levels. There are other nurse leaders who are concerned that the mandated staffing levels would soon become the maximum staffing levels rather than the minimum.

The Joint Commission (JC), formerly known as the Joint Commission on Accreditation of Healthcare Organizations (JCAHO), surveys hospitals on the quality of care provided. The JC does not mandate staffing levels, but does assess staffing effectiveness. The JC standards (2006) regarding staffing require organizations to monitor at least four indicators, including two human resource indicators and two clinical indicators. An example of a human resource indicator is NHPPD. An example of a clinical indicator is skin breakdown occurrence. There are 21 indicators from which to choose. Those indicators chosen must be analyzed and staffing levels adjusted based on the resulting information (White, 2006).

SKILL MIX

Skill mix is another critical element in nurse staffing. **Skill mix** is the percentage of RN staff compared to other direct care staff, LPNs, and nursing assistive personnel (NAP). For example, in a unit that has 40 FTEs budgeted, with 20 of them being RNs and 20 FTEs of other skill types, the RN skill mix would be 50%. If the unit had 40 FTEs, with 30 of them being RNs, the RN skill mix would be 75%. The skill mix of a unit should vary according to the care that is required and the care delivery model utilized. For example, in a critical care unit, the RN skill mix will be much higher than in a nursing home where the skills of an RN are required to a much lesser degree.

STAFF SUPPORT

Another important factor to consider in developing a staffing pattern is the support in place for the operations of the unit or department. For instance, does your organization have a systematic process to deliver medications to the department or do unit personnel have to pick up patient medications and narcotics? Does your organization have staff to transport patients to and from ancillary departments? The less support available to your staff, the more nursing hours have to be built into the staffing pattern to provide care to patients.

HISTORICAL INFORMATION

As you consider the many variables that affect staffing, it helps to ask the following questions: What has worked in the past? Were the staff able to provide the care that was needed? How many patients were cared for? What kind of patients were they? How many staff were utilized and what kind of staff were they? This kind of information can help to identify operational issues that would not be apparent otherwise. For example, it is important to review any data on quality or staff perceptions regarding the effectiveness of any previous staffing plans. This information will allow you to calculate previous NHPPD and outcomes for comparison to your current staffing plans. History is a valuable tool that we often overlook as we plan for the future.

ESTABLISHING A STAFFING PATTERN

A staffing pattern is a plan that articulates how many and what kind of staff are needed by shift and day to staff a unit or department. There are

basically two ways of developing a staffing pattern. It can be generated by determining the required ratio of staff to patients; nursing hours and total FTEs are then calculated. It can also be generated by determining the nursing care hours needed for a specific patient or patients and then generating the FTEs and staff-to-patient ratio needed to provide that care. In most cases, you would use a combination of methods to validate your staffing plan.

STAFFING AN INPATIENT UNIT

An inpatient unit is a hospital unit that is able to provide care to patients 24 hours a day, 7 days a week. Establishing a staffing pattern for this kind of unit utilizes all the data discussed in the previous sections. Using data from all your sources, you can build a staffing plan that you believe will meet the needs of the patients, the staff, and the organization. To illustrate the concept of calculating a staffing plan, we will use a typical medical unit with 24 beds and an average daily census (ADC) of 20. (Figure 9-6). Average daily census (ADC) is calculated by taking the total number of patients at census time, usually midnight, over a period of time (for example, weekly, monthly, or yearly) and dividing by the number of days in the time period. Many institutions budget their staffing based on ADC and then adjust for patient census and acuity changes. To fully understand the complexity of decisions involved in staffing, you must review the "Models of Care Delivery" section later in this chapter. Allocating FTEs cannot be separated from an intelligent understanding of how patient care is delivered and how to use the right mix of staff to accomplish that patient care.

SCHEDULING

Scheduling of staff is the responsibility of the nurse manager. The nurse manager must ensure that the schedule places the appropriate staff on each shift for safe, effective patient care. There are

Scenario: A 24-bed medical unit where the ADC is 20 and NHPPD is budgeted at 8.

Step 1:

Formula: Number of patients × NHPPD = care hours per day = shifts needed per 24 hours

Example: $20 \times 8 = \dfrac{160 \text{ care hours per 24 hour day}}{8} = 20$ eight-hour shifts needed per 24 hours

Step 2:

Allocate 20 staff to the unit by shift and skill mix, based on when and how care is provided.

	% of Staff Per Shift	# of Staff	RN	Tech/Unit Clerk
Days	40	8	4	4
Evenings	35	7	4	3
Nights	25	5	$\dfrac{4}{12}$	$\dfrac{1}{8}$ (Total 20)

Step 3:

Calculate FTE to cover staff days off. (Calculations are in parentheses in the matrix below.)

Formula: $\dfrac{\text{Number of staff needed per shift} \times \text{Days of needed coverage}}{\text{Number of shifts each FTE works}}$

Example: $\dfrac{4 \times 7}{5} = 5.6$

	% of Staff Per Shift	# of Staff	RN	Tech/Unit Clerk
Days	40	8	4 (5.6)	4 (5.6)
Evenings	35	7	4 (5.6)	3 (4.2)
Nights	25	5	$\dfrac{4\ (5.6)}{12\ (16.8)}$	$\dfrac{1\ (1.4)}{8\ (11.2)} = 20\ (28)$

Step 4:

Provide coverage for benefit time off, e.g., vacation, educational time, etc. Managers and other support staff are often not replaced on their days off.

Formula: Productive hours/budgeted nonproductive hours = percent of nonproductive hours × total FTE = additional FTE needed to cover benefits;

Productive + nonproductive FTE to cover each week = Grand Total FTE

Example: 2080/232 = 0.11 × 28 = 3.08;

   3.08 + 28 = 31.08 Grand Total FTE

Figure 9-6 Staffing plan template for an inpatient unit. (Delmar/Cengage Learning).

many issues to consider as staff are scheduled: patient needs and acuity, the number of patients, the experience of your staff, and the supports available to the staff. The combination of these factors determines the number of staff to be scheduled on each shift.

PATIENT NEED

Patient classification systems do not tell you when the nursing activity will take place over the next 24 hours. In addition to planning for the acuity of the patients, the staffing plan must support having staff working when the work needs to be done. A good example of this would be an oncology unit in which chemotherapy and blood transfusions typically occur on the evening shift. In this scenario, staffing in the evening may need to be higher than for other shifts to support these nurse-intensive activities.

EXPERIENCE AND SCHEDULING OF STAFF

Each nurse is different regarding his or her knowledge base, experience level, and critical thinking skills. A novice nurse takes longer to accomplish the same task than an experienced nurse. An experienced RN can handle more in terms of workload and acuity of patients. If a nursing unit requires special skills or competencies, you would also want to plan for additional nursing hours, so that staff with those skills are scheduled when the patient care needs may arise. The underlying principle of good staffing is that those you serve come first. This may dictate some undesirable shifts, but there must be appropriate numbers and kinds of staff on hand to care for the patients you serve. Staff are plotted out across a staffing sheet (Figure 9-7).

The scheduled days should be assigned so that there are an even number of staff available across the week. Typically, the spread of FTEs across the 24-hour period falls within the following guidelines: days 33% to 50%, evenings 30% to 40%, and nights 20% to 33%. The spread is based on patient need.

SHIFT VARIATIONS

To attract and retain employees, organizations offer traditional schedules and flexible schedules to meet organizational and employee needs. Traditional staffing patterns are generally 8-hour shifts, 7 A.M. to 3:30 P.M., 3 P.M. to 11:30 P.M., and 11 P.M. to 7:30 A.M. A full-time employee works 10 8-hour shifts in a 2-week period. The start time of 8-hour shifts may vary by organization or by unit and patient need. For example, emergency departments are typically busiest during the evening into the night hours. An 8-hour shift for the ED may be 7 P.M. to 3 A.M. to cover the peak activity times.

NEW OPTIONS IN STAFFING PATTERNS

Twelve-hour shifts have become very popular across the country. In many organizations, employees can work less than 40 hours per week and get full-time benefits. In one example, a nurse could work three 12-hour shifts per week and have 4 days off and be full time. Another popular option is weekend programs. Weekend program staff work two 12-hour shifts every weekend and are paid a rate that would make the 24 hours of work equal to 40 hours of work. Some of these programs include full-time benefits as well. These programs are expensive, but they can be helpful. See Figure 9-8. Note that any time you implement a scheduling plan, it is critical to assess what the effect will be on the care of patients.

The number of staff shift handoff reports per day also affects patient care. A shift handoff report occurs any time the nurse caring for a group of patients reports off to the nurse on an oncoming shift. Such shift handoff reports are opportunities for missed communication and errors in patient care. In eight-hour shifts, there are three shift handoff reports per 24 hours; whereas, in twelve-hour shifts, there are only two shift handoff reports.

SELF-SCHEDULING

Self-scheduling is a process in which unit staff take leadership in creating and monitoring the work schedule while working within defined

Name	Monday 04	Tuesday 05	Wednesday 06	Thursday 07	Friday 08	Saturday 09	Sunday 10	Monday 11	Tuesday 12	Wednesday 13	Thursday 14	Friday 15	Saturday 16	Sunday 17
Melinda	A		D	A		D	D			D	D	D	A	
Carlos		8.00 1900			N	N	N		8.00 1900		A	N		
Tabitha	12.00 0900		A		D	12.00 0900	12.00 0900	12.00 0900		A		N		
Susan	D	8.00 1100		E	E	E	P	vac		8.00 1100	E	E	P	E
Barbara		14.00 2400	13.00 2400	13.00 2400	A				14.00 2400	13.00 2400	13.00 2400		D	A
Rosemary	D	D	D	D		E			A	N	N		E	N
Robert	N	N	N	N			N	N	N	N	N		E	P
Jacqueline	E	E	P		E	E	E	E	E	E	E	P	P	P
Marcella		D		D	D	D	A	P	D			D	D	
Nirmala	P			E	8.00 0800		E	E			E	8.00 0800	E	E
Gary		E	E		E	N	E	E	E	E		12.00 1500	D	
Irma	N	N	N	N	N	P	P	N	N	P	E	P		
Toni	8.00 0730	8.00 0730	8.00 0730	8.00 0730	8.00 0730			8.00 0730	8.00 0730	P	8.00 0730	A	N	

The 1st number in a square is the number of hours scheduled; the second number is the shift start time in military time.

Standard Work Assignments

D 0700–1500
E 1500–2300
N 2300–0700
A 0700–1900
P 1900–0700

Figure 9-7 Excerpt from schedule for an emergency department showing great variation in shift design. (Delmar/Cengage Learning).

Weekend staff working at $42 an hour × 24 hours = $1,008 per weekend

Regular staff working at $25 an hour × 24 hours = $600 per weekend
_____

Difference in cost = $408 per weekend option FTE

Six weekend option staff members at $1,008 would cost $2,448 more than regular staff per weekend; $2,448 × 52 weekends a year would cost $127,296 more than regular staff annually.

Figure 9-8 Annual cost of a weekend option program for one nursing unit. (Delmar/Cengage Learning).

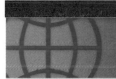

REAL WORLD INTERVIEW

We have developed a nursing practice quality scorecard. The scorecard is a tool to display data on our three organizational priorities: mission, customer orientation, and cost-effectiveness. By looking at measures in all three arenas, we can see how we are doing in these areas. We also can see if changes made in one arena positively or negatively affect the other measures. To look at nursing's mission for nursing practice, we track and trend several of the American Nurses Association national indicators. We track medication errors, patient falls, restraints, nosocomial pressure ulcers, and urinary tract infections. For customer satisfaction, we measure overall satisfaction with nursing care provided and how well patients' pain was controlled. For cost-effectiveness, we track nursing hours per patient day. All of these measures are tracked and trended on control charts every three months. The specific data is trended, and measures that are greater than two standard deviations from the target are identified as potential points to be reviewed for identification of opportunities for improvement.

One of the areas we chose to target for improvement was medication errors. It became evident that the most prominent reason for medication errors was delayed and omitted medications. Further investigation proved that the procedures for obtaining medications were unclear and outdated. We have written new procedures to specify responsibilities of the nursing staff and the pharmacy staff. We are now monitoring our rate of medication errors to see if our changes have made any improvement in the error rate.

Another example of use of the scorecard was in review of our pressure ulcer rate. We found there was an increase in the incidence of pressure ulcers. In review of causes, we found that the reporting system had been revised to include all stages of skin breakdown. Since the reporting change, we have seen an increase in the number of pressure ulcers reported. This is a positive change, as we now have accurate data on which to target our improvement efforts.

Lessons that we have learned in the development of the scorecard is that we needed to set improvement targets earlier in the process to push the search for opportunities for improvement. We also learned that many of these measures are not well defined, and, therefore, benchmarking to other organizations is difficult. We continue to strive for further improvement and utilize the scorecard to measure our success and look for opportunities for improvement. Reviewing nursing outcome data for the entire nursing division has been a powerful tool to ensure that care provided is meeting expected outcomes, and it allows us to benchmark our outcomes to other organizations.

Louann Villani, RN, BSN
Nursing Quality Specialist
Albany, New York

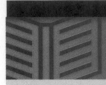

EVIDENCE FROM THE LITERATURE

Citation: Aiken, L. H., Clarke, S. P., Cheung, R. B., Sloane, D. M., & Silber, J. H. (2003). Education levels of hospital nurses and surgical patient mortality. *Journal of the American Medical Association, 290*(12), 1617–1623.

Discussion: This study looked at whether the proportion of RNs with a baccalaureate or higher level of nursing education is associated with risk-adjusted mortality and failure to rescue of surgical patients in Pennsylvania. "Nurses constitute the surveillance system for early detection of complications and problems in care, and they are in the best position to initiate actions that minimize negative outcomes for patients" (p. 1617). It stands to reason that the level of education of an RN might impact the nurse's clinical judgement and ability to serve as a detector and minimizer of complications, although impact on patient outcomes has not been studied before.

Outcomes data from hospital discharges from 168 adult acute-care hospitals were compared to American Hospital Association (AHA) administrative data on the hospitals and a survey of Pennsylvania nurses. There was a statistically significant relationship between the proportion of RNs with a baccalaureate or higher level of nursing education and patient mortality and failure to rescue. Each 10% increase in the RN BSN or higher proportion resulted in a 5% reduction of mortality and failure to rescue, after adjusting for both patient and hospital characteristics. Nurses' years of experience were not found to be a significant factor in the statistical models developed by the team.

Implications for Practice: The conventional idea that nursing experience is more important than the underlying educational preparation for the RN role is refuted by this study. These findings are additive to our knowledge that nurse-to-patient staffing ratios for medical-surgical nursing of more than 1:4 are associated with increased mortality and failure to rescue. Although further studies are needed to control for additional variables, this study strongly supports the need for leaders to encourage RNs to advance their education for the sake of patients and to set goals that increase the proportion of their nurses who hold a BSN or higher level degree.

guidelines. Often, there is a staffing committee that is part of unit-shared governance, which is a unit model where staff manage professional practice through unit committees. Increasing staff control over their schedule is a major factor in nurse job satisfaction and retention and has been associated with reductions in sick time usage. The nurse manager retains an important role in self-scheduling through mentoring, providing open communication, and holding everyone to equal expectations. To ensure that patient care needs are met, there must be structure to a self-scheduling program. This is often achieved by a unit committee, made up of staff that reports to the nurse manager. It is important to spell out the roles and responsibilities of all—the unit-based committee, the chairperson if there is one, the staff, and the manager. Generic boundaries need to be established regarding fairness, fiscal responsibility, evaluation of the self-scheduling process, and the approval process. Table 9-2 spells out specific issues that must be addressed.

NURSE-SENSITIVE PATIENT OUTCOMES

Nurse-sensitive patient outcomes such as patient length of stay and incidence of pneumonia, post-operative infections, pressure ulcers, urinary

TABLE 9-2	ISSUES TO BE SPELLED OUT IN SELF-SCHEDULING GUIDELINES

1. Scheduling period: Is the scheduling period 2, 4, or 6 week intervals?

2. Schedule time line: What are the time frames for both staff and per diem workers to sign up for regular work, special requests, and overtime?

3. Staffing pattern: Will 8 or 12 hour shifts, or both, be used?

4. Weekends: Are staff expected to work every other weekend? If there are extra weekends available, how are they distributed?

5. Holidays: How are they allocated?

6. Vacation time: Are there restrictions on the amount of vacation during certain periods?

7. Unit vacation practices: How many staff from one shift can be on vacation at any time?

8. Requests for time off: What is the process for requesting time off?

9. Short-staffed shifts: How are shifts that are short-staffed handled?

10. On call, if applicable: How do staff get assigned or sign up for on-call time?

11. Cancellation guidelines: How and when do staff get canceled for scheduled time if they are not needed?

12. Sick calls: What are the expectations for calling in sick, and how are these shifts covered?

13. Military/National Guard leave: What kind of advance notice is required?

14. Schedule changes: What is the process for changing one's schedule after the schedule has been approved?

15. Shifts defined: What are the beginnings and endings of available shifts?

16. Committee time: When does the self-scheduling committee meet and for how long?

17. Seniority: How does it play into staffing and request decisions?

18. Staffing plan for crisis/emergency situations: What is the plan when staffing is inadequate?

19. Job sharing: Who can participate? When?

tract infections, and "failure to rescue" i.e, death of a patient with one of five life-threatening complications—pneumonia, shock or cardiac arrest, upper gastrointestinal bleeding, sepsis, or deep vein thrombosis, for which early identification can influence the risk of death (Needleman, Buerhaus, Mattke, Stewart, Zelevinsky, 2002) are negatively affected when nurse staffing or the skill mix is inadequate.

Professional organizations are also weighing in on staffing and patient outcomes. For example, the American Association of Critical-Care Nurses (AACN) considers appropriate staffing to be one of six key measures of sustaining healthy work environments for nurses (AACN, 2005), and the Emergency Nurses Association (ENA) has issued guidelines for determining appropriate ED nurse staffing (Ray et al., 2003).

CASE STUDY 9-1

You are working on a patient care unit that is planning to begin doing its own scheduling. Using Figure 9-7, make a schedule for your unit. Identify the number of nurses budgeted for each day. Develop a plan to allocate these nurses to cover 24 hours a day, 7 days a week of patient care for 2 weeks.

NURSE STAFFING AND NURSE OUTCOMES

In addition to patient outcomes, nurse outcomes should also be measured. Staff's perception of the adequacy of staffing should be tracked. Kramer and Schmalenberg (2005) recommend an instrument to measure Perception of Adequacy of Staffing (PAS) as a proxy measure of acceptable staffing levels. Nurse perception of staffing effectiveness must be monitored by hospitals seeking magnet status. Initiating such measures might lead to comparisons for benchmarking best practice in the future and linking RN staffing perception to patient outcomes (Shirey & Fisher, in press). There should be the ability for staff to communicate both in written and verbal form regarding staffing concerns. In addition, actual staffing compared to recommended staffing should be tracked. This will give clues to other staffing issues. Medication errors is another measure that has been linked with inadequate NHPPD. When resources are scarce, data are imperative to drive needed changes. The outcomes of ineffective staffing patterns and nursing care can be devastating to patients, staff, and the organization.

MODELS OF CARE DELIVERY

To ensure that nursing care is provided to patients, the work must be organized. A **nursing care delivery model** organizes the work of caring for patients. The decision about which nursing care delivery model is used is based on the needs of the patients and the availability of competent staff in the different skill levels.

CASE METHOD AND TOTAL PATIENT CARE

In the case method, the nurse has one patient whom the nurse cares for exclusively. Total patient care is the modern-day version of the case method. In **total patient care**, the nurse is responsible for the total care for the nurse's patient assignment for the shift the nurse is working. The RN is responsible for several patients. The RN may have some support from LPNs or NAP, but the LPNs and NAP are not assigned to a specific group of patients.

ADVANTAGES AND DISADVANTAGES

The advantage of total patient care and the case method for patients is the consistency of one individual caring for patients for an entire shift. This enables the patient, nurse, and family to develop a relationship based on trust. This model provides a higher number of RN hours of care than other models. The nurse has more opportunity to observe and monitor progress of the patient. A disadvantage is that these models utilize a high level of RN nursing hours and are more costly to deliver care. This level of RN intensity is not always warranted in patients with low acuity.

FUNCTIONAL NURSING CARE

Functional nursing divides the nursing work into functional duties. These duties are then assigned to one of the team members. In this model, each care provider has specific duties or tasks he or she is responsible for. For instance, a typical assignment of labor for RNs is medication nurse or admission nurse and so on. Decision making is usually at the level of the head nurse or charge nurse (Figure 9-9).

ADVANTAGES AND DISADVANTAGES

In this model, care can be delivered to a large number of patients. This system utilizes other types of less skilled health care workers when there

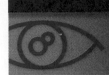

CRITICAL THINKING 9-1

Recently, you have been part of a unit committee that is reviewing data on your unit's pressure ulcer rates. In researching further, you discover that your unit's rates are significantly higher than those of other units. Staffing on your unit has been stable and in accordance with the staffing plan. The staff are experienced, and, in fact, they include some of the longest tenured staff in the hospital.

Why is the pressure ulcer rate higher than that of other units? What could your committee do to investigate this nurse-sensitive outcome further?

Surgical Unit

```
                    ┌──────────────┐
                    │ Charge nurse │
                    └──────────────┘
        ┌──────────┬──────────┴──────────┬──────────┐
   ┌─────────┐ ┌─────────┐         ┌──────────┐ ┌──────────┐
   │   RN    │ │   RN    │         │   LPN    │ │   NAP    │
   │Medication│ │Admission│         │Treatment │ │Vital signs│
   │  nurse  │ │  nurse  │         │  nurse   │ │ Bathing  │
   └─────────┘ └─────────┘         └──────────┘ └──────────┘
   ┌─────────────────────────────────────────────────────┐
   │                      Patients                        │
   └─────────────────────────────────────────────────────┘
```

Figure 9-9 Functional nursing model. (Delmar/Cengage Learning).

is a shortage of RNs. Patients are likely to have care delivered to them in one shift by several staff members. To a patient, care may feel disjointed. Staff must be aware of this disadvantage and work to eliminate this outcome.

TEAM NURSING

Team nursing is a care delivery model that assigns staff to teams that then are responsible for a group of patients. A unit may be divided into two teams, and each team is led by a registered nurse. The team leader supervises and coordinates all the care provided by those on his team. The team is most commonly made up of LPNs and NAP, but occasionally there is another RN. Care is divided into the simplest components and then assigned to the appropriate care provider. In addition to supervision duties, the team leader also is responsible for providing professional direction to those on the team regarding the care provided (Figure 9-10).

A **modular nursing** delivery system is a kind of team nursing that divides a geographic space into modules of patients, with each patient module cared for by a team of staff led by an RN. The modules may vary in size, but typically there is one RN with an LPN and nursing assistant to make up the module. In this case, the RN is responsible for the overall care of the patients in her module.

ADVANTAGES AND DISADVANTAGES

In team nursing and modular nursing, the RN is able to get work done through others, but patients sometimes receive fragmented, depersonalized care. Communication in these models is complex. There

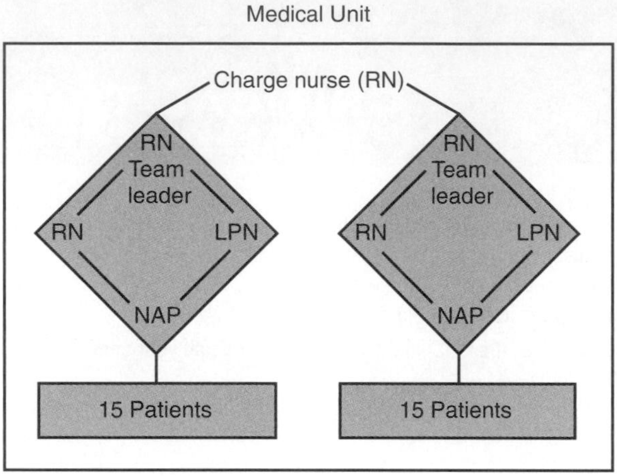

Medical Unit

Figure 9-10 Team nursing model. (Delmar/Cengage Learning).

is shared responsibility and accountability, which can cause confusion and lack of accountability. These factors may contribute to RN dissatisfaction with these models. These models require the RN to have very good delegation and supervision skills.

PRIMARY NURSING

Primary nursing is a care delivery model that clearly delineates the responsibility and accountability of the RN and designates the RN as the primary provider of care to patients. Primary nursing is a form of the case model that consists of four elements. These are allocation and acceptance of individual responsibility for the decision making to one individual; assignments of daily care by the case method; direct person-to-person communication; and operational responsibility of one person for the quality of care administered to patients on a unit 24 hours a day, 7 days a week (Manthey, 1980). Patients are assigned a primary nurse, who is responsible for developing with the patient a plan of care that is followed by other nurses caring for the patient. Nurses and patients are matched according to needs and abilities. Patients are assigned to their primary nurse regardless of unit geographic considerations. In the primary nursing model, the role of the head nurse changes to one of leader by empowering the staff RNs to be knowledgeable about their patients and to direct the care of

their primary patients. The primary nurse has the authority, accountability, and responsibility to provide care for a group of patients. Associate nurses care for the patient when the primary nurse is not working. Several associate nurses are assigned to each patient (Figure 9-11).

ADVANTAGES AND DISADVANTAGES

An advantage of this model is that patients and families are able to develop a trusting relationship with one primary nurse. There is defined accountability and responsibility for the nurse to develop a plan of care with the patient and family. The approach to care is holistic, which facilitates continuity of care rather than a shift-to-shift focus. Nurses, when they have adequate time to provide necessary care, find this model professionally rewarding because it gives the authority for decision making to the nurse at the bedside. Disadvantages include a high cost because there is a higher RN skill mix. With no geographical boundaries within the unit, nursing staff may be required to travel long distances at the unit level to care for their primary patients. Nurses often perform functions that could be completed by other staff. And finally, nurse-to-patient ratios must be realistic to ensure there is enough nursing time available to meet the patient care needs.

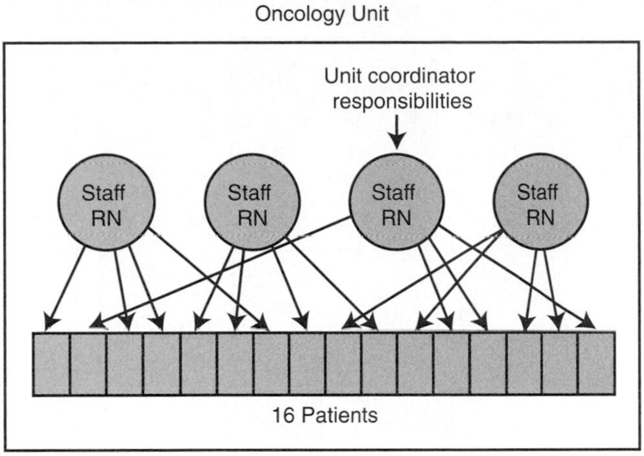

Oncology Unit

Figure 9-11 Primary nursing model. (Delmar/Cengage Learning).

PATIENT-CENTERED OR PATIENT-FOCUSED CARE

Patient-centered care or **patient-focused care** is designed to focus on patient needs rather than staff needs. In this model, required care and services are brought to the patient. In the highest evolution of this model, all patient services are decentralized to the patient area, including radiology and pharmacy services. Staffing is based on patient needs. In this model, there is an effort to have the right person doing the right thing. Care teams are established for a group of patients. The care teams may include other disciplines such as respiratory or physical therapists. In these teams, disciplines collaborate to ensure that patients receive the care they need. Staff are kept close to the patients in decentralized work stations. For example, on a rehabilitation unit, physical therapists may be members of the care team and work at the unit level rather than in a centralized physical therapy department (Figure 9-12).

ADVANTAGES AND DISADVANTAGES

The pros of this system are that it is most convenient for patients and expedites services to patients. But it can be extremely costly to decentralize major services in an organization. A second disadvantage is that some staff have perceived the model as a way of reducing RNs and cutting costs in hospitals. In fact, this has been true in some organizations, but many other organizations have successfully used the patient-centered model to have the right staff available for the needs of the patient population.

PATIENT CARE REDESIGN

In the 1990s, pressure to reduce health care costs was significant. Hospitals bore the brunt of this pressure. During this decade, patient care redesign was an initiative to redesign how patient care was delivered. The industry learned a lot about how care is delivered as it struggled with the redesign process. In addition to cost reduction, the redesign movement goals included making care more patient centered and not caregiver centered. This was accomplished by reducing the number of caregivers with which each patient had to interface and by organizing care around the patients, thus encouraging greater patient satisfaction. The concept is one of having caregivers cross-trained so they can intervene in more patient situations without having additional resources from outside the care team to assist. Examples include having the team members, for example, RNs and cross-trained care technicians,

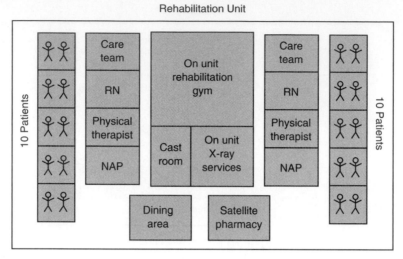

Figure 9-12 Patient-centered care model. (Delmar/Cengage Learning).

draw lab specimens instead of having a phlebotomy team come to the unit, or team members doing their patients' breathing treatments instead of calling respiratory therapy to come to the unit. Team control of these functions allowed the functions to occur when patients needed them and not at the convenience of outside departments. Work flow analysis is a tool used to determine what activities are value-added and how to streamline or eliminate those that do not contribute to improved patient outcomes (Capuano, Bokovoy, Halkins, & Hitchings, 2004). The term *value-added* refers to activities that possess the following characteristics:

- The customer is willing to pay for this activity.
- The activity must be done right the first time.
- The activity must somehow change the product or service in some desirable manner (Six Sigma, 2006).

Many of these value-added changes in care attributed to the patient care redesign movement of the 1990s continue to this day as good practices within patient-centered care. Other aspects of redesign have not survived. Those redesign projects that failed to assist caregivers to change their roles or

failed to consider unit culture in the patient care redesign were frequently not successful.

CARE DELIVERY MANAGEMENT TOOLS

In 1983, the federal government established diagnostic-related groups (DRGs) as a payment system for hospitals. In DRGs, the national average **length of stay (LOS)** for a specific patient type is used to determine payment for that grouping of Medicare patients. Length of stay (LOS) refers to the average number of days a patient is hospitalized from day of admission to day of discharge. In DRGs, hospitals are paid the same amount for caring for a DRG patient group regardless of the actual LOS of the specific patient. This prompted initiatives in hospitals to reduce LOS and reduce hospital costs. There are further adjustments to costs based on patient co-morbidities, that is, additional conditions (such as diabetes or hypertension) that add to the complexity of care needed by, for example a patient with heart disease. Hospitals were able to benchmark their LOS for specific patient populations against a national database published through the Medicare DRG system. As hospitals looked for opportunities to reduce costs through reduction in the LOS, clinical pathways and case management surfaced as significant strategies.

CLINICAL PATHWAYS

Clinical pathways are a major initiative to come out of the efforts to reduce LOS and are widely used to enhance outcomes and contain. **Clinical pathways** are care management tools that outline the expected clinical course and outcomes for a specific patient type. Clinical pathways take a different form in each organization that develops them. Typically they are pathways that outline the normal course of care for a patient. Pathways are often done by day, and expected outcomes are articulated for each day. It is the expected outcomes that patient progress is measured against. In some organizations, the pathways include multidisciplinary orders for care, including orders from nursing, medicine, and other allied health professionals such as physical therapy and dietary services. This serves to further expedite care for patients. Figure 9-13 provides an excerpt from a clinical pathway.

These pathways can be used by nursing and medical practitioners and case managers to care for the patient and measure the patient's progress against expected outcomes. Any variance in outcome can then be noted and acted upon to get the patient back on track.

CASE MANAGEMENT

Case management is a second strategy to improve patient care and reduce hospital costs through coordination of care. Typically a case manager is responsible for coordinating care and establishing goals from preadmission through discharge. In the typical model of case management, a nurse is assigned to a specific high-risk patient population or service, such as cardiac surgery patients. The case manager has the responsibility to work with all disciplines to facilitate care. For example, if a postsurgical hospitalized patient has not met ambulation goals according to the clinical pathway, the case manager would work with the physician and nurse

to determine what is preventing the patient from achieving these goals. If it turns out that the patient is elderly and is slow to recover, they may agree that physical therapy would be beneficial to assist this patient in ambulating. In other models, the case management function is provided by the staff nurse at the bedside. This works well if the population requires little case management, but if the patient population requires significant case management services, there needs to be enough RN time allocated for this activity. In addition to facilitating care, the case manager usually has a data function to improve care. In this role, the case manager collects aggregate data on patient variances from the clinical pathway. The data are shared with health care clinicians who participate in the clinical pathway and are then used to explore opportunities for improvement in the pathway or in hospital systems.

DISEASE MANAGEMENT

Increasingly, health care centers are developing disease management (DM) programs. **Disease management** is a "systematic, population-based approach to identify persons at risk, intervene with specific programs of care, and measure clinical and other outcomes" (Epstein & Sherwood, 1996). An objective of disease management is cost containment, and research indicates that this is occurring. A study of nurses who managed patients with congestive heart failure in an aged population showed significantly lower numbers of patient readmissions and costs (Rich et al., 1995).

DM can be as simple as a pharmaceutical pamphlet describing how best to use a medication, or as complex as nurse managers developing individualized care plans and regularly contacting patients to ensure compliance with the plans.

Disease management strategies use a variety of methods, including telephone, the Internet, and in-person visits, to keep high-risk, high-cost patients out of the hospital. These DM strategies collect data from and send reminders to patients who need constant monitoring. They also provide information systems that help caregivers develop care plans and gather data for clinical improvement initiatives.

Clinical Pathway: Lower Extremity Revascularization EXCERPT

ADDRESSOGRAPH

DAILY ANTICIPATED OUTCOMES

POD2	Date/Time /Init When met	POD3	Date/Time /Init When met	POD4	Date/Time /Init When met	POD5	Date/Time /Init When met
Patient rates pain 0-2 on pain scale 0-10 using po analgesia.		Graft signal present with doppler.		Graft signal present with doppler.		Graft signal present with doppler.	
Graft signal present with doppler.		Incisional edges will be approximated without drainage.		Able to participate in self-care and adjunct therapies.		Ambulates independently.	
Patient will verbalize knowledge of plan of care, testing and treatment.		Site of invasive devices without signs of infection.		Patient viewed diet video.		Patient/significant other will verbalize understanding of activity/diet restrictions, medication use, wound management.	
Ambulate in hall Q I D.		Ambulates in hall Q I D.					
Tolerates po solids.		Patient/significant other will describe appropriate problem-solving skills to decrease anxiety.				Completed nutrition posttest.	
Voiding without difficulty.		Rehab referral started: _yes _no					
		Family support available at discharge, specify _____					

TO BE KEPT IN PROGRESS NOTE SECTION OF CHART AT ALL TIMES.

Figure 9-13 Example of a clinical pathway. (*Source:* Courtesy of Albany Medical Center, Albany, NY).

KEY CONCEPTS

■ To plan nurse staffing, you must understand and apply the concepts of full-time equivalents (FTEs) and nursing hours per patient day (NHPPD).

■ Determination of the number of FTEs needed to staff a unit requires review of patient classification data, NHPPD, regulatory requirements, skill mix, staff support, historical information, and the physical environment of the unit.

- In developing a staffing pattern, additional FTEs must be added to a nursing unit budget to provide coverage for days off and benefited time off.

- Scheduling of staff is the responsibility of the nurse manager, who must take into consideration patient need and acuity, volume of patients, budget, and the experience of the staff.

- Self-scheduling can increase staff morale and professional growth, but requires clear boundaries and guidelines to be successful.

- Evaluating the outcomes of your staffing plan for patients, staff, and the organization is a critical activity that should be done regularly.

- Case management and clinical pathways are care management tools that have been developed to improve patient care and reduce hospital costs.

KEY TERMS

benchmarking

case management

clinical pathways

diagnostic-related groups (DRGs)

direct care

disease management

full-time equivalent

functional nursing

indirect care

inpatient unit

length of stay (LOS)

modular nursing

nonproductive hours

nursing care delivery model

patient acuity

patient-centered care

patient classification system

patient-focused care

primary nursing

productive hours

self-scheduling

skill mix

staffing pattern

team nursing

total patient care

REVIEW QUESTIONS

1. Patient classification systems measure nursing workload required by the patient. The higher the patient's acuity, the more care the patient requires. Which of the following statements is a weakness of classification systems?
   A. Patient classification data are useful in predicting the required staffing for the next shift and for justifying nursing hours provided.
   B. Patient classification data can be utilized by the nurse making assignments to determine what level of care a patient requires.
   C. Classification systems typically focus on nursing tasks rather than a holistic view of a patient's needs.

   D. Aggregate patient classification data are useful in costing out nursing services and for developing the nursing budget.

2. If your RN staff members receive 4 weeks of vacation and 10 days of sick time per year, how many productive hours would each RN work in that year if she utilized all of her benefited time?
   A. 2,080 productive hours
   B. 1,840 productive hours
   C. 1,920 productive hours
   D. 1,780 productive hours

3. Patient outcomes are the result of many variables, one being the model of care delivery that is utilized. From the following scenarios, select which is the *worst* fit between patient need and care delivery model.
   A. Cancer patients being cared for in a primary nursing model
   B. Rehabilitation patients being cared for in a patient-centered model
   C. Medical intensive care patients being cared for in a team nursing model
   D. Ambulatory surgery patients with a wide range of illnesses being cared for in a functional practice model

4. The medical-surgical unit provides 200 hours of care daily to 20 patients. Their NHPPD is which of the following?
   A. 1
   B. 10
   C. 20
   D. 200

REVIEW ACTIVITIES

1. How do you know whether the outcomes of your staffing plan are positive? What measures do you have available in your organization that indicate your staffing is adequate or inadequate?

2. You are a nurse on a new unit for psychiatric patients. What should be considered in planning for FTEs and staffing for this unit?

3. You are a new nurse and you have increasing concerns regarding the staffing levels on your unit. You are becoming increasingly anxious each time you go to work. What should you do?

EXPLORING THE WEB

- Mandated staffing levels:
  www.nursingworld.org
  Go to *staffing issues* on the menu and review the legislative agenda for the ANA regarding staffing. Also review data on the ANA's latest staff survey.

- Nursing quality measures:
  www.mriresearch.org
  Search for *quality measures*.

- Staffing effectiveness:
  www.jointcommission.org
  Type *staffing effectiveness* into the search box, and read about staffing effectiveness standards issued by the JC.

- Staffing and quality:
  www.ahrq.gov
  This government site of the Agency for Healthcare Research and Quality provides evidence-based analysis of clinical issues. Look in the section on Quality and Patient Safety. You can also search using the term *safe staffing*.

REFERENCES

Adomat, R., & Hewison, A. (2004). Assessing patient category/dependence systems for determining the nurse/patient ratio in ICU and HDU: A review of approaches. *Journal of Nursing Management, 12*(5), 299–308.

Aiken, L. H., Clarke, S. P., Cheung, R. B., Sloane, D. M., & Silber, J. H. (2003). Education levels of hospital nurses and surgical patient mortality. *Journal of the American Medical Association, 290*(12), 1617–1623.

American Association of Critical-Care Nurses. (2005). *AACN standards for establishing and sustaining healthy work environments.* Aliso Viego, CA: AACN.

Beglinger, J. E. (2006). Quantifying patient care intensity: An evidence-based approach to determining staffing requirements. *Nursing Administration Quarterly, 30*(3), 193–202.

Capuano, T., Bokovoy, J., Halkins, D., & Hitchings, K. (2004). Work flow analysis: Eliminating nonvalue-added work. *Journal of Nursing Administration, 34*(5), 246–256.

Epstein, R. S., & Sherwood, L. M. (1996). From outcomes research to disease management: A guide for the perplexed, *Annals of Internal Medicine, 124,* 835–837.

Gran-Moravec, M. B., & Hughes, C. M. (2005). Nursing time allocation and other considerations for staffing. *Nursing & Health Science, 7*(2), 126–133.

Joint Commission (JC). (2006). Staffing standards. Retrieved November 9, 2006, from www.jointcommission.org.

Kramer, M., & Schmalenberg, C. (2005). Revising the essentials of magnetism tool: There is more to adequate staffing than numbers. *Journal of Nursing Administration, 35*(4), 188–198.

Manthey, M. (1980). *The practice of primary nursing.* Boston: Blackwell Scientific.

Needleman, J., Buerhaus, P., Mattke, S., Stewart, M., & Zelevinsky, K. (2002). Nurse-staffing levels and the quality of care in hospitals. *New England Journal of Medicine, 346*(22), 1715–1722.

Ray, C. E., Jagim, M., Agnew, J., Inglass-McKay, J., & Sheehy, S. (2003). ENA's new guidelines for determining emergency department nurse staffing. *Journal of Emergency Nursing, 29*(3), 245–253.

Rich, M. W., Beckham, V., Wittenberg, C., Leven, C. L., Friedland, K., & Carney, R. M. (1995). A multidisciplinary intervention to prevent readmission of elderly patients with congestive heart failure. *New England Journal of Medicine, 333,* 1190–1195.

Shirey, M., & Fisher, M. L. (in press). Leadership agenda for change: Toward healthy work environments for the 21st century. *AACN Journal.*

Six Sigma. (2006). Value added. Retrieved December 1, 2006, from www.sixsigma.com/dictionary/value-added-134.htm.

Unruh, L. Y., & Fottler, M. D. (2006). Patient turnover and nursing staff adequacy. *Health Services Research, 41*(20), 599–612.

White, K. M. (2006). Policy spotlight: Staffing plans and ratios. *Nursing Management, 37*(4), 18–24.

SUGGESTED READINGS

Harrison, J. (2004). Addressing increasing patient acuity and nursing workload. *Nursing Management (Harrow), 11*(4), 20–25.

Lang, T. A., Hodge, M., Olson, V., Romano, P. S., & Kravitz, R. L. (2004). Nurse-patient ratios: A systematic review on the effects of nurse staffing on patient, nurse employee, and hospital outcomes. *Journal of Nursing Administration, 34*(7–8), 326–337.

Mangold, K. L., Pearson, K. K., Schmitz, J. R., Loes, J. L., & Specht, J. P. (2006). Perceptions and characteristics of registered nurses' involvement in decision making. *Nursing Administration Quarterly, 30*(3), 266–272.

Rischbieth, A. (2006). Matching nurse skill with patient acuity in the intensive care units: A risk management mandate. *Journal of Nursing Management, 14*(5), 397–404.

CHAPTER 10

Budgeting for Patient Care

The purpose of creating and analyzing records of what transpires in hospitals is to know how the money is being spent; whether it is, in fact, doing good, or whether it is doing mischief.

(Florence Nightingale, 1859)

OBJECTIVES

Upon completion of this chapter, the reader should be able to:

1. Discuss national and international perspectives on the cost of health care.
2. Discuss budgets commonly used for planning and management.
3. Describe key elements that influence budget preparation.
4. Identify revenue and expenses associated with the delivery of nursing service.
5. Discuss budget monitoring.
6. Illustrate a scope of service.

You are assigned to a patient care unit for your clinical experience. You are wondering what types of services are provided to patients on this unit. You talk with your instructor and the nursing manager of the unit. Together, you review the unit's scope of service and budget.

What kinds of nursing services are provided to patients on this unit?

How does the unit's budget help ensure provision of care for patients on this unit?

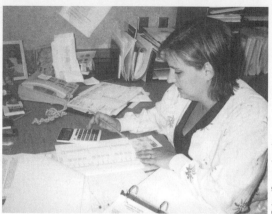

Delmar/Cengage Learning

Regardless of how expert, creative, collaborative, and altruistic a health care system may be, it cannot function without money. Securing the bottom line is basic to achieving the mission of providing health care. Nurses need to understand concepts of budgeting and economics to help secure this bottom line. **Economics** is the study of how scarce resources are allocated among possible uses in order to make appropriate choices among the increasingly scarce resources.

The study of economics is based on three general premises: (1) scarcity—resources exist in finite quantities and consumption demand is typically greater than resource supply; (2) choice—decisions are made about which resources to produce and consume among many options; and (3) preference—individual and societal values and preferences influence the decisions that are made. In a traditional market economy, the sellers sell to the buyers who buy, with each trying to maximize their gains from the transactions. Health care does not fit well in this model. For example, consider the concept of price elasticity, which is related to the price that an individual is willing to pay for a given item. Normally, as the price goes up, the demand goes down. When the purchase is health care, however, the price may be viewed as irrelevant to the decision to purchase. Think of a wristwatch that you might always purchase for $10, would likely not buy at $100, and would never consider at $1,000. Now, imagine that instead of a wristwatch, the item

in question is a medication or therapy needed to save your sick child. Now the consideration of price in the decision-making process is likely quite different. Thus, health care is much less "elastic" with reference to price than many other consumer goods.

Another aspect of health care's difference from the traditional economic model relates to the knowledge of options and payment mechanisms available to the consumer. In a typical market, the buyer is also the payer. In health care, the health care provider (buyer) ordering a hospitalization or treatment is a doctor or nurse. The provider is not the payer, nor is the patient (buyer) who is using the hospital or treatment the payer. The actual payer is the third-party reimburser (insurance company or government). Consequently, the financial impact of the decision on the provider (buyer) and the patient user (buyer) is skewed. Neither of these buyers is the payer.

This chapter presents basic health care budgeting and economics concepts that are important to the novice nurse entering clinical practice. Included are perspectives on the role cost has played and will play in directing health care delivery, the methods for determining the cost of delivering nursing care, and the effect of health care policy on the delivery of nursing care.

Common financial language and tools are discussed so nurses can understand the elements of cost-effective care.

SOME PERSPECTIVES ON THE COST OF HEALTH CARE

Socialized systems of providing health care are in place around the world. Philosophically, under such systems, complete health care and hospital care are provided to all the citizens in a community, district, or nation (universal access). However, it is important to realize that the term **socialized health care** refers to a variety of health care programs, each specific about what coverage is provided and how it is funded.

Savage, Hoelscher, and Walker (1999) studied seven industrialized European countries and Canada for commonalities in coverage and funding. Their work reveals both centralized and decentralized compulsory single-payer systems with fee-for-service components, as well as some private insurance components. Funding for the programs under study also varied. In general, care is funded through public taxation of citizens, who are then eligible for care but who may or may not use it. Programs in Canada, Sweden, and the United Kingdom are funded from income taxes and selected other taxes. Germany and the Netherlands rely on payroll taxes for funding. (Table 10-1).

The authors of the 1999 study pointed out that the countries studied face similar challenges of aging populations with chronic disease, the need to ration costly technology, severe budget shortages, managed competition, decentralization, and vertical integration. Compare the 1999 study findings to the 16% of the gross domestic product ($6,280 per capita) spent in 2004 by the United States, more than any other country in the world and nearly twice that of many of the European countries studied, as shown in Table 10-1. Still, there are nearly 47 million people in the United States without health insurance, and the United States continues to experience a stubbornly high infant mortality rate.

TABLE 10-1	PROJECTED COMPARISON OF HEALTH CARE SPENDING, INFANT MORTALITY RATE, AND LIFE EXPECTANCY ACROSS FOUR INDUSTRIALIZED COUNTRIES			
Country	% GDP	Infant Mortality Rate	Male Life Expectancy (years)	Female Life Expectancy (years)
United States	16.0	6.50	72.95	79.67
Germany	10.7	4.16	74.1	80.5
Canada	9.7	4.75	76.2	82.8
United Kingdom	6.9	5.16	74.7	80.2

Source: Percent of GDP and Infant Mortality Rate retrieved June 20, 2006, from www.en.wikipedia.org. Life Expectancy retrieved March 31, 2006, from www.photius.com.

THE COST EQUATION: MONEY = MISSION = MONEY

The mission statement of any health care business or unit describes the purpose for existence of the business or unit and the rationale that justifies that existence. The mission directs decision making about what is or is not within the purview of the business or unit. The vision statement is a logical extension of the mission into the future and establishes long-range goals for the business or unit. Once the vision is established and the business can articulate where it wants to go, a strategic plan that identifies how to achieve the vision or how to accomplish the

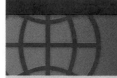

REAL WORLD INTERVIEW

During my many experiences over the past years with the Ontario, Canada, Health Care System and Ontario Health Insurance Program (OHIP), I have had annual visits to my General Practitioner (GP) with referrals to specialists for various tests, including x-rays, blood work, and hospital stays as needed. All my medical expenses while in these doctors' care are covered completely by the OHIP funds. Medications, glasses, and dental work are not covered unless one's gross annual income is a very minimal amount, in which case, some of them are covered.

My husband was a diabetic, and he had a stroke 20 years ago at the age of 53. His GP met us at the hospital and assessed him through triage. My husband lost the use of his right arm and leg and his ability to comprehend language. The supreme care and compassion of his doctors and nurses helped my husband and family cope with the severity of this horrific disease. We paid for an upgrade to a semiprivate room. All other expenses while he was in the hospital were covered by OHIP. His rehabilitation began two weeks after his stroke, and he was transferred to the rehabilitation center, where he stayed for three months. All expenses while he was there were funded by OHIP.

After his acute illness, my husband saw a specialist every three months to monitor his blood sugar levels. He saw his GP every three months for his hypertension and saw his optometrist every year. He went for speech therapy once a week, physical therapy three times a week, and went to a nutritionist twice a year. This was all covered by OHIP.

He had several episodes of congestive heart failure through the years. Each time, I called 911, and the fire department came within minutes, administered oxygen, and inquired about his medical problems and medications while waiting for the ambulance medics to arrive. The medics took his vitals, gave him nitro, and called the admitting hospital.

We have four hospitals in Hamilton, Ontario, where I live. In the emergency department (ED), my husband was always processed immediately. When a heart specialist was called in, it took about an hour for him to arrive. Then the heart specialist would decide whether my husband was to be admitted to Intensive Care or a ward. There were times when a bed was not available until the next day, and we had to wait in the ED.

All emergencies in our ED are taken care of fairly promptly, the most severe first. Elective surgery such as knee or hip replacements, eye cataracts, etc., require a longer waiting period, sometimes up to six months. Hospital and emergency patients are on the priority list for magnetic resonance imaging (MRI) and CT scans. Other patients may have to wait for a couple of months for these tests. I also have the option, if I can afford it, of visiting the Buffalo, New York area clinics for MRIs, etc., if it is not an emergency, and I want to do it quicker. I would have to pay for these visits and tests out of pocket. All in all, I have been fairly pleased with our Canadian health system.

Flo Paradisi
Hamilton, Ontario, Canada

goals is developed. There must be cohesion and consistency across the mission, vision, and strategic plan for the business or unit to successfully achieve its mission. There must also be money, for without it no mission can be accomplished.

BUSINESS PROFIT

Revenue (income) minus cost (expense) equals profit. Profit is not restricted to for-profit businesses. Profit is not a dirty word. All businesses must realize a profit to remain in business. In for-profit businesses, a portion of the profit is distributed to stockholders in appreciation for their investing in the business and the remainder is used to maintain and grow the organization. In nonprofit businesses, there are no stockholders to share the profit, so all of it is fed back into the business for maintenance and growth.

Not-for-profit organizations desiring a purer image than the term *profit* engenders refer to their profit as a contribution to **margin**, with the rule of thumb being to secure 4% to 5% of the total budget as profit or margin. A truism of business is: no margin, no mission. Mission and margin are strategically and operationally linked by the reality that resources are required to carry out the organization's strategic plan and achieve its mission. Without margin, or with limited margin, there would be a lack of money to replace worn-out equipment, to establish new services or enlarge existing services in response to changing community needs for health care, to purchase state-of-the-art technology, to

improve salaries, to maintain existing buildings or undertake new construction, and to replace heating and lighting systems. Failure to maintain such infrastructure can impair the organization's ability to be competitive, resulting in failure to meet its mission and eventual organizational failure.

INFORMATION TECHNOLOGY, SALARY AND MEDICATION COSTS

Close examination of a health care budget often reveals that although the nursing payroll is the most expensive payroll item and the most expensive operating budget item, the most expensive item on the total budget is often diagnostic, therapeutic, and information technology.

The high cost of technology has been recognized by regulatory agencies for many years. In pursuit of cost control in hospitals, the states independently established laws more than 30 years ago creating Certificate of Need (CON) agencies to oversee, regulate, and approve major technology and construction expenditures. A secondary goal was to ensure equitable distribution of and access to high-end technology across the state. The CON approach was not successful because it focused only on hospitals and provided no incentives to change either physician or patient behavior. Hospitals were given spending limits, but there was no incentive for physicians to change their practice, so they didn't. Without incentives, patients' expectations and demands for care also remained unchanged. More recently, managed care programs have exerted oversight of the use of complex, expensive technology by requiring justification and approval prior to its use for payment to occur. Also, there has been a movement toward rationing the most expensive technology to those with the ability and willingness to pay it over and above their health insurance coverage. The best-selling book *Who Lives? Who Dies? Ethical Criteria in Patient Selection* by John Kilner (1992) underscores public and professional concern about rationing. We have begun to see managed care programs become more lenient in response to a public and professional outcry

CRITICAL THINKING 10-1

You notice that a colleague frequently does not record patient charge items for elderly patients. When you inquire about it, you are told that your colleague feels sorry for those on fixed incomes and wants to save them money. Who pays when your colleague does this?

about who possesses the appropriate expertise to make clinical decisions.

COST OF MEDICATIONS AND HEALTH CARE EXECUTIVE SALARIES

Medications are a significant item in the overall budget. A recent health care Web site visit identified these drug charges. See Table 10-2. Also note the health care compensations shown in Table 10-3.

PAY-FOR-PERFORMANCE PROJECTS

An example of a Pay-for-Performance health care demonstration project is one that the Centers for Medicare and Medicaid Services (CMS) is doing in conjunction with Premier, Inc., a nationwide organization of not-for-profit hospitals. CMS will reward participating top-performing hospitals by increasing their payment for Medicare patients. Top-performing hospitals will receive bonuses based on their performance on evidence-based quality measures for inpatients with heart attack, heart failure, pneumonia, coronary artery bypass graft, and hip and knee replacements. This is a three-year demonstration project that is expected to cost roughly $7 million a year for each of the

three years. CMS has indicated that financial awards will be paid as follows:

- Hospitals in the top decile of hospitals for a given diagnosis will be provided a 2% bonus of their Medicare payments for the measured condition.
- Hospitals in the second decile will be paid a 1% bonus.
- In year three, hospitals that don't achieve performance improvements above the demonstration baseline will have their payments adjusted.
- Hospitals will receive 1% lower Diagnosis Related Group (DRG) payments for clinical conditions that score below the ninth decile and 2% lower if they score below the tenth decile. **Diagnosis Related Group (DRG)** is a Medicare system used to classify hospital patients into one of approximately 500 groups that are expected to use similar hospital resources and have similar needs and outcomes. (Diagnosis-related Group, 2009).

NURSING COST

Fiscally, most organizations view nursing as a cost center that does not independently generate revenue. Although some deviation from that fiscal philosophy may occur when selected nursing practitioners are permitted by law to bill directly

TABLE 10-2	COST OF SELECTED MEDICATIONS
Drug and Doses Cost	
Acyclovir-90	$43.49
Advair Diskus-180	$555.95
Lipitor-90	$237.99
Lisinopril-90	$31.99
Lorazepam-90	$43.99
Nexium-90	$429.97

Source: Compare drug prices. (2009). Available at www.drugstore.com/

TABLE 10-3	HEALTH CARE COMPENSATION

	Annual Salary
Jeff Barbakow, Executive, Tenet Healthcare	$35 million
Miles White, Executive, Abbott Laboratories	$30.4 million
Richard Jay Kagan, Executive, Schering-Plough	$24.4 million
Chief Executive Officer (CEO)–Non-MD	$231,404
Chief Executive Officer (CEO)–MD	$275,123
Director of Human Resources	$82,690
Medical Director	$241,670
Director of Nursing	$82,138
Nurse Practitioner	$82,513
Physical Therapist	$63,117
Cardiologist	$370,295
Anesthesiologist	$344,691
General Surgeon	$327,902
Family Medicine MD	$185,740
Emergency Care MD	$255,530
Dentist	$165,599

Source: Useem, J. (2003, April 28). Have they no shame? *Fortune, 147*(8), 56–64, and 2007 American Medical Group Association Compensation Data available at www.cejkasearch.com/compensation/amqa_administrative_compennsation_survey.htm.

for their unique professional services, the cost of providing nursing care (wages, benefits, selected supplies and equipment, overhead) is commonly bundled into a catchall, room, or per diem, cost that assumes that every patient consumes identical nursing resources each day. Such a view is not only antiquated, it is incorrect. Nursing care is not an identical product delivered in assembly-line fashion. It varies remarkably in intensity, in depth, and in breadth across patients, consistent with their unique, individual dependency needs.

Access to a high degree of nursing care is an important reason for hospitalization. When access to both nursing care and medical technology is needed, hospitalization is unquestionably appropriate. Consequently, the revenue generated from hospitalization is, in fact, payment primarily for consumption of medical technology and nursing services and should be recognized as such.

TYPES OF BUDGETS

Health care organizations use several types of budgets to help with future planning and management. A **budget** is a plan that provides formal quantitative expression for acquiring and distributing funds over the ensuing time period (generally one year). A budget is based on what is known about how much was spent in the past and how that will inevitably change in the coming year. The types of budgets are operational, capital, and construction.

OPERATIONAL BUDGET

An **operational budget** accounts for the income and expenses associated with day-to-day activity within a department or organization. Revenue generation is based on billable services and expenses associated with equipment, supplies, staffing, and other indirect costs. Revenue may be based on the number of days that a patient stays on an inpatient unit or the number of hours spent in a procedure room. Revenue may also be based on the types of procedures delivered to a patient. Depending on reimbursement rates and requirements, expenses are sometimes bundled or included into a procedure or room charge, for example, an admission packet that includes a washbasin, cup, soap holder, and so on. In other situations, supply items may be billed separately, such as IV start kits, leukocyte removal filters, and so on.

CAPITAL BUDGET

A **capital budget** accounts for the purchase of major new or replacement equipment. Equipment is purchased when new technology becomes available or when older equipment becomes too expensive to maintain because of age-related problems such as inefficiencies resulting from the decreased speed of equipment or increased downtime (amount of time it is out of service for repairs). Sometimes equipment maintenance is cost-prohibitive due to the expense and limited availability of replacement parts. Other times equipment may become antiquated because of its inability to deliver service consistently, meet industry or regulatory standards, or provide high-quality outcomes.

CONSTRUCTION BUDGET

A **construction budget** is developed when renovation or new structures are planned. The construction budget generally includes labor, materials, building permits, inspections, equipment, and so on. If it is anticipated that a department will need

to close during construction, then projected lost revenue is accounted for in the budget. Revenue and expenses may also be shifted to another department that absorbs the services on a temporary basis.

BUDGET OVERVIEW

An operational budget is a financial tool that outlines anticipated revenue and expenses over a specified period. A process called **accounting**, which is an activity that managers engage in to record and report financial transactions and data, assists with budget documentation. Budgets serve as standards to plan, monitor, and evaluate the performance of a health care system. Budgets account for the income generated as compared to the expenses needed to deliver the service. **Profit** is determined by the relationship of income to expenses. Profitability results when the income is higher than the expenses.

Budgets make the connection between operational planning and allocation of resources. This is especially important because health care organizations measure multiple key indicators of overall performance. These key indicators can be illustrated in a dashboard. A **dashboard** is a documentation tool providing a snapshot image of pertinent information and activity at a particular point in time. A dashboard or balanced scorecard identifies any of four perspectives of an organization: finances, customer satisfaction and services, internal operating efficiency, and learning and growth (Norton & Kaplan, 2001). Figure 10-1 shows the dashboard of two separate units: gastrointestinal laboratory (GI lab) and a medical unit. **Variance**, or the difference between what was budgeted and the actual result, can be tracked.

BUDGET PREPARATION AND SCOPE OF SERVICE

Formulating a budget involves a systematic approach that begins with preparation. Budgets are generally developed for a 12-month period and are monitored monthly. The yearly cycle can be based on a

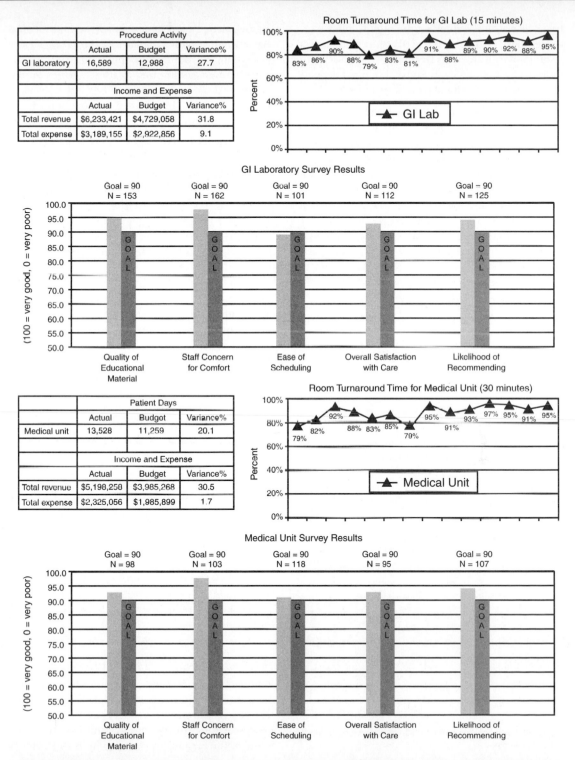

Figure 10-1 Patient satisfaction, turnaround time, and budget activity. (*Source:* Adapted with permission of Northwestern Memorial Hospital, Chicago, IL).

fiscal year as determined by the organization (e.g., September 1 through August 31) or a calendar year (e.g., January 1 through December 31). Shorter- or longer-term budgets may also be developed depending on the organizational planning process.

Prior to the beginning of the budget year, most organizations devote approximately six months to preparing and developing the operational budget. To prepare a budget, organizations gather fundamental information about a variety of elements that influence the organization, including patient demographic and marketing information such as age, race, sex, and income; competitive analysis; regulatory influences; strategic plans; goals; and history. Additionally, it is helpful to review the department's scope of service. See Figure 10-2.

MARKETING

Pulling together demographic information relative to the population that the organization serves is most helpful because it identifies unique market

A medical nursing unit provides primarily inpatient care to patients with acute or chronic medical problems, such as congestive heart failure, diabetes, pulmonary disease, and cancer. The unit, equipped with 30 private beds, a full kitchen, a lounge, and conference/consultation rooms, is operational 24 hours per day, 7 days per week. Patient education and support groups are held routinely in the library located directly on the unit. Team nursing is employed as the model of care. Nurses, patient care technicians, and unit secretaries are employed, with a social worker and diabetes educator providing additional patient support. Patients admitted to the unit for longer than 48 hours are discussed during daily multidisciplinary rounds. The rounds include case management personnel; psychosocial counselors; and nutrition, nursing, and medical staff. Staff discuss patient problems to facilitate future care, including discharge planning.

Figure 10-2 Medical nursing unit, scope of service. (Delmar/Cengage Learning).

characteristics, such as age, race, sex, and income that influence patient behavior. Marketing strategies are built around the population types that an organization is attempting to attract. For example, if a hospital is opening an open heart or transplant department, then outreach activities might be developed to attract those patients that can benefit from the specialty screening, prevention, or treatment services.

Marketing is the process of creating a product or health care service for patients and it uses the four P's of marketing, that is, Patient, Product, Price, and Placement, to place desirable health care services or products in desirable locations at a price that benefits both patients and the health care facility. In this way, the health care facility, the patient, and the community benefit. Marketing of services does have a price tag, such as the cost of advertising campaigns on television and radio. Using printed materials, mailing information to patient residences, and advertising in journals, magazines, and newspapers are all examples of ways to educate and stimulate the public for future referrals for health care services. Once marketing strategies are implemented, most organizations attempt to measure their effectiveness, or return on investment.

COMPETITIVE ANALYSIS

A competitive analysis is important because it probes how the competition is performing as compared to other health care organizations. A competitive analysis examines other hospitals or practices' strengths and weaknesses, in addition to details such as location and new or existing services and technology. Figure 10-3 presents a competitive analysis of three different hospitals.

REGULATORY INFLUENCES

Regulatory requirements and reimbursement rates have an effect on financial performance. Regulatory changes are influenced by several governing bodies. A government agency that has high visibility in the area of reimbursement is the Centers

Competitive Analysis: Hospital A

Location: Rural—100 miles from metropolitan area

Affiliation: Currently negotiating with three academic hospitals

General clinical description:
- Scattered bed approach to inpatient oncology
- Ambulatory chemotherapy clinic
- Many of the same physicians on staff at Hospital J

Radiation capability: None—refers to Hospital J

Support services: Cancer screenings offered sporadically

Miscellaneous:
- Tumor board
- Cancer committee

Competitive Analysis: Hospital B

Location: Suburb of large metropolitan city

Affiliation: University hospital

General clinical description:
- Dedicated oncology inpatient unit
- Ambulatory chemotherapy department
- Comprehensive breast center
- Head and neck oncology team

Radiation therapy:
- Linear accelerator—two units
- High dose rate
- Intraoperative radiation therapy
- Stereotactic radiosurgery

Support services:
- Home infusion and home care program
- Hospice care program
- Annual cancer awareness fair
- Support group—general cancer patients

Miscellaneous:
- Tumor registry
- Tumor board
- Committee on cancer
- Head and neck patient conferences
- Stereotactic radiosurgery conferences

Competitive Analysis: Hospital C

Location: Urban city with a population of 150,000

Affiliation: For-profit corporation
- Medical oncology affiliation with University K
- Radiation Therapy Department affiliation with University K Radiation Therapy Department

General clinical description:
- Dedicated inpatient medical oncology unit
- Dedicated inpatient surgical oncology unit
- Four-bed autologous and stem cell bone marrow transplant unit (Eastern Cooperative Oncology Group Referral Center for autologous bone marrow transplants)
- Coagulation laboratory
- Therapeutic pheresis
- Pain clinic
- Oncology clinic
- Oncology rehabilitation
- Breast cancer rehabilitation program
- Ambulatory care chemotherapy unit
- Medical oncologist on staff at two hospitals

Radiation therapy:
- Linear accelerator
- Stereotactic radiosurgery
- Hyperthermia
- Brachytherapy

Support services:
- Home health and hospice program
- Cancer registry
- Cancer committee
- Physician update—quarterly cancer newsletter
- Cancer information line
- Cancer advisory council
- Cancer Survivor's Day offered annually
- Cancer screenings offered routinely
- Cancer support group—general cancer patients

Figure 10-3 Competitive analysis of three hospitals. (Delmar/Cengage Learning).

for Medicare and Medicaid Services (CMS), whose mission is to ensure health care security for beneficiaries. CMS (www.cms.hhs.gov) administers federal control, quality assurance, and fraud and abuse prevention for Medicare, Medicaid, and the State Children's Health Insurance Program (SCHIP). Under the aegis of the Department of Health and Human Services, it is also responsible for coordinating health care policy, planning, and legislation.

CASE STUDY 10-1

The manager from an inpatient unit asks for staff input into identifying ways to decrease use of health care supply and paper items. These items have been identified as being in excess of the budget by 10% to 20% during the past three months. This is the first time that the staff have been involved in helping with cost containment. Clinical nurses and assistants have been invited to participate.

When approaching an analysis of health care supply use, what might be the first step in the process? If you were to break the staff into work groups, which members should be chosen to analyze the use of clerical supplies? How would you proceed if you were trying to determine the supply costs associated with starting an IV with continuous intravenous infusions and medications? Would nursing and pharmacy be helpful in this process?

Other regulatory bodies play a role in reimbursement by ensuring that federal and state laws are adhered to through approval and accreditation. For example, the Food and Drug Administration (www.fda.gov) regulates the use of drugs, food products, and medical devices in the United States. If equipment or drugs under its jurisdiction are not approved, then organizations cannot bill for their use, by law. The Joint Commission (JC) (www.jointcommission.org) accredits hospitals and health care agencies to ensure that they meet specific standards. Medicare and Medicaid will not reimburse for services unless a hospital is accredited by the JC.

Regulatory requirements may change regarding who may deliver a specific service and in what type of setting; for example, a procedure may have to be done in the hospital rather than in a practitioner's office if it is to be reimbursed by the insurance company. Medicare and Medicaid change their reimbursement rates periodically. Total and partial coverage of specific procedures can change and may not be predictable from year to year.

Managed care organizations and insurance companies typically negotiate rates on a yearly basis, which can affect hospital revenue. Consumers' willingness to pay out of pocket when not covered by insurance affects revenue as well.

STRATEGIC PLANS, GOALS, AND HISTORY

During the budget preparation phase, it is important to examine the history of an individual nursing or hospital department or section thoroughly. Hospital systems are frequently divided into sections, departments, or units to compartmentalize them for organizational purposes. These subsections or units, commonly called **cost centers**, are used to track financial data. Each department or cost center defines its own scope of service, goals, and strategic plans. This is an ongoing, ever-changing process.

REVENUE PROJECTIONS

Revenue is income generated through a variety of means, including billable patient services, investments, and donations to the organization. Specific unit-based revenue is generated through billing for services such as x-rays, invasive diagnostic or therapeutic procedures, drug therapy, surgical procedures, and physical therapy. Revenue can also be generated through the delivery of multiple services over time, such as hourly rates for chemotherapy administration or blood transfusions. The specific number and types of services and procedures have to be projected for the budget. The payments received by hospitals often do not equal the actual hospital or unit charges for the services rendered. For example, there may be a fixed or flat reimbursement rate per case regardless of how long the patient stays in the hospital or how much the hospital pays for the service. If the costs exceed the reimbursement rate, then the provider absorbs the remaining costs.

It is important to note that the reimbursement rates of third-party payers affect revenue and can change from year to year. Uniform rates are often used, which transfers significant financial risk to the provider. Medicare, Medicaid, managed care companies, and insurance companies dictate or negotiate rates with health care organizations that may include discounts or allowances. Payers determine what costs are allowable for procedures, visits, or services. Payment schedules vary from state to state and among plans. Additionally, the rates can change monthly such as with the ambulatory payment classification (APC) system from Medicare, which applies to the outpatient setting. The reimbursement rates or payments received by hospitals often do not equal the actual hospital or unit charges for the services rendered. For example, there may be a fixed or flat reimbursement rate per case regardless of how long the patient stays in the hospital or how much the hospital pays for the service. If the costs exceed the reimbursement rate, then the provider absorbs the remaining costs.

Another payment classification system called diagnosis-related groups (DRGs) is used to group inpatients into categories based upon the number of inpatient days, age, complications, and so on. Reimbursement covers room and board, tests, and therapy during a predetermined length of stay.

Some patients will not have health care insurance nor the ability to pay their bills. Therefore, the hospital may receive only a portion of the payment for services, if any.

Typically, organizations will review their payer mix to determine the percentage of patients carrying different types of health care coverage (Figure 10-4). The proportions help measure the anticipated dollars to be received for services delivered and projections for the coming year.

If charges for patient care are negotiated with a third-party payer, such as insurance companies and managed care corporations, they are preestablished

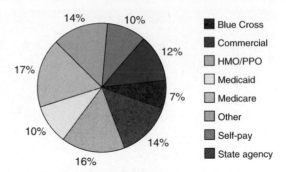

The reimbursement rates vary depending upon the payer. For example, Medicare may reimburse 40% of charges, Medicaid's rate may be 30%, and managed care may be at 60%. Factoring in reimbursement rates leads to profit and loss calculations for an organization.

Figure 10-4 Inpatient payer mix. (Delmar/Cengage Learning).

and are not negotiable once established. Third-party payers often impose a penalty fee, as a disincentive, if a health care organization changes a charge under contract. The penalty often exceeds the charge amount and will usually create a loss for the organization.

The following illustrates the differences in reimbursement related to a procedure. The charge for a central line placement is $2,500, which includes the use of the fluoroscopy equipment, supplies, nursing, and technical time. If a hospital places 200 central lines per year, then the anticipated total revenue is $500,000. The breakdown of third-party payers becomes important because the total revenue does not mean that the hospital will be reimbursed for the full amount of $500,000. Third-party payers typically contract with health care organizations for the amount that the third-party payer is willing to pay or reimburse. Table 10-4 demonstrates the potential reimbursement rates based upon varying third-party payers.

EXPENSE PROJECTIONS

Expenses are determined by identifying the costs associated with the delivery of service. Budget expenditures are resources used by an organization to deliver services and may include supplies, staffing, labor, equipment, utilities, and miscellaneous items. See Figure 10-5.

TABLE 10-4	TOTAL CHARGES—CENTRAL LINE PLACEMENT $500.000	
Third Party Payer Reimbursement	**Rate (Measured in Percent of Charges)**	**Expected Reimbursement**
Managed Care	60%	$300,000
Medicare	40%	$200,000
Medicaid	30%	$150,000

	Budget	Actual	% Variance	Comments/Actions
Revenue				
Inpatient	21,171,760	22,011,344	4	Patient days increasing
Outpatient	393,863	412,318	4.7	Clinic visits are increasing
	List all line items over or under budget			
Overall Expenses	3,370,828	3,400,795	(.1)	Expenses in line with budget
Salary	3,071,298	3,034,483	(1.2)	Salary is over budget consistently with added FTEs
Full-time equivalent employees (FTEs)	56.5	55.5	(1.2)	Increasing FTEs to accommodate volume and census
RN	46.6	45.4	(1.2)	
Assistive Staff	10.1	10.0	0.0	
Overall Medical Supplies	120,223	129,742	(9)	Supplies are over budget due to volume
IV Sets	80,000	85,000	(9)	Higher acuity patients requiring multiple IVs
Surgical Instruments	20,000	18,008	9	
Phlebotomy Supplies	21,742	17,722	8	
Clerical Supplies	1,629	2,460	(6.6)	Implementation of electronic medical record delayed Increasing paper expense
Paper Supply	1,300	1,800	(7.2)	Patient education materials are increasing, causing higher expense
Purchased Service	183,752	193,790	(5.5)	Consultant expense for bed and board
Transportation	75,000	72,000		
Maintenance	150,800	125,700	8.3	
Continuing Education	1,500	1,500	0	
Staff Training	1,985	1,900	9	

Figure 10-5 Cardiovascular nursing step down unit budget (CVT step down). (*Source:* Used with permission of Northwestern Memorial Hospital, Chicago, IL).

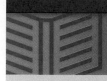

EVIDENCE FROM THE LITERATURE

Citation: Needleman, J., Buerhaus, P., Mattke, S., Stewart, M., & Zelevinsky, K. (2002). Nurse-Staffing Levels and the Quality of Care in Hospitals. *New England Journal of Medicine, 346*(22), 1714–1722.

Discussion: Administrative data from 799 hospitals in 11 states (covering 5,075,969 discharges of medical patients and 1,104,659 discharges of surgical patients) was examined to note the relationship between the amount of care provided by nurses at the hospital and patients' outcomes.

The mean number of hours of nursing care per patient day was 11.4, of which 7.8 hours were provided by registered nurses, 1.2 hours by licensed practical nurses, and 2.4 hours by nurses' aides. Among medical patients, a higher proportion of hours of care per day provided by registered nurses and a greater absolute number of hours of care per day provided by registered nurses were associated with a shorter length of stay ($P = 0.01$ and $P < 0.001$, respectively), and lower rates of both urinary tract infections ($P < 0.001$ and $P = 0.003$, respectively) and upper gastrointestinal bleeding ($P = 0.03$ and $P = 0.007$, respectively). A higher proportion of hours of care provided by registered nurses was also associated with lower rates of pneumonia ($P = 0.001$), shock or cardiac arrest ($P = 0.007$), and "failure to rescue," which was defined as death from pneumonia, shock or cardiac arrest, upper gastrointestinal bleeding, sepsis, or deep venous thrombosis ($P 5 0.05$). Among surgical patients, a higher proportion of care provided by registered nurses was associated with lower rates of urinary tract infections ($P = 0.04$), and a greater number of hours of care per day provided by registered nurses was associated with lower rates of "failure to rescue" ($P = 0.008$). No associations existed between increased levels of staffing by registered nurses and the rate of in-hospital death or between increased staffing by licensed practical nurses or nurses' aides and the rate of adverse outcomes.

Implications for Practice: A higher proportion of hours of nursing care provided by registered nurses and a greater number of hours of care by registered nurses per day are associated with better care for hospitalized patients and improved outcomes.

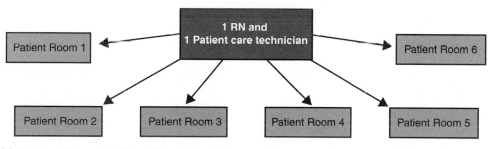

Figure 10-6 Inpatient staffing model. (Delmar/Cengage Learning).

STAFFING The amount and types of staff are often accounted for in a staffing model. The model outlines the number of staff required based upon a primary statistic such as procedures or patients. Figure 10-6 illustrates a sample staffing model.

Staffing ratios and salary data are particularly important because of the cost factor. Specialty salaries fluctuate, depending upon supply and demand. When there are shortages of certain staff, the salary tends to increase. Additionally, a health

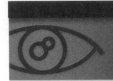

CRITICAL THINKING 10-2

You work in an Emergency Department (ED) that sees 6,000 patients a month. Patients are charged $200.00 per visit plus charges for tests and medications. Thus, these 6,000 patients can generate $1,200,000 in gross revenue for the hospital. Consider that there are 15 RNs making $30.00 per hour and 6 MDs making $150.00 per hour working each shift. Salaries for the RNs total $324,000. Salaries for the MDs total $648,000. The total monthly salary for these two groups is $972,000. Of the 6,000 patients, 50% have Medicare/Medicaid, 45% are covered by managed care or insurance, and 5% have no insurance. Thus, just 95% of patients can pay their bills. The other 5% of patients' bills are written off by the hospital as bad debt.

Medicare/Medicaid/Managed Care/Insurance companies often only pay 55% of the bills for these patients. They may deny payment for 45% of the bills. Thus, for the $1,140,000 billed (95% of $1,200,000), the hospital will receive approximately $627,000 (55% of the $1,140,000 billed). Approximately $513,000 of the bill will not be paid by Medicare/Medicaid/ Managed Care/Insurance. Consider the following:

What other expenses besides salary must the hospital pay out of the $627,000 that it receives? Consider hospital space, liability insurance, technology costs, and so on. Consider that the hospital will also be partially reimbursed for all services delivered during the patient's visit.

Notice the effect that increasing the volume of patients has on your budget figures. What happens to your budget if the patient volume goes to 8,000 patient ED visits per month and staffing stays the same?

Are patients receiving useful information about future illness prevention and healthy living practices in the ED?

Is this a cost-effective way to deliver health care?

How could we better serve the health care needs of Americans?

care organization may change its benefits, offering a more attractive package that includes continuing education; paid time off for education, vacation, sick time, or personal needs; or professional membership expenses. Institutions may also look for alternative ways to supplement or deliver services during staff shortages. This means that supplemental staff—professional agency nurses, nurses from in-house registries, or patient care technicians—may be hired at a different salary rate. It is important to note whether a unit has had historical difficulty retaining or recruiting staff. Recruitment and retention, especially attracting, interviewing, hiring, and orienting staff, require dollars. For example, it has been estimated that the turnover cost

per nurse, including advertising, recruitment, orientation, and time to fill the vacancy, can equate to $67,000 (Jones, 2005). The average cost to educate a nurse during a 6-week orientation period is more than $5,000. Not only the salary but also benefits and unproductive time are frequently factored into a salary package, and they need to be included in the budget. See Table 10-5.

DIRECT AND INDIRECT EXPENSES

Expenses can be further broken down into direct and indirect. **Direct expenses** are those expenses directly associated with the patient, such as medical and surgical supplies, wages, and drugs. **Indirect expenses** are expenses for items such as

TABLE 10-5	UNPRODUCTIVE TIME	
Unproductive Time	**Number of Days**	**Salary***
Vacation	21	$4,200
Holiday	7	$1,400
Sick	5	$1,000
Personal	3	$ 600
Education	1	$ 200
Total	37	$7,400

*Salary dollars are based upon an average rate of $25.00 per hour. Remember to calculate the number of days times eight hour shifts. The salary dollars change depending upon pay rate and shifts, for example, day shift versus evening shift differential or ten and twelve hour shift rates.

utilities—gas, electric, and phones—that are not directly related to patient care but are necessary to support care. Other support functions frequently charged to a department that are not specifically related to patient care delivery are housekeeping, maintenance, materials management, and finance.

FIXED AND VARIABLE COSTS. **Fixed costs** are those expenses that are constant and are not related to productivity or volume. Examples of these costs are building and equipment depreciation, utilities, fringe benefits, and administrative salaries. **Variable costs** fluctuate depending upon the volume or census and types of care required. Medical and surgical supplies, drugs, laundry, and food costs often increase the volume.

BUDGET APPROVAL AND MONITORING

Once developed, budgets are submitted to administration for review and approval, and the entire health care team is then responsible for ensuring that expenses are kept within the budgeted amount. The manner in which this is accomplished depends on the organization. Some institutions request that budget dashboards (see Figure 10-7) be developed reflecting monthly departmental activity at a glance. Note that one can review patient volume/access, patient satisfaction, human resources staffing, expenses, and budget monthly using this dashboard. Variance reports or dashboards may be posted so that all staff members have an opportunity to review the budget and participate in any needed improvement.

Staff can meet to discuss implementation or reinforcement of strategies that can positively affect the dashboard. Following are examples of such strategies:

- Analyze time efficiency of staff involved in patient care.
- Plan for supplies needed for every patient encounter and consciously eliminate unnecessary items.
- Learn how a department is reimbursed for services delivered, identifying covered and excluded expenses.

Year to Date Volume/Access					
Department	**Cost Center**	**Volume Year to Date**	**Percentage Budget Variance**	**Percentage Variance from Last Year**	**Days to Next Appointment/ Available Bed**
GI Laboratory	1265	6,706	16	23	3
Medical Unit	7095	9,705	18	28	1
Patient Satisfaction					
	Overall Score		Percentile	Percentile	Results Reporting
Department	**Actual**	**Target**	**Actual**	**Target**	**Average Report Turnaround Time** / **Reports > 24**
GI laboratory	90.5	91.70	90	95	28 / 20%
Medical unit	89	90.00	88	92	NA / NA
Human Resources					
					Employee Performance
		Actual	**Vacancies**	**Turnover**	**Staff Performance Reviews on Time**
Department	**Manager**	**FTEs Year to Date**	**Year to Date**	**Rate**	**> 30 Days**
GI laboratory	1	33.00	0.4	8%	0
Medical unit	1	45.00	6	12%	1
Expenses					
				Supply	Productivity
		Percentage of Budget Compared to Actual	**Percentage Variance from Budget Year to Date**	**Variance from Budget Year to Date**	**Variance from Last Year**
Department					
GI laboratory	250	(5.00)	11.00	unfavorable	unfavorable
Medical unit	118	8.00	12.00	favorable	unfavorable
Capital Budget					
Line Items	**Number**	**Year**	**Budgeted**	**Expensed**	**Balance**
GI lab					
7 Video endoscopes	10002895	2001	112,550.00	109,389.19	14,226.00
Endoscopy travel cart	30256409	2001	2,750.00	0.00	32,750.00
Scopes	89756452	2001	38,255.00	35,225.00	1,199.00
Comments					
Financial improvement plan ongoing in GI lab: Interventional charges have been adjusted and cost reduction/inventory control is being explored with materials management.					
Medical nursing unit has achieved highest overall patient satisfaction goal. Multidisciplinary conferences are being held every other day to focus on patient care issues.					

Figure 10-7 G1 laboratory and medical unit dashboard. (*Source:* Adapted with permission of Northwestern Memorial Hospital, Chicago, IL).

- Explore new products with vendor representatives, and network with colleagues who have tried both new and modified products.
- Reduce the length of stay by troubleshooting early.
- Enhance productivity through rigorous process improvement.
- Ensure that staff have the right tools and that the tools are ready when needed.

- Track various steps in patient care that are time consuming or problematic for a unit (e.g., communication from front desk to recovery room, staff response to patient call lights, number of staff responding to an emergency code).
- Acquire a working knowledge of how a department/unit monitors financial and quality indicators, and participate in the development of action plans to increase patient satisfaction or to create the "best patient experience."

KEY CONCEPTS

- Nurses play an integral role in the development, implementation, and evaluation of a unit or department budget.

- Hospitals use several types of budgets to help with future planning and management. These include operational, capital, and construction budgets.

- The budget preparation phase is one of data gathering related to a variety of elements that influence an organization, including demographic information, marketing, competitive analysis, regulatory influences, and strategic plans. Additionally, it is helpful to understand the department's scope of service, goals, and history.

- Once background data have been gathered, the development of the budget can follow. This includes projecting revenue and expenses.

- Expenses are determined by identifying the cost associated with the delivery of service. Expenditures are resources used by an organization to deliver services and may include labor, supplies, equipment, utilities, and miscellaneous items.

- Once developed, budgets are submitted to administration for review and final approval. The approval process may take several months as the unit budgets are combined to determine the overall budget for the health care organization.

- Health care economics is grounded in past values and culture. Nearly 150 years ago, Florence Nightingale recognized that the resources being used to care for sick people ought to be tracked and analyzed to improve clinical and business outcomes.

- In the United States, multiple programs exist to pay for health care.

- Industrialized countries around the world offer tax-supported socialized health care to every citizen through centralized or decentralized programs at about half of the U.S. per capita cost.

- The ability to track and manage both cost and quality is critical to achieve an organization's economic and quality goals.

KEY TERMS

accounting

budget

capital budget

construction budget

cost centers

dashboard

Diagnosis Related Group (DRG)

direct expenses

economics

fixed costs

indirect expenses

margin

marketing

operational budget

profit

revenue

socialized health care

variable costs

variance

REVIEW QUESTIONS

1. An operational budget accounts for
   A. the purchase of minor and major equipment.
   B. construction and renovation.
   C. income and expenses associated with daily activity within an organization.
   D. applications for new technology.
2. Economics is the study of
   A. the cost:quality interface.
   B. cost accounting.
   C. the cost of doing business.
   D. how to manage scarcity of resources.
3. Profit is synonymous with
   A. dividends.
   B. billing privileges.
   C. margin.
   D. certificate of need.
4. The following should be done immediately after an operational budget has been put into place:
   A. Demographic information
   B. Regulatory influences
   C. Competitive analysis
   D. Budget monitoring

REVIEW ACTIVITIES

1. Review Figure 10-3. Construct a competitive analysis for two nursing units where you are doing your clinical experience. What did you observe?
2. Look around your clinical agency. Do you see any dashboards? What do they reveal about your agency?
3. Interview the nurse manager of a health care organization to gain an understanding of how various costs are managed. Use the following questions to guide the interview:

What method is used to measure nursing cost?
How are contracts with various insurers such as Medicare, Medicaid, Blue Cross, and managed care discounted?
What percentage of profit did the organization make last year, and how was it allocated?
Which professional services are billed directly?

EXPLORING THE WEB

- Go to the site for the Joint Commission and look for budgeting-related information: *www.jointcommission.org*
- Review the site for the American Organization of Nurse Executives: *www.aone.org*
- Visit the site for nurse-sensitive outcomes at: *www.nursingworld.org*
- Review these sites for helpful information. What did you find there? Healthcare Financial Management Association: *www.hfma.org*

American College of Healthcare Executives:
www.ache.org
Centers for Medicare and Medicaid Services:
www.cms.hhs.gov
Agency for Healthcare Research and Quality:
www.ahrq.gov

■ Search an alternate government bureau site to
see what professionally relevant information you
can find:
www.bls.gov

■ Search the following sites for information of
interest to nurses:
www.florence-nightingale.co.uk
www.aahn.org
www.webmd.com
www.medexplorer.com
www.healthology.com
www.medicarerights.org

REFERENCES

American Medical Group Association Compensation Data. (2007). Available at www.cms.hhs.gov/AcuteInpatientPPS/Downloads/AMGA_2007%20Report.pdf.

Compare drug prices. (2009). Available at www.drugstore.com/. Click on Compare drug prices.

Diagnosis-related Group. (2009). Available at en.wikipedia.org/wiki/Diagnosis-related_group#References.

Jones, C. B. (2005). The Costs of Nurse Turnover, Part 2. *Journal of Nursing Administration, 35*(1), 41–49.

Kilner, J. F. (1990). Who lives? Who Dies? Ethical Criteria in Patient Selection. New Haven: Yale University Press.

Needleman, J., Buerhaus, P., Mattke, S., Stewart, M., & Zelevinsky, K. (2002). Nurse-Staffing Levels and the Quality of Care in Hospitals. *New England Journal of Medicine, 346*(22), 1714–1722.

Nightingale, F. (1859). *Notes on hospitals; being two papers read before the National Association for the Promotion of Social Science, at Liverpool in October, 1858. With evidence given to the Royal Commissioners on the State of the Army in 1857* (2nd ed.). London: Parker.

Norton, D., & Kaplan, R. (2001). *The strategy-focused organization: How balanced scorecard companies thrive in the new business environment.* Boston: Harvard Business School Press.

Savage, G., Hoelscher, M., & Walker, E. (1999). International health care: A comparison of the United States, Canada, and Western Europe. In L. Wolper (Ed.), *Health care administration: Planning, implementing, and managing organized delivery systems* (3rd ed). Gaithersburg, MD: Aspen.

Useem, J. (2003, April 28). Have they no shame? *Fortune, 147*(8), 56–64.

SUGGESTED READINGS

Joint Commission. (JC). (2006). *Comprehensive Accreditation Manual for Hospitals (CAMH): The Official Handbook.* Oakbrook Terrace, IL: Joint Commission.

Vonderheid, S., Pohl, J., Schafer, P., Forrest, K., Poole, M., Barkauskas, V., et al. (2004). Using FTE and RVU performance measures to assess financial viability of academic nurse-managed centers. *Nursing Economics, 22*(3), 124–134.

Wagner, C., Budreau, G., & Everett, L. (2005). Analyzing fluctuating unit census for timely staffing intervention. *Nursing Economics, 23*(2), 85–90.

CHAPTER 11

Planning Care

OBJECTIVES

Upon completion of this chapter, the reader should be able to:

1. Discuss assessment of the external and internal environment of health care.
2. Review SWOT analysis.
3. Articulate the importance of aligning the organization's strategic vision with the organization's mission, philosophy, and goals.
4. Review common organizational structures.
5. Discuss shared governance.
6. Identify the Fourteen Forces of Magnetism.

The patient care manager of an acute care surgical unit has been informed that there are plans to merge that unit with an ambulatory surgery unit that currently cares for patients requiring 24-hour observation. The patient care manager has been recommended to oversee the development of the new work unit. The institution believes the creation of this new unit will enhance revenue, staff productivity, and outcomes of patient care. Therefore, resources are available to design and staff the new work unit in a manner that is congruent with the institution's mission, with the understanding that the investment will bring added value to the organization.

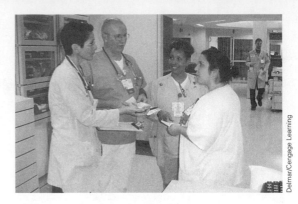

What are your reactions as a new nurse on this unit?

What unit structures and patient care processes need to be put in place?

What outcomes should you monitor?

How will you ensure your competency and continued professional growth on this new unit?

Planning patient care requires care delivery structures, processes, and measures of the outcome of care delivery. Planning must be consistent with the needs of the patients, the community, and the mission and vision of the organization. Planning is built on values and a philosophy of professional nursing practice.

The seminal (1999) Institute of Medicine (IOM) report *To Err Is Human* states that preventable adverse events cause between 44,000 and 98,000 deaths each year at an annual cost of between $37.6 billion to $50 billion. That report and the follow-up IOM report, *Crossing the Quality Chasm* (2001), have changed the way we view quality and patient safety. It is now generally understood that patient safety is dependent on the implementation of collaborative teams and interdisciplinary focused care-delivery systems that address the realities of practice and patient care. Recent research studies stress that the way a nurse's work is organized is a major determinant of patient welfare. Consequently, nurses in leadership positions must be educationally prepared to be able to develop and implement sound models for the effective

delivery of patient care. Although many health care organizations collect large sets of data and are beginning to use scientific methods to improve the services they render, these activities are typically fragmented, isolated from day-to-day nursing management, and lack alignment with organizational strategy.

This chapter discusses assessment of a health care organization's external and internal environment; identifies the importance of the philosophy and values, mission, and vision to achieving goals; and then reviews common organizational structures and work processes. The importance of monitoring outcomes is also discussed.

ASSESSMENT OF EXTERNAL AND INTERNAL ENVIRONMENT

As outlined in Figure 11-1, planning patient care involves clarifying the organization's philosophical values or what is important to the organization; identifying the mission of why the organization exists; articulating a vision statement of what the organization wants to be; and utilizing an environmental assessment, or SWOT analysis, which examines the organization's Strengths, Weaknesses, Opportunities, and

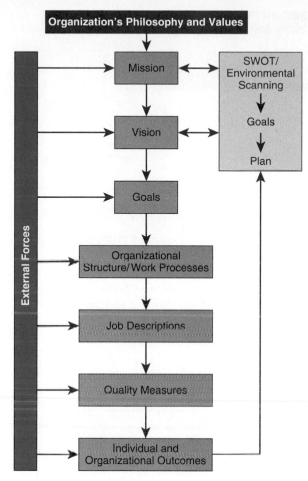

Figure 11-1 Planning care. (Delmar/Cengage Learning).

COMMUNITY AND STAKEHOLDER ASSESSMENT

A frequently overlooked but highly important area for analysis is the stakeholder assessment. A stakeholder is any person, group, or organization that has a vested interest in the program or project under review. Stakeholders in health care include people such as patients, nursing and medical practitioners, community representatives, insurance companies, hospital administrators, accreditation agencies, pharmaceutical companies, and technology and equipment companies, etc. A **stakeholder assessment** is a systematic consideration of all potential stakeholders to ensure that the needs of each of these stakeholders are incorporated in the planning phase. For a program to be successful, the involvement of all those who will be affected is essential.

DEVELOPMENT OF VALUES AND PHILOSOPHY, MISSION, VISION, AND GOALS

Every organization has a guiding philosophy and values. Most often, the philosophy is explicitly stated and detailed in a formal mission statement.

THE MISSION STATEMENT

The **mission statement** is a formal expression of the purpose or reason for existence of the organization. It is the organization's declaration of its primary driving force and the manner in which it believes care should be delivered. Most health care organizations have mission statements that speak to providing high quality or excellence in patient care. Some mission statements focus exclusively on providing care, whereas others assume a broader view and consider such elements

Threats. (Figure 11-2) This information provides data that then drive the development of one- to five-year goals for the organization. Tactics are then created and prioritized. The organizational structure and work processes are developed into annual operating work plans for the organization, which can be measured. This same process is used for unit or departmental planning. In developing a plan, unit staff must also examine their organization's mission, vision, and goals. Unit plans should be congruent with and support the mission and vision of the organizational system of which they are a part.

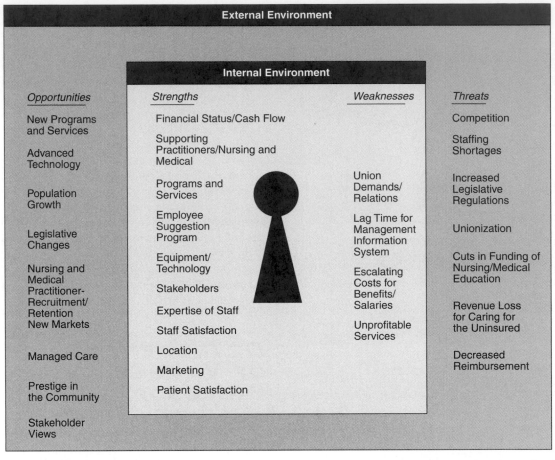

Figure 11-2 Key to success in strategic planning: SWOT analysis. (*Source:* Compiled with information from Jones, R., & Beck, S. [1996] *Decision Making in Nursing.* Clifton Park, NY: Delmar Cengage Learning).

as the education of health care professionals and/or the promotion of research as contributing to their broader mission.

For the mission statement to mean the most, all members of the organization should participate in its development and it should be written and easily available to all staff to encourage the development of an organization that is focused on meeting its mission.

Questions to be answered by the group charged with development of the mission statement include the following:

- What do we stand for?
- What principles or values are we willing to defend?
- Who are we here to help? (www.csuchico.edu)

A mission statement should be written according to the following three guidelines:

1. It should be no longer than a couple of sentences.
2. It should state the organization's purpose using action words.
3. It should be simple and from the heart.

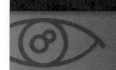

CRITICAL THINKING 11-1

Examine these two mission statements and then respond to the questions that follow.

Hospital A: "Our mission is to ensure the highest quality of care for the patients in our community. We believe that each patient has the right to the most innovative care that current science and technology can provide. To that end, we have assembled a world-renowned medical staff who will strive to ensure that the latest developments in medical science are used to combat disease."

Hospital B: "Our mission is to provide excellence in care to all. Our health care staff, nursing and medical practitioners, and other professionals believe that care can best be provided in an atmosphere of collaboration and partnership with our patients and community. We believe in education—for our patients, for our staff, and for future health care providers. At all times we strive for optimal health promotion and the prevention of disease and disability."

Which of these institutions do you think would be more likely to have a patient lecture series on living with diabetes? Value the contributions of nursing? Provide experimental therapy for cancer? Be open to scheduling routine patient care visits for uninsured patients?

VISION STATEMENT

The unit vision statement reflects the organization's vision for the future. A unit vision statement then exemplifies how the mission and vision of the unit will be actualized within the organization's mission and vision.

Following are four elements of a vision for the future:

1. It is written down.
2. It is written in present tense, using action words, as though it were already accomplished.
3. It covers a variety of activities and spans broad time frames.
4. It balances the needs of providers, patients, and the environment. This balance anchors the vision to reality. (Wesorick et al., 1998)

GOALS AND QUALITY MEASURES

The next step in the planning process is for the organization and the work unit to develop goals and quality measures that reflect the mission. A **goal** is a specific aim or target that the unit wishes to attain within the time span of one year. Measures of the goal may reflect finances, customer satisfaction and services, internal operating efficiency, and learning and growth (Norton & Kaplan, 2001). See Table 11-1.

STRUCTURES, PROCESSES, AND OUTCOMES

As discussed in the chapter on Quality Improvement, an organization or patient care unit must structure the unit's environment and develop work processes to achieve quality outcomes. For example, if an organization seeks to improve all patient care outcomes, the post-operative surgical unit in that organization may develop environmental structures and work processes to improve outcomes similar to Table 11-2.

Each nurse and nursing assistive personnel on the surgical unit must review patient care routines/standards to achieve the organization and unit goals. See Tables 11-3 and 11-4.

TABLE 11-1	MISSION, GOALS, AND QUALITY MEASURES

Mission

The People's Choice Health care Center provides excellent health care to all patients through partnerships with patients and the community and collaboration with nursing and medical practitioners and other health care staff. We believe in continuous education for patients, health care staff, and future health care providers. We are committed to optimal health care promotion and prevention of disease and disability.

Goals

1. Collaborate with all health care staff to improve patient care
2. Increase customer satisfaction scores
3. Increase number of emergency room visits
4. Increase the number of patient days
5. Increase use of computers by all staff
6. Increase funding for staff's continued education
7. Encourage all staff to attend one education program yearly
8. Increase number of specialty certifications of staff
9. Monitor nurse-sensitive patient outcomes, such as incidence of cardiac arrest, UTI, upper GI bleeding, thrombophlebitis, and failure to rescue
10. Decrease medication errors
11. Improve evidence-based care delivery
12. Achieve national patient safety goals
13. Improve all patient care outcomes

Quality Measures for Emergency Department

Customer/Patient

1. Increase in patient satisfaction
2. Increase in customer returns, when required
3. Decrease in patient complaints
4. Increase in market share
5. Decrease in repeat asthma patient visits
6. Develop patient education materials explaining norms for ER stays, well and ill child care, and so on

(continues)

TABLE 11-1	MISSION, GOALS, AND QUALITY MEASURES (CONTINUED)

7. Develop evidence-based standards for care of patients with cardiac arrest, UTI, upper GI bleeding, and thrombophlebitis

8. Review all Emergency Department deaths

Financial

1. Increase use of computers on all units

2. Monitor budget compliance

3. Improve nurse staffing ratios

4. Develop computerized order entry system for medications

Internal Processes

1. Achieve 90% on key Performance Improvement measures

2. Decrease sick time and overtime by 10%

3. Increase number of nursing research projects

4. Achieve Magnet status

5. Increase use of Best-Practice Educational Materials for all patients and staff

6. Increase participation of nursing, medicine, nursing assistive personnel, and pharmacy staff in quality improvement activities

7. Arrange for all staff to attend one outside conference yearly

8. Set up nursing journal club meetings monthly

9. Set up interdisciplinary committee on medication administration safety

10. Review policies for adherence to Evidence-Based Practice standards.

Employee Growth and Learning

1. 50% of the nursing department joins a professional nursing association

2. All nurses working in the emergency room are certified in ACLS, PALS, and so forth

3. One-third of nurses are continuing their nursing education

4. 50% of all staff are cross-trained and can work in the ICU and ER

5. 90% of employees are very satisfied

6. 90% of staff are retained

7. All nurses are able to use the computer to access and record patient information, to search literature, and so forth

8. 20% of nursing staff present a community program on topics such as stroke yearly

9. Each staff member compiles a professional portfolio, including evidence of Quality Patient Outcomes, Evidence-Based Practice, etc.

TABLE 11-2	STRUCTURE AND WORK PROCESS EXAMPLES TO DECREASE NEGATIVE POST-OPERATIVE OUTCOMES

Structure	Process
1. Increase RN staffing on the unit	Review patient care routines/standards for pre-op care, e.g., teaching about coughing and deep breathing exercises, early ambulation, etc., to decrease negative outcomes.
2. Increase number of incentive spirometers	Review patient care routines/standards for teaching about incentive spirometer use to decrease negative outcomes.
3. Etc.	Etc.

TABLE 11-3	SURGICAL UNIT, INDIVIDUAL RN'S DAILY ROUTINES/STANDARDS EXCERPT

0700	Shift handoff report
0715	Patient rounds
0730	Review post-operative care routines/standards and patient care with Nursing Assistive Personnel (NAP). See Table 11-4.
0800	Give patient Medications
0900	Document/monitor care and assist NAP. Use additional patient care standards, as needed.
Etc.	

TABLE 11-4	SURGICAL UNIT, NURSING ASSISTIVE PERSONNEL (NAP) ROUTINES/STANDARDS EXCERPT

0700	Monitor patient call lights during shift handoff report
0715	Take vital signs/pass fresh water
0730	Review post-operative routines/standards and patient care with RN to include
	• ambulating assigned patients at 0800, 1200
	• turning, coughing, and deep breathing patients at 0800, 1000, 1200, 1400
	• giving all baths and linen changes to assigned patients, by 1100
Etc.	

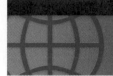

REAL WORLD INTERVIEW

I'm a new graduate nurse. I understand how tough it is adjusting straight out of school into a "real" job. My fellow new graduates and I did some brainstorming and came up with a few things to help make your transition at Bassett an easier one. Here goes!

- Ever wonder where all the Carpujets are? Just when you need to flush an IV, you can't find one anywhere. Guess what, Carpujets are located at the pharmacy! Just give them a call, and they will send you a bunch.

- How about all those tabs on the edge of the charts? It took me two months to find out what they mean on surgery! Red is for STAT orders. Blue is for medicine orders. Yellow alerts the unit clerk. Green alerts the RN.

- How to make your shift run smoother: It's always a good idea to round with the doctors. They know all kinds of information you need to know, and it's a great time to give your input. Collaboration!

- Know what team your patient is on and what doctor is on that specific team and who is coming onto the shift and who is leaving. Nothing is worse than trying to page a doctor before you realize he or she isn't there! That can be a little embarrassing, not to mention time consuming.

- Words of Wisdom: Write things down, it helps you remember.

- Just one more tidbit. Always bring any documentation and information such as medication lists and vital signs with you to the phone before you page the doctor. Then, you'll have the answers to his or her questions.

I hope that this information will be useful to you.

Christina Denton, RN, Surgery Unit
Bassett Healthcare
Cooperstown, New York

ORGANIZATIONAL STRUCTURE

Organizations are structured or organized to facilitate the execution of their mission, goals, reporting lines, and communication within the organization. This is true of entire organizations as well as individual nursing units. There are a number of ways to describe organizational structures.

TYPES OF ORGANIZATIONAL STRUCTURES

Usually, the existing organizational structures are communicated by means of an organizational chart. Figure 11-3 is an example of an organizational chart for a typical acute care general hospital. This organization has a tall bureaucratic structure with many layers in the hierarchy or chain of command and a centralized formal authority in the board of trustees. It represents a formal, top-down reporting structure. (Shortell & Kaluzny, 2006)

MATRIX STRUCTURE

Today, given the greater complexity of the health care system, more organizations are using matrix structures. Note that in this structure, a person may report to two or more managers. Figure 11-4 shows a matrix design (Shortell & Kaluzny, 2000).

FLAT VERSUS TALL STRUCTURE

Organizations are considered flat when there are few layers in the reporting structure. A tall organization would have many layers in the chain of command. An example of a flat organizational

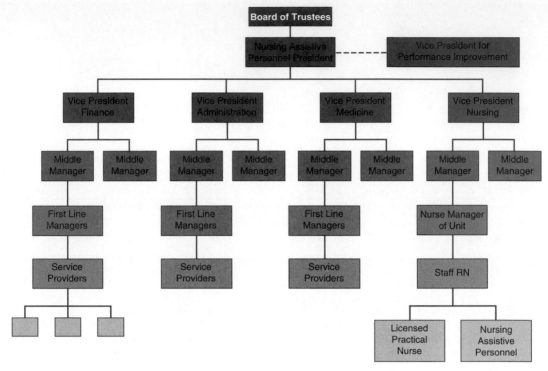

Figure 11-3 Organizational chart, formal authority structure: acute care general hospital. (*Source:* Shortell, S., & Kaluzny, A. [2000]. *Health care management: Organization design and behavior* [4th ed.]. Clifton Park, NY: Delmar Cengage Learning).

structure is a department of nursing that has no divisions and has many unit managers reporting to one director of nursing. (Figure 11-5)

DECENTRALIZED VERSUS CENTRALIZED STRUCTURE

The terms *centralized* and *decentralized* refer to the degree to which an organization has spread its lines of authority, power, and communication. A tall, bureaucratic design like that in Figure 11-3 would be considered highly centralized. A matrix design like that in Figure 11-4 would be on the decentralized end of the continuum. As can be seen in Figure 11-4, the nursing manager can interface with the Alzheimer's disease program manager without going through a central, hierarchical core, as would happen in a bureaucratic structure like that in Figure 11-3.

Other characteristics or attributes can be used to review organizations. Many typologies exist that

may be used for this purpose. For example, Shortell and Kaluzny (2006) suggest using such things as external environment, mission/goals, work groups/work design, organizational design, interorganizational relationships, change/innovation, and/or strategic issues to review different health service organizations.

DIVISION OF LABOR

The way the labor force is divided or organized has an effect on how the mission is accomplished. The organizational chart in Figure 11-3 graphically depicts how the formal authority in this organization is functionally structured. At the highest level, the board of trustees delegates authority to the president, who delegates to the vice presidents, and so on. At the vice presidential level, there are four department vice presidents. The vice presidents each report to the president. The middle managers report to their

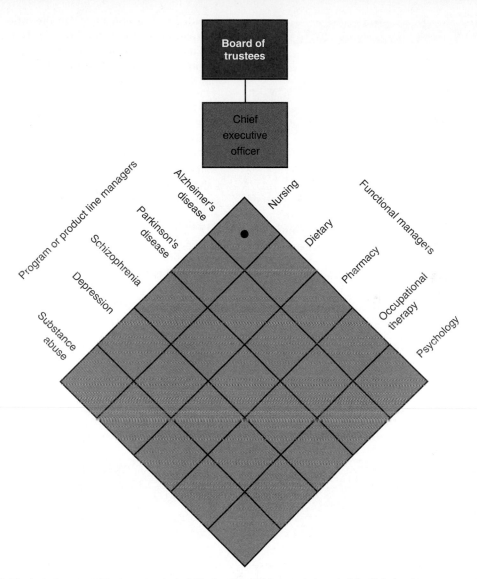

Figure 11-4 Matrix design: a psychiatric center. An individual worker in this example is part of the Alzheimer's program, as well as a member of the nursing department. (*Source:* Shortell, S., & Kaluzny, A. [2000]. *Health care management: Organization design and behavior* [4th ed.]. Clifton Park, NY: Delmar Cengage Learning).

vice president. The first line managers or unit nurse manager reports to the middle managers. The service providers or staff nurse reports to the first line managers or unit nurse manager, respectively. In this design, the division of labor is quite efficient and specialized. A danger with this division of labor is that each individual may be so focused on a specific area that he or she

has little perspective on the overall picture. For example, a service provider may focus on one area of a nursing unit and have little information about other areas.

In the matrix structure shown in Figure 11-4, the structure is less important and the workforce roles and reporting relationships are based on the

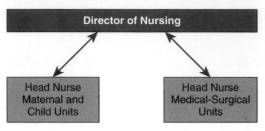

Figure 11-5 Example of a flat organizational structure. (Delmar/Cengage Learning).

project or task to be accomplished, rather than on a rigid hierarchy. An example of this is the planning involved in the preparation for a Joint Commission planning (JC) review. The team could be comprised of various individuals at varying levels of responsibility and from programs across the organization, but they could interact with staff at all levels and report as a task force at a high level in the organization.

SPAN OF CONTROL   The term *span of control* is used to designate the number of individuals who report to one person. If the span of control is too narrow, an organization may become "top heavy," and much time may be wasted in unnecessary communications up and down the chain of command,

resulting in lost efficiency. On the other hand, if the span of control is too broad, it is difficult for one manager to give adequate attention to the support and development of all the individuals that report to him or her.

DIVISION OF LABOR BY GEOGRAPHIC AREA.   Care delivery divided according to geography or location can be efficient. It might consist of the North Team and the West Team. For example, each nursing team may consist of an RN team leader, a licensed practical nurse (LPN), and a nursing assistive personnel (NAP).

DIVISION OF LABOR BY PRODUCT OR SERVICE.   Sometimes, care delivery is organized around product lines or service lines. This is based on a patient's diagnosis or the specialty care required by a patient. For example, there might be a cardiology service line, a woman's health service line, and an oncology service line. Figure 11-6 demonstrates a product line design (Shortell & Kaluzny, 2006).

ROLES AND RESPONSIBILITIES

Note that exact roles and responsibilities within each level and division are not defined on the organizational charts beyond specifying the given

CASE STUDY 11-1

A patient developed a rash from a new medication, unbeknownst to the medication nurse, who never asked about any signs of problems. The treatment nurse noticed the rash during a routine dressing change, but never thought to inquire about any new dietary or medication changes. It was not until the time of discharge when the patient read the drug information sheet advising that any skin changes be reported that the patient asked the discharge planning nurse if the week-old rash was significant.

What could have been done differently?

Was anyone at fault? Who?

Why is good communication especially important in a situation in which there is a division of labor by function?

What types of problems could you expect if staff members focused on their own tasks and failed to communicate with each other about the patient's physical, emotional, psychosocial, educational, and discharge needs?

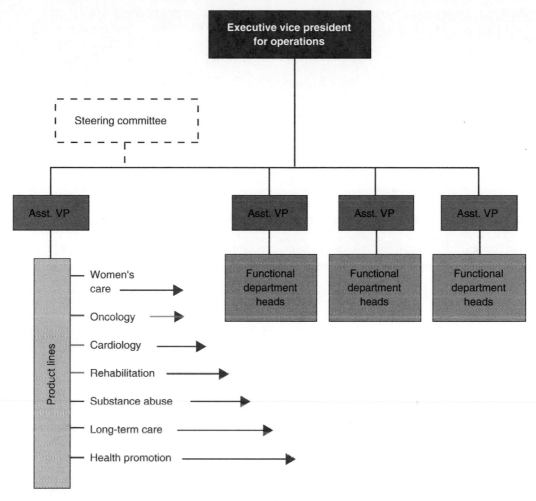

Figure 11-6 Product line design. (*Source:* Shortell, S., & Kaluzny, A. [2000]. *Health care management: Organization design and behavior* [4th ed.]. Clifton Park, NY: Delmar Cengage Learning).

division, for example, nursing. Scope of responsibilities, specific duties, and specific job requirements are found in documents such as individual job or position descriptions.

REPORTING RELATIONSHIPS

An organizational chart, such as the one that appears in Figure 11-3, allows one to determine the formal reporting relationships. These are shown with a solid line. Sometimes dotted lines are used in an organizational chart to depict dual or

secondary reporting relationships. An example of this might be the role of the Vice President for Performance Improvement. This individual might directly report to the President, but also have position accountabilities to the board of trustees. The formal reporting relationships may or may not reflect the actual communications that occur within the institution. For example, information may be communicated outside the formal reporting relationships. This method of information sharing is often referred to as the "grapevine". An example

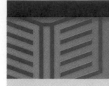

EVIDENCE FROM THE LITERATURE

Citation: Parsons, M. L. et al. (Oct.–Dec. 2004). Capacity building for magnetism at multiple levels: A healthy workplace intervention, part 1; An emergency department's health workplace process and outcomes, part 2. *Topics in Emergency Medicine, 26*(4), 287–295; 296–304.

Discussion: Parsons outlines a theoretical model that guides an intervention to build capacity for magnetism to create healthy workplaces. The theoretical model and intervention addressed an existing gap. The gap existed between the hospital-wide shared governance organizational level and the nursing unit level. A unit-based capacity-building intervention promoted collaboration and communication, enhancing patient care and workplace empowerment through staff organization and clinical decision making. The intervention was implemented using principles of participatory action research with infrastructure support.

Staff called the phases of the intervention "The Creating Our Future Program." Tangible practice and process improvements resulted from four action planning teams focused on (1) organized patient care, (2) rapid patient disposition, (3) diagnostics, and (4) initiation of care. Outcomes included the elimination of RN vacancies and agency use and improvements in patient and employee satisfaction, including interaction between staff and practitioners. Staff reported feeling empowered to continuously improve the emergency department.

Implications for Practice: A culture of shared governance on a nursing unit facilitates process improvements with outcomes of increased patient and staff satisfaction, resulting in enhanced staff retention.

---

of grapevine communication is when a nurse has a personal friend who is in a high administrative position who shares confidential information about pending budget cuts with her.

SHARED GOVERNANCE

Shared governance is an organizational framework grounded in a philosophy of decentralized leadership that fosters autonomous decision making and professional nursing practice (Porter-O'Grady et al. 1997). Shared governance, by its name, implies the allocation of control, power, or authority (governance) among mutually (shared) interested vested parties (Stichler, 1992).

In most health care settings, the vested parties in nursing fall into two distinct categories: (1) nurses practicing direct patient care, such as staff nurses, and (2) nurses managing or administering the provision of that care, such as managers. In shared governance, a nursing organization's management assumes the responsibility for organizational structure and resources. Management relinquishes control over issues related to clinical practice. In return, staff nurses accept the responsibility and accountability for their professional practice.

Unit-based shared governance structures are most successful if there is an organization-wide structure of shared governance in place that unit-based functions can coincide with. Organizational shared governance structures are usually council models that have evolved from preexisting nursing or institutional committees. In a council structure, clearly defined accountabilities for specific elements of professional practice have been delegated to five main arenas: clinical practice, quality, education, research, and management of

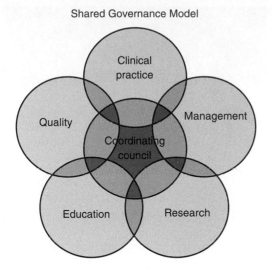

Shared Governance Model

Figure 11–7 A shared governance model. (Delmar/Cengage Learning).

resources (Porter-O'Grady et al. 1997). Figure 11-7 illustrates a shared governance model.

PURPOSE OF THE COUNCILS

The purpose of the clinical practice council is to establish nursing practice standards for a unit. The purpose of the quality council is to make recommendations about hiring, promoting, and credentialing nursing staff, and to oversee the unit quality management initiatives.

The purpose of the nursing education council is to assess the learning needs of the unit staff and develop and implement evidence-based programs to meet these needs.

The research council advances research utilization with the intent of incorporating evidence-based findings into the clinical nursing standards of practice. The research council may also coordinate research projects if advanced practice nurses practice at the institution.

The purpose of the management council is to ensure that the standards of nursing practice and governance agreed upon by unit staff are upheld and that adequate resources are available to deliver patient care.

The purpose of the nursing coordinating council is to facilitate and integrate the activities of the other councils.

MAGNET HOSPITALS

In 1983, the American Academy of Nursing (AAN), an organization affiliated with the ANA, appointed a Task Force on Nursing Practice in Hospitals. The purpose of the task force was to identify workplace characteristics that were successful in recruiting and retaining hospital nurses. Of the 163 hospitals studied, 41 (25%) were described as magnet hospitals (McClure, Poulin, Sovie, & Wandelt, 1983). A magnet designation was earned through demonstrated high nurse satisfaction, low nurse turnover, and low nurse vacancy rates. The AAN's landmark study concluded that the 41 original magnet hospitals shared a set of core organizational attributes that were desirable. The study stimulated additional independent research that provided further evidence to highlight the achievement of superior outcomes in magnet hospitals.

By June 1990, the ANA established the American Nurses Credentialing Center (ANCC) as a separate, incorporated, nonprofit organization that was to serve as the credentialing arm for magnet hospitals. The initial proposal for the Magnet Hospital Recognition Program was approved by the ANA Board of Directors in December 1990. The Magnet Program proposal indicated that the program would be built upon the 1983 AAN magnet hospital study. Further, the Magnet Program would use the 1999 *ANA Scope and Standards for Nurse Administrators,* now in its second revision (ANA, 2004), as a baseline for program development.

THE MAGNET RECOGNITION PROGRAM

The Magnet Recognition Program (ANCC, 2004) was created to achieve three major goals:

1. Promote quality in a milieu that supports professional nursing practice.

2. Identify excellence in the delivery of nursing services to patients.
3. Provide a mechanism for the dissemination of best practices in nursing services.

Many benefits come from magnet nursing services including improved patient quality outcomes, enhanced organizational culture, improved nurse recruitment and retention, enhanced safety outcomes. and enhanced competitive advantage (American Nurses Credentialing Center. (2006).

There are fourteen forces of Magnetism (ANCC, 2004) (Table 11-5).

CRITICAL THINKING 11-2

To learn more about some of the most important questions that must be addressed at the beginning of the magnet application process, access and complete the document entitled "Staff Nurse Opinion Questionnaire" (ANCC, 2008) at www.nursingworld.org. Click on *American Nurses Credentialing Center*. Click on *Calling All Staff Nurses*. Complete the Nurse Opinion Questionnaire that you find there.

TABLE 11-5	THE FOURTEEN FORCES OF MAGNETISM
Forces of Magnetism	**Definition**
Quality nursing leadership	■ Nurse leaders are perceived as knowledgeable, strong risk-takers who follow an articulated philosophy of nursing.
	■ Nurse leaders are strong staff advocates and supporters.
	■ The outcomes of quality nursing leadership are evident in nursing practice at the patient's bedside.
Organizational structure	■ Organizational structures are flat with decentralized, unit-based decision making.
	■ Strong nursing representation is evident in the organizational committee structure.
	■ Chief nursing officer reports to the organization's chief executive officer and is a member of the executive team.
Management style	■ Nursing and hospital administrators share a participative management style that incorporates feedback from staff at all levels of the organization.
Personnel policies and programs	■ Organization offers competitive salaries and benefits.
	■ Flexible staffing models are utilized.
	■ Personnel policies reflect staff involvement and clinical promotional opportunities.

(continues)

TABLE 11-5	THE FOURTEEN FORCES OF MAGNETISM (CONTINUED)
Professional models of care	■ Nurses have accountability for their nursing practice. ■ Practice model reflects nurses as coordinators of care.
Quality of care	■ Providing quality of care is seen as an organizational priority. ■ Nurse leaders develop the work environment so that quality of care can be delivered, and nurses perceive they are able to provide high-quality care.
Quality improvement	■ Staff nurses participate in quality improvement processes, and they perceive the processes as educational and beneficial to quality patient care.
Consultation and resources	■ Knowledgeable experts, including advanced practice nurses, are available and utilized. ■ Adequate consultation with other health care human resources are available within the organization.
Autonomy	■ Nurses engage in autonomous practice consistent with professional standards. ■ Independent professional judgment is expected within the context of interdisciplinary collaboration in patient care.
Community and the hospital	■ The hospital maintains a strong community presence, with the community perceiving the hospital as a productive and positive corporate citizen.
Nurses as teachers	■ Nurses are expected to incorporate teaching in all aspects of their professional practice.
Image of nursing	■ Nurses are seen as crucial to the hospital's capability to provide patient care services, a perception also held by other members of the health care team.
Interdisciplinary relationships	■ Positive interdisciplinary relationships are present, with a sense of mutual respect exhibited among all disciplines.
Professional development	■ Significant emphasis is placed on the professional development of the staff, including orientation, inservice education, continuing education, formal education, and ongoing competency maintenance. ■ Value is given to personal and professional growth, including emphasis on employee career development. *Source:* ANCC, 2004 and Urden and Monarch, 2002.

Source: American Nurses Credentialing Center. (2004). *Magnet recognition program: Application manual 2005.* Washington, DC: American Nurses Credentialing Center. Urden, L. D., & Monarch, K. (2002). The ANCC Magnet Recognition Program: Converting research into action. In M. L. McClure & A. S. Hinshaw (Eds.), *Magnet hospitals revisited: Attraction and retention of professional nurses* (pp. 103–115). Washington, DC: American Nurses Publishing.

KEY CONCEPTS

- Nurses have increasing opportunities to become involved in planning for the delivery of health care services in their organizations and communities. To do so effectively, however, they will need a basic understanding of how organizations are structured, how organizational systems function, and how to engage in the planning process.

- Successful orchestration of a patient care unit in today's health care environment is achieved through vision-driven professional practice.

- Shared governance is an organizational framework grounded in a philosophy of decentralized leadership that fosters autonomous decision making and professional nursing practice.

- The mission statement reflects an organization's values and provides the reader with an indication of the behavior and actions that can be expected from that organization.

- A health care organization needs to have a good idea of where it fits into its environment and what types of programs and services are needed and demanded by its customers or stakeholders.

- The purpose of planning is twofold. First, it is important that everyone has the same idea or vision of where the organization is headed; second, a good plan can help to ensure that the needed resources are available to carry out the initiatives that have been identified as important to the unit or agency.

- Organizations are structured or organized in a manner that is designed to facilitate the execution of their mission and their strategic plans.

- The Fourteen Forces of Magnetism define a quality nursing organization.

KEY TERMS

goal
mission statement

philosophy
shared governance

REVIEW QUESTIONS

1. The below figure is an example of what type of organizational structure?
   A. Tall
   B. Matrix
   C. Product Line
   D. Flat

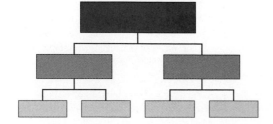

2. A document that describes the institution's values and philosophy is
   A. the organizational chain of command.
   B. the organizational chart.
   C. the mission statement.
   D. the strategic plan.

3. Which of the following is the outcome of the processes by which an organization engages in environmental analysis, goal formulation, and strategy development with the purpose of organizational growth and renewal?
   A. Stakeholder assessment
   B. SWOT analysis
   C. Strategic planning
   D. Mission development

4. The most formal and hierarchical organizational structure would be expected to have an organizational chart with
   A. a matrix design.
   B. many layers of command.
   C. a product line design.
   D. a number of dotted lines representing reporting relationships.

5. SWOT means
   A. strengths, weaknesses, opportunities, threats.
   B. strengths, worries, outcomes, threats.
   C. strengths, weaknesses, opportunities, treatment.
   D. structures, worries, outcomes, threats.

REVIEW ACTIVITIES

1. Having a plan in place can help an organization to make a decision about one alternative over another. For example, an institution whose plan calls for positioning itself as the leading cancer care provider in the area would be well served to advertise for nurses in the clinical journal of *Oncology Nursing* rather than in a local newspaper, even if the costs of advertising in the journal were higher. Identify another situation in which a plan could guide an organization in its choices among alternative actions.

2. Write a beginning mission statement for your professional nursing career. Do you plan to care for vulnerable populations in the community, become an expert in critical care nursing, or seek advanced education to become a midwife? Once you have identified your mission, outline a plan with objectives to attain your goal. For example, you might want to conduct a SWOT analysis, looking at the external environment; your internal environment (your skills, talents, and preferences); and the strengths, weaknesses, threats, and opportunities that exist in each. Once you have completed this exercise, you will have a better idea of which opportunities to pursue. For example, if you know that you want to work in pediatrics, you might ask for a pediatric journal subscription for your birthday. Additionally, you may be able to select or have input into the selection of your final clinical rotation in school, or you may be able to look for meetings, conferences, or educational sessions in your area of interest.

3. Examine the organizational structure of an organization or institution with which you are familiar. How would you characterize it using the types of structures that were discussed in this chapter? Is the organization a hierarchy, a matrix, or some other design? Does the way that the institution or organization is structured assist it in meeting its goals? Why or why not?

EXPLORING THE WEB

- You have been asked by your nurse manager and members of the credentialing committee to revamp the current clinical promotion ladder so that it more clearly differentiates and rewards nurses for their education level and expertise. Visit: *www.uchsc.edu*
  Note the University of Colorado's nursing differentiated practice model that can be accessed there.

- Upon completion of your nursing degree, you plan to interview for a position at an area hospital. In preparation for your interview, you want to understand the mission as well as other information about that institution. Today that information is readily available on the Web. For example, if you were planning to apply at Loyola University Chicago (*www.luc.edu*), you would go to *www.luhs.org*. By clicking the Learn About Us tab (on the home page) and then the

Mission Statement tab, you can view the mission statement.

- What impressions do you form about health care organizations and their missions? Does the stated mission seem to fit with the general "feel" that you get from the Web site? Could you easily find information about positions available? About the institution? Try this exercise with your local hospital or medical center.

- Go to the magnet hospitals site: *www.nursingworld.org.* Type in *magnet*, and then click *search*. What information do you find here?

- Visit the Web site for the nursing profession's honor society: *www.nursingsociety.org* This site provides weekly information from Sigma Theta Tau International. What did you see there that may be helpful to you in your practice?

REFERENCES

American Nurses Association. (2004). Nursing Administration: Scope and Standards of Practice. (2nd ed.). Washington, DC.

American Nurses Credentialing Center. (ANCC). (2004). *Magnet recognition program: Application manual 2005.* Washington, DC: American Nurses Credentialing Center.

American Nurses Credentialing Center. (ANCC). (2006). *Benefits of becoming a magnet-designated facility.* Retrieved May 6, 2006, from nursingworld.org/ancc/magnet/benes.html.

American Nurses Credentialing Center. (ANCC). (2008). Nurse opinion questionnaire. Available at www.nursecredentialing.org/magnetorg/snsurvey.cfm.

Institute of Medicine. (IOM). (1999). *To err is human.* Washington, DC: National Academies Press.

Institute of Medicine. (IOM). (2001). *Crossing the quality chasm.* Washington, DC: National Academies Press.

Jones, R., & Beck, S. (1996). *Decision Making in Nursing.* Clifton Park, NY: Delmar Cengage Learning.

McClure, M., Poulin, M., Sovie, M., & Wandelt, M. (1983). *Magnet hospitals: Attraction and retention of professional nurses.* American Academy of Nursing Task Force on Nursing Practice in Hospitals. Kansas City, MO: American Academy of Nursing.

Norton, D. P., & Kaplan, R. S. (2001). *The strategy focused organization.* Boston, MA: Harvard Business School.

Parsons, M. L., Cornett, P. A., Sewell, S., & Wilson, R. W. (2004, Oct–Dec). Capacity building for magnetism at multiple levels: A healthy workplace intervention, part 1; An emergency department's health workplace process and outcomes, part 2. *Topics in Emergency Medicine, 26*(4), 287–295; 296–304.

Porter-O'Grady, T. (1997). *Implementing shared governance: Creating a professional organization.* St. Louis, MO: Mosby-Year Book.

Porter-O'Grady, T., Hawkins, M. A., & Parker, M. L. (1997). Whole-systems shared governance. Gaithersburg, MD: Aspen Publishers, Inc.

Shortell, S., & Kaluzny, A. (2000). *Health care management: Organization design and behavior* (4th ed.). Clifton Park, NY: Delmar Cengage Learning.

Shortell, S., & Kaluzny, A. (2006). *Health care management: Organization design and behavior* (5th ed.). Clifton Park, NY: Delmar Cengage Learning.

Stichler, J. F. (1992). A conceptual basis for shared governance. In N. D. Como & B. Pocta (Eds.), *Implementing shared governance: Creating a professional organization* (pp. 1–24). St. Louis, MO: Mosby.

Urden, L. D., & Monarch, K. (2002). The ANCC Magnet Recognition Program: Converting research into action. In M. L. McClure & A. S. Hinshaw (Eds.), *Magnet hospitals revisited: Attraction and retention of professional nurses* (pp. 103–115). Washington, DC: American Nurses Publishing.

Wesorick, B., Shiparski, L., Troseth, M., & Wyngarden, K. (1998). *Partnership council field book.* Grandville, MI: Practice Field Publishing.

SUGGESTED READINGS

Buerhaus, P., Donelan, K., Ulrich, B., Norman, L., Williams, M., & Dittus, R. (2005). Hospital RNs' and CEOs' perceptions of the impact of the nursing shortage on the quality of care. *Nursing Economics, 23*(5), 214–221.

Doyle, V., & Turkie, W. (2006). Transforming the organization of care. *Nursing Management—UK, 13*(2), 18–21.

Institute of Medicine. (IOM). (2004). Keeping patients safe: Transforming the work environment of nurses. Washington, DC: National Academies Press.

Institute of Medicine. (IOM). (2006). *Keeping patients safe: Transforming the work environment of nurses.* Retrieved August 21, 2006, from www.iom.edu/Default.aspx?id=16173.

Jones, C. B., & Mark, B. A. (2005). The intersection of nursing and health services research: An agenda to guide future research. *Nursing Outlook, 53*(6), 324–332.

Personality Pathways. (2006). *Introduction to type.* Retrieved August 22, 2006, from www.personalitypathways.com/ MBTI_intro.

Porter-O'Grady, T. (2003). A different age for leadership, part 2: New rules, new roles. *Journal of Nursing Administration, 33*(3), 173–178.

Scott, L., & Caress, A. (2005). Shared governance and shared leadership: Meeting the challenges of implementation. *Journal of Nursing Management, 13*(1), 4–12.

Turkel, M. (2004). Magnet status: Assessing, pursuing, and achieving nursing excellence. *Journal of Nursing Administration, 29*(2), 14–20.

Wesorick, B. (2006). *Clinical practice model resource center.* Retrieved August 22, 2006, from www.cpmrc.com.

CHAPTER 12

Time Management and Setting Patient Care Priorities

Time is the coin of your life. It is the only coin you have, and only you can determine how it will be spent.

(Carl Sandberg)

OBJECTIVES

Upon completion of this chapter, the reader should be able to:

1. Discuss concepts of time management.
2. Describe strategies for setting priorities.
3. Discuss shift hand-off report.
4. Apply time management strategies to enhance personal productivity.

Inez has just completed her medical-surgical orientation as a new graduate registered nurse. This evening is her first solo shift, but she is frightened and feels like she is holding up the world on her new graduate shoulders. Although she feels that everything rests on her, she is not really alone. Inez and Carole, the other RN, along with one certified nursing assistant, are responsible for 12 possible patients on this section of the unit. Currently, 10 patients are in this section, but a new admission is on the way, another patient is returning from surgery, the dinner trays are arriving, and Inez has medications to pass. Just as the dinner trays arrive, a patient's family member runs out to Inez and states that her mom is confused and incontinent and has pulled out her IV.

What would you do if you were Inez?

What would you do first?

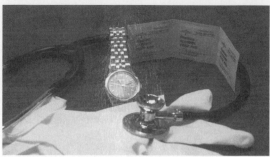

Many nurses become nurses out of idealism. They want to help people by meeting all their needs. Unfortunately, most new graduates find it impossible to meet all or even most of their patients' needs. Needs tend to be unlimited, whereas time is limited. In addition to the direct patient care responsibilities, there are shift responsibilities, charting, doctors' orders to be transcribed or checked, medications to be given, and patient reports to be given.

New graduates often go home feeling totally inadequate. They wake up remembering what they did not accomplish. One young nurse shared with tears in her eyes that once, when she answered a call bell late in her shift, the patient requested a pain medication. She went to the narcotics cabinet to get the medication, but was interrupted by an emergent situation. When she arrived home, she was so exhausted that she fell asleep rapidly, only to awaken with the realization that she had not returned with her patient's medication. Her guilt was tremendous. She had gone into nursing to relieve pain, not to ignore it.

Time management allows the novice nurse to prioritize care, decide on outcomes, and perform the most important interventions first. Time management skills are important not just for nurses on the job, but for nurses in their personal lives

as well. They allow nurses to make time for fun, friends, exercise, and professional development. This chapter discusses concepts of time management and strategies for setting priorities when delivering nursing care. Strategies to enhance personal productivity are also discussed.

TIME MANAGEMENT CONCEPTS

Time management has been defined as "a set of related common-sense skills that helps you use your time in the most effective and productive way possible" (Mind Tools, 2006a). In other words, time management allows us to achieve more with our time. Time management requires self-examination of what pursuits are really important, analysis of how time is currently being used, and assessment of the distractions that have been siphoning time from more important pursuits (Maloney, 2008).

A simple principle, the **Pareto Principle**, states that 20% of focused effort produces 80% of results, or, conversely, that 80% of unfocused effort produces 20% of results (Pareto Principle, 2008) (Figure 12-1).

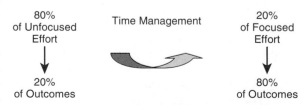

Figure 12-1 The Pareto Principle. (Delmar/Cengage Learning).

The Pareto principle reminds us to focus our efforts on the most important outcomes and develop plans to achieve them to maximize the results we get. For example, when a nurse begins a shift, it is good to pause immediately after the hand-off shift report and prioritize the outcomes and activities for the shift. On a busy unit, it is possible to overlook important activities needed to achieve key outcomes if the nurse does not focus on priorities.

ANALYSIS OF NURSING TIME

Analysis of nursing time use is an important step in developing a plan to effectively use time. Nurses often undervalue their time. Consider salary and benefits. Benefits are frequently forgotten, but they add 15% to 30% to salary. If a nurse is making $26 an hour, benefits add $3.90 to $7.25 to the hourly cost of a nurse's time. The value of nursing time in this example, excluding what the organization is paying in workers' compensation and payroll taxes, is $29.90 to $33.25 an hour. The organization has also invested in nurse recruitment, orientation, and development, which easily can exceed $20,000 per nurse. Nursing time is a valuable commodity. Keeping this in mind will be invaluable when considering work that can be delegated to personnel who receive less compensation or when considering spending time on completing a task that does not support achieving an outcome.

USE OF TIME

Numerous studies have shown how nurses use their time (Scharf, 1997; Upenieks, 1998; Urden & Roode, 1997).

Fitzgerald, Pearson, Walsh, Long, and Heinrich (2003) found a distribution similar to previous studies—34% of nursing time was spent giving direct care; 38% in indirect support activities including documentation, obtaining supplies, and professional communication; 8% on unit activities—cleaning and tidying; 7% on other activities such as looking for other personnel, setting up equipment, and completing professional reading; and 13% on personal time for breaks, personal conversations, and reading (Figure 12-2).

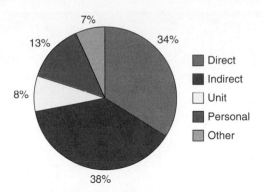

Figure 12-2 Use of nursing time. (*Source:* Compiled with information from Fitzgerald, M., Pearson, A., Walsh, K., Long, L., & Heinrich, N. [2003]. Patterns of nursing: A review of nursing in a large metropolitan hospital. *Journal of Clinical Nursing, 12*[3], 326–332).

How do you use your time? Memory and self-reporting of time have been found to be unreliable. (Pelletier and Duffield, 2003).

An **activity log** is a time management tool that can assist the nurse in determining how both personal and professional time is used. The activity log (Table 12-1) should be used for several days. Behavior should not be modified while keeping the log. The nurse should record every activity, from the beginning of the day until the end.

After filling out the activity log for several days, a nurse needs to review it and ask herself how the Pareto principle would apply. Has 20% of the effort resulted in 80% of the outcome achievement? If the activities have not achieved the desired outcomes, the nurse needs to change activities and focus on priorities. She should start by noticing her most energetic time of day. Activities that take focus and creativity should be scheduled at high-energy times and dull, repetitive tasks at low-energy times. Scheduling time for proper rest, exercise, and nutrition allows for quality time.

CREATE MORE TIME

There are three major ways to create time. One is to delegate work to others or hire someone else to do work. Another is to eliminate chores or

TABLE 12-1 | WORK ACTIVITY LOG

Time	Name of Activity (Medication administration, vital signs, bed-making, patient transport, and so on)	Time Required and Feelings (Energetic, bored, and so on)	Could be better done by someone else? Who? (LPN, nursing assistant, housekeeper, and so on)	Toward what outcome achievement? (Increase in patient's functional status, prevention of complications, and so on)
0500	Treadmill	30 min – energetic	Keep for self	Fitness
0530	Shower and breakfast	45 min – energetic	Keep for self	Health
0630	Drive to work	10 min – alert	Keep for self	Get to work
0700	Hand-off shift report	15 min – alert	Keep for self	Patient identification
0730	Patient rounds/planning	15 min – alert	Keep for self	Prioritize patients
0730				
0800				
0830				
0900				
0930				
1000				
1030				
1100				
Etc.				

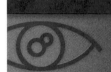

CRITICAL THINKING 12-1

The relationship between personal lifestyle and the incidence of several diseases has been demonstrated. Many health promotion programs include the expectation that people invest in themselves. Do you invest in yourself with your daily activities to promote higher education; planned savings; healthy eating; regular exercise; deferred gratification; avoidance of smoking, tanning booths, drugs, and excessive alcohol consumption; and regular physical checkups? Do you know people who seem to live only from one day to the next because their perspective of time is in the immediate and they do not seem to recognize the benefits of setting priorities and doing long-term planning?

tasks that add no value. The last way is to get up earlier in the day. When a person delegates a task, he or she cannot control when and how the task is completed. Initially, it may take more time to get others to do the chore than to just do it, but this investment of time should save the investor time and energy in the future. If a chore is boring and mundane, it makes more sense to work an hour more at a job one enjoys in order to pay for someone else to do unrewarding, boring work.

Getting up one hour earlier in the day for a year can free up 365 hours, or approximately nine weeks a year, extra time that can be used to enrich life. After several days of rising an hour earlier, an individual may feel tired and respond to the fatigue by going to bed a little earlier (Mind Tools, 2006b). This may be a good strategy for many people, especially those who are not productive in the evening and spend time doing activities that are minimally rewarding such as watching television. If a person does not get to bed earlier, though, and the end result of getting up early is fatigue, the strategy is not beneficial (Maloney, 2008).

SETTING PRIORITIES

To plan effective use of time, nurses must understand the big picture and decide on priority outcomes. Start by reviewing the big picture. No nurse works in isolation. Nurses should know what is expected of their coworkers, what is happening on the other shifts, and what is happening in the agency and the community. If the previous shift was stressed by a crisis, a shift may not get started as smoothly (Hansten, Washburn & Jackson 2004). If areas outside of the unit are overwhelmed, someone might be moved to assist on the overwhelmed unit. When nurses take the big picture into consideration, they are less likely to be frustrated when asked to assist others. They can also build into their time management plan the possibility of giving and receiving assistance.

FIRST PRIORITY: LIFE-THREATENING PROBLEMS WITH ABCS

Life-threatening conditions include patients at risk to themselves or others and patients whose vital signs and level of consciousness indicate potential for respiratory or circulatory collapse (Hansten, Washburn & Jackson, 2004). A patient whose condition is life-threatening is the highest priority and requires monitoring until transfer or stabilization. Life-threatening conditions can occur at any time during the shift and may or may not be anticipated.

A quick guide to assessing life-threatening emergencies is as simple as ABC. A stands for Airway.

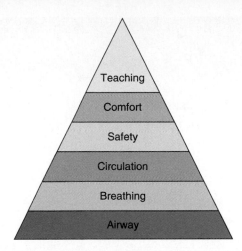

Figure 12-3 Prioritization triangle. (Delmar/Cengage Learning).

Is the airway open and patent or in danger of closing? This is the highest priority for care. B stands for Breathing. Is there respiratory distress? C stands for circulation. Is there any circulatory compromise? This method is a way of prioritizing actions. Although there is clearly an order of importance, ABC is often assessed simultaneously while observing the patient's general appearance and level of consciousness (Figure 12-3 and Table 12-2 and 12-3). Patients with life-threatening conditions usually have an IV access line and receive continuous monitoring of their cardiac rhythm, blood pressure, pulse, respiration, and oxygen saturation level. Their temperature and urinary output is monitored closely as well.

SECOND PRIORITY: ACTIVITIES ESSENTIAL TO SAFETY

Activities that are essential to safety are very important and include those responsibilities that ensure the availability of life-saving monitoring, medications, and equipment, and that protect patients from infections and falls. They include asking for assistance or providing assistance during two-people transfers or turning and movement of heavy patients (Hansten, Washburn & Jackson, 2004). They also include monitoring the patient for the prevention of nurse-sensitive outcomes.

TABLE 12-2	TOP-PRIORITY PATIENT CARE GROUPS

Top-priority patient care groups

Respiratory	■ Airway compromise
	■ Severe respiratory distress, inadequate breathing
	■ Critical asthma
	■ Chest trauma with respiratory distress
Cardiovascular	■ Cardiac arrest
	■ Shock or hypotension
	■ Exsanguinating hemorrhage
Neurological	■ Major head injury
	■ Unconscious or unresponsive
	■ Active seizure state
Musculoskeletal (MSK)	■ Major trauma
	■ Traumatic amputation—extremity
	■ Major cold injury—hypothermia
Skin	■ Burn, >25% body surface area (BSA) or airway involvement
Gastrointestinal (GI)	■ Difficulty swallowing, with airway or respiratory compromise
	■ Abdominal trauma, penetrating or blunt
Gynecological (GYN)	■ Vaginal bleeding, patient with abnormal vital signs
Hematologic/Immunologic (HEM/IMMUN)	■ Anaphylaxis
Endocrine (ENDO)	■ Hypoglycemia—altered consciousness
Infection (INF)	■ Septic shock
Child or elder abuse	■ Unstable situation or conflict

Source: Compiled with information from Warren, D., Jarvis, A., Leblanc, L.; the National Triage Task Force members. (2001). Canadian Paediatric Triage and Acuity Scale: implementation guidelines for emergency departments. CJEM;3 (suppl), S1–27.

THIRD PRIORITY: COMFORT AND TEACHING

Activities that provide Comfort and Teaching lead to outcomes that relieve symptoms and/or lead to healing. They are the activities that, if omitted, will hinder the patient's recovery. These essential activities include those that provide comfort and relieve symptoms, such as pain, nausea, and so on—and those activities that promote healing, such as providing nutrition, ambulation, positioning, medication administration, and teaching.

TABLE 12-3	SETTING PRIORITIES FOR SAFE PATIENT OUTCOMES

- First Priority—ABCs. Remember Maslow's (1970) Hierarchy of Human Needs. Assess physiological needs first. See high-priority unstable patients who have any threats to their ABCs first (i.e., airway, breathing, and circulation). These patients require nursing assessment, judgment, and evaluation until transfer or stabilization. Life-threatening conditions can occur at any time during the shift and may or may not be anticipated. Notice your patient's level of consciousness and general appearance. Remember that all equipment and observations used to support and monitor the status of patients' ABCs are also a high monitoring priority (e.g., monitoring suicide threats, vital signs, level of consciousness, neurological status, skin color and temperature, pain, IV access, cardiac monitor, oxygen, suction, and urine output).

- Second Priority—Safety. Next, assess Maslow's second level of human needs (i.e., safety and security). Are there any threats to patient safety and security such as threats of violence, need for fall prevention, infection control, and so on? See these patients next.

- Third Priority—Comfort, Teaching, and other needs. Assess the patients' other needs and prioritize using Maslow's hierarchy. These patient needs may also include love and belonging, self-esteem, and self-actualization. What do the nursing and medical standards of care include, e.g., comfort, ambulation, positioning, and teaching etc.? Stable patients who need standard, unchanging procedures and have predictable outcomes are seen last. Monitoring ABCs and patient safety is always top priority!

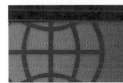

REAL WORLD INTERVIEW

I am sometimes assigned to work in the triage section where patients are seen when they first enter the Emergency Department (ED). It can be really nerve-wracking at times, with everyone needing or wanting to be cared for immediately. The principles of setting priorities really come in handy in this situation. I decide which patient will be cared for in the ED first based on priorities. If a patient has a life-threatening attack on their ABCs, such as an asthma attack, chest pain, significant alteration in vital signs, or significant bleeding, I arrange for this patient to be cared for immediately. My next priority is to ensure safety for my patients. I constantly monitor all the patients in the triage area of the ED until they can be seen. I want to be sure that their condition remains stable and that they are safe while waiting to be seen. I also think it is important to keep the patients who are waiting informed as to how patients are seen and cared for in the ED. When patients see that we care for them based on how ill they are, they don't seem to mind waiting as much when someone who is sicker than them is cared for first. Of course, they all want to be cared for reasonably quickly. That is my goal also!

Patricia Kelly, RN
Chicago, Illinois

Vaccaro (2001) states that prioritizing has several traps that nurses should avoid.

Frequently, nurses act on the "doing whatever hits first" trap. This means that a nurse may respond to things that happen first. For example, a nurse at the beginning of the day shift chooses to fill out the preoperative checklist for a patient going to surgery the next day, rather than assess the rest of his or her patients first.

The second trap is "taking the path of least resistance." In this trap, nurses may make the flawed assumption that it is easier to do a task rather than delegate it when they could be completing another task that only nurses can complete. For example, a nurse who is admitting a patient needs the patient's vital signs and weight, baseline assessment, and patient orders. The first two tasks can be delegated to Nursing Assistive Personnel (NAP) so that the nurse may complete the baseline assessment of the patient and then call the Nursing or Medical Practitioner for orders.

The third trap is "responding to the squeaky wheel," wherein nurses feel compelled to respond to whatever need has been vocalized the loudest. In this case, the nurse may choose to respond to a family member who has come to the nursing station every half hour with some concern. To appease the family member, the nurse may take time to focus on one of his or her many verbal concerns and overlook a more pressing patient need elsewhere.

The fourth trap is called "completing tasks by default." This trap occurs when nurses feel obligated to complete tasks that no one else will complete. A common example of this trap is emptying the garbage when it is full instead of asking housekeeping to do it.

The last trap is "relying on misguided inspiration." The classic example of this trap is when nurses feel "inspired" to document findings in the chart and avoid taking care of a higher priority responsibility. Unfortunately, some tasks will never become inspiring and need discipline, conscientiousness, and hard work to complete them.

CONSIDERATIONS IN SETTING PRIORITIES

Priorities are established by nurses using Maslow's Hierarchy of Needs while considering patients' immediate, short-, and long-term goals and the importance and urgency of each patient care activity.

Covey, Merrill, and Merrill (2002) have developed another way of setting priorities, Activities are classified as:

- Urgent or not urgent
- Important or not important

If an activity is neither important nor urgent, then it becomes the lowest priority.

Some activities that are often thought of as important may not be. Sometimes laboratory data, vita signs, and intake and output reports are ordered more frequently than the status of the patient indicates. Frequent monitoring of these parameters when a patient is stable may make no significant difference in patient outcomes. When nurses begin their shifts, they should question the activities that make no difference in outcomes (Hansten, Washburn & Jackson, 2004). If a practitioner orders these activities, a nurse should work to get the order changed. Similarly, if there is a nursing policy or procedure that does not make a difference in patient care, the nurse should work to change it. Nurses should give priority to the activities that they know are most likely to make a difference in patient outcomes.

SHIFT HAND-OFF REPORT AND ASSIGNMENTS

Before a plan is made for a shift, the shift hand-off report, at best, can lead to a smooth and effective start to the new shift. At worst, it can leave the on-coming shift members with inadequate or old data on which to base their plan. The Joint Commission included a standardized approach to shift hand-off reporting as one of its patient safety goals for 2006 (Kirkpatrick, 2006). The end of shift hand-off report *can* be given in a face-to-face seated report or during walking rounds.

Whether the report is relayed face to face or during walking rounds, information must be transmitted to allow for the effective and efficient implementation of care. If the outgoing nurse fails to cover all pertinent points, the oncoming shift must ask for the appropriate information. See Table 12-4 for a tool for taking and giving reports.

During or after report, the oncoming nurse can complete an assignment sheet or a written or computerized action plan that sets the priorities for the shift and makes assignments to team members. Assignments should include specific reporting guidelines and deadlines for accomplishment of the tasks (Figure 12-4). When a nurse makes an assignment,

TABLE 12-4	TOOL FOR END-OF-SHIFT HAND-OFF REPORT

Notes

Demographics	■ Room number
	■ Patient name
	■ Sex
	■ Age
	■ Practitioner
Diagnoses	■ Primary
	■ Secondary
	■ Nursing and medical
	■ Admit date
	■ Surgery date
Patient Status	■ Do Not Attempt Resuscitation (DNAR) status
	■ Current vital signs
	■ Problem with ABC's, level of consciousness, or safety
	■ Oxygen saturation
	■ Pain score
	■ Skin condition
	■ Ambulation
	■ Fall risk
	■ Suicide risk
	■ Presence/absence of signs and symptoms of potential complications
	■ New orders/changes in treatment plan

(continues)

TABLE 12-4	TOOL FOR END-OF-SHIFT HAND-OFF REPORT (CONTINUED)

Notes

Fluids/tubes/oxygen Laboratory tests and treatments	■ IV fluid, rate, site
	■ Tube feedings—type of tube, solution, rate, and patient toleration
	■ Oxygen rate, route; other tubes, e.g., chest tube, NG tube, foley, and so on, type and drainage
	■ Abnormal lab and test values
	■ Labs and tests to be done on oncoming shift
	■ Treatments done on your shift, include dressing changes (times, wound description) and other procedures
	■ Identify treatments to be done during next shift
Expected shift outcomes	Priority outcomes for one or two nursing diagnoses
	Patient learning outcomes
Plans for discharge	Expected date of discharge
	Referrals needed
	Progress toward self-care and readiness for home
Care support	Availability of family or friends to assist in ADL (activities of daily living)
Priority Interventions	Interventions that must be done this shift

he or she plans patient care by reviewing several factors, e.g., patient needs, agency organizational systems, and staffing. See Table 12-5.

MAKE PATIENT CARE ROUNDS

If the end-of-shift hand-off report does not include walking rounds, the oncoming nurse needs to make initial rounds on the patients at risk for life-threatening conditions or complications first. As the nurse makes rounds, he or she performs rapid assessments. These assessments may vary from the information given during the shift hand-off report, so the information gathered on rounds may change the shift plan. A patient with asthma who had been calm and without respiratory distress on the previous shift may have experienced a visitor who wore perfume and delivered bad news. As the oncoming nurse makes initial rounds and uses the quick ABC assessment, he or she may quickly determine that

ASSIGNMENT SHEET EXCERPT

Unit __2   South__

Date_ October 2, 2008	Notify RN immediately if:
	T <97 or >100
Shift _____Days_____	P <60 or >110
	R <12 or >24
Charge nurse____Mary____	SBP <90 or >160
	DBP <60 or >100
RNs Break/Lunch	BS <70 or >200
Steve 0900 and 1100	Pulse oximetry <95%
Lakeisha 0930 and 1130	Urine output <30 cc/hour
Colleen 1000 and 1200	

NAPs Break/Lunch	Notify RN one hour prior to end of shift:	Narcotic Count _____Steve_____
Juan 0900 and 1100	I and O	Glucometer Check ____Colleen____
	Patient goal achievement	Stock Pyxis _____Lakeisha_____
Pat 0930 and 1130		Pass Water _____Juan_____
		Stock Linen _____Pat_____
		Other ___Colleen attend in-service at 1300

Room and Initials	Patient	Staff	AM/PM Care	Weight I & O	IV	Activity	Accu-check	Tests	NPO	Comments
501, Mr. M. M.	27-year-old with newly diagnosed AIDS, left lower lobe pneumonia	Steve, RN	Complete care	0715 1400	KVO	Bedrest		Lab		Vitals Q4H
502, Mr. M. G.	61-year-old with acute congestive heart failure (CHF)	Lakeisha, RN	Partial care	0715 1400	KVO	BRP	1100	Lab	Yes	Vitals Q4H
503, Ms. S. C.	92-year-old with new right hip fracture, in Bucks traction	Juan, NAP	Complete care	I & O at 1400	KVO	Bedrest		Lab and xray	Yes	Vitals Q4H
504, Ms. N. J.	48-year-old, with new cholelithiasis	Pat, NAP	Self care		KVO	Up ad lib		Ultra-sound	Yes	
505, Ms. L. G.	89-year-old with new onset CVA with right side paralysis	Colleen, RN	Complete care	0715 1400	NS @ 125 cc/hr.	Bedrest	1100	Lab		Vitals Q4H

Figure 12-4 Assignment sheet excerpt. (Delmar/Cengage Learning).

TABLE 12-5	FACTORS CONSIDERED IN MAKING ASSIGNMENTS

- Priority of patient needs
- Geography of nursing unit
- Complexity of patient needs
- Other responsibilities of staff
- Attitude and dependability of staff
- Need for continuity of care by same staff
- Agency organizational system
- State laws, e.g., state nurse practice act
- In-service education programs
- Need for fair work distribution among staff
- Need for lunch/break times
- Need for isolation

- Need to protect staff and patients from injury
- Skill, education, and competency of staff, that is, RN, LPN, NAP
- Hospital policy and procedure
- Patient care standards and routines for surgical, medical, maternal child, and/or mental health patients
- Environmental concerns
- Equipment checks, medication checks
- Accreditation regulations
- Needs of other units in hospital, number of staff, problems left over from earlier shifts, etc.
- Desired patient outcomes

the patient has suddenly developed respiratory distress. The patient may have been initially prioritized as requiring only comfort activities directed at healing, but the patient is now experiencing a life-threatening reaction and requires appropriate nursing interventions as well as continuous monitoring. While assessing the patient, the nurse must check all the patient's IV lines to make sure that the correct fluid is infusing and the infusion site is without complication. The nurse must also check the patient's drains, tubes, and continuous treatments. The nurse should listens to the patient's concerns and desires. It is important to remember that plans are just that—plans—and have to be flexible based on ever-changing patient care needs. Times for treatments and medications may have to be changed. Often nurses believe that the times for administering medication are inflexible, yet practitioners usually write medication orders as daily, twice a day, three times a day, or four times a day. These kinds of orders give nurses flexibility in administration times. Although unit policy dictates

when these medicines are given, unit policy is under nursing control.

EVALUATE OUTCOME ACHIEVEMENT

At the end of the shift, the nurse must reexamine the shift action plan. Did he or she achieve the desired outcomes? If not, why? Were there staffing problems or patient crises? What was learned from this for future shifts?

If, at the end of a shift, the nurse did not accomplish the desired intended outcomes, he or she might review the shift activities to see what time wasters interfered with outcome achievement. Marquis and Huston (2005) described time wasters as procrastination, inability to delegate, inability to say no, management by crisis, haste, and indecisiveness. Sullivan and Decker (2004) add interrupting telephone calls and socialization to the list. Reed and Pettigrew (2006) include complaining, perfectionism, and disorganization as well.

CASE STUDY 12-1

Y ou are working the day shift on a medical-surgical unit. You are responsible for six patients with the assistance of NAP and an LPN. What are the outcomes you want to achieve? Please use the criteria previously given for prioritizing, i.e., ABC, safety, etc. Which patients will you give to each care provider? Make out an assignment sheet building on the format in Figure 12-5. Discuss your rationale.

Patient	Priority Nursing Assessments
Ms. J. D. is a 68-year-old patient who is post-op day 1 after a total shoulder replacement following a traumatic fall. She is confused and on multiple medications and has a history of hypertension and multiple falls. She is anxious and frightened by the "visiting spirits."	ABCs, level of consciousness, vital signs, safety, distal pulse, incision/dressing check, breath sounds. See this patient second during rounds.
Mr. D. B. is a 55-year-old patient with insulin-dependent diabetes mellitus, juvenile onset at age 12. He is post-op day 2 after a right below-the-knee amputation. He complains of severe right leg pain and is restless. Mr. D. B. has a history of noncompliance with diet and is on sliding scale insulin administration.	ABCs, symptoms of hypoglycemia, glucoscan at 4 P.M. and 9 P.M., vital signs, safety, incision/dressing check, pain, DB teaching. See this patient third during rounds. You may need to check his glucose level STAT.
Mr. J. K. is a 35-year-old patient with a history of alcohol abuse admitted for severe abdominal pain. He is throwing up coffee-ground-like emesis.	ABCs, level of consciousness, seizure and shock potential, hematemesis, DTs, safety, vital signs, CBC, hematocrit, type and cross-match, 16-gauge IV line for possible blood transfusion, oxygen, cardiac monitor. See this patient first during rounds.

Now, identify the priority nursing assessments for this next group of patients. See table 12-6.

TABLE 12-6 PRIORITY PATIENT ASSESSMENTS, GROUP II

Patient	Priority Nursing Assessments
Ms. H. M. is an 85-year-old patient who was transferred from a nursing home because of dehydration. She is vomiting and has abdominal pain of unknown etiology. Intravenous hydration continues and a workup is planned. Ms. H. M. is alert and oriented.	
Mr. A. B. is a 72-year-old patient who is status post cerebrovascular accident. He is to be transferred to rehabilitation. He needs his belongings gathered and a nursing summary written.	
Ms. V. G. is an 82-year-old patient who is postop day 5 after an open reduction of a femur fracture. She has a history of congestive heart failure, hypertension, and takes multiple medications. Her temperature is elevated. She is confused.	

FIND PERSONAL TIME FOR LIFELONG LEARNING

Finding time for lifelong learning and maintaining a balance with family, school, and work is a struggle for recent graduates, and even for more-seasoned nurses.

Nurses can achieve their dreams, work, and have a personal life via many ways. Flaherty (1998) offers tips for balancing school, family, and work in Table 12-7.

TABLE 12-7	MAINTAINING BALANCE IN LIFE WHEN RETURNING TO SCHOOL

1. Let your employer know that you are interested in returning to school. Most employers are supportive of additional education and will be flexible with your schedule. But they will continue to expect a competent, dedicated employee.

2. Develop computer skills. By using a computer, you can e-mail professors and classmates at any time. You can do online research. You can easily incorporate constructive criticisms into papers and build on previous work. Technology is the working student's friend.

3. Choose a flexible educational program. Many programs offer several classes in a row on a single day, weekend and night classes, or weeklong immersion classes. Some programs offer distance-learning opportunities.

4. Do not be surprised by the demands of school. Courses will be difficult and demanding of time. Remember that you have faced difficult demands and challenges before. Use the same techniques that helped you in the past.

5. Solicit support from family and friends. They can offer emotional support, as well as child care.

6. Use all available resources at the school and at work. Develop mentors and role models. Establish relationships with faculty. Discover and use academic support services such as writing centers and tutors. Read syllabi and course instructions carefully.

7. Focus on the outcome. Keep the end in sight and do not give up. Take it one course at a time. Reward yourself along the way. When a course is completed, celebrate.

8. Be careful of the sacrifices. You may replace some hobbies with school. But save some time for the things that are really meaningful to you and your family and friends.

9. Manage time. Ten minutes spent on planning saves time and energy later. Keep your sense of humor.

10. Take care of yourself and your responsibilities. Set aside a day to take care of personal chores and errands.

11. If you need a break, take one. Take time to reflect on what you are accomplishing. If you are feeling overwhelmed, take only one course or take a semester off.

12. Study on the run. Taping lectures and listening to them as you commute is a great way to study on the run.

Source: Adapted from Flaherty, M. (1998). The Juggling Act: 10 Tips for Balancing Work, School, and Family. *Nurseweek.* Retrieved on December 7, 2008, from www.nurseweek.com/features/98–5/juggle.html.

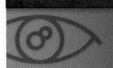

CRITICAL THINKING 12-2

Four of Jose's patients were discharged today by 10:00 A.M. The nursing supervisor asked Jose to help out in the Emergency Room. Jose agreed and was assigned to help the triage nurse. Identify the order in which the following patients should be seen in the ER.

Group 1

- A 2-year-old boy with chest retractions
- A 1-year-old girl choking on a grape
- A 5-year-old boy with a knee laceration

How about Group II? Which patient would you see first?

Group II

- A 60-year-old female who is nonresponsive and drooling
- A 30-year-old male trauma patient who has absent breath sounds in the right side of his chest
- A 15-year-old female who cut her wrist in an attempted suicide

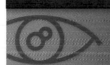

CRITICAL THINKING 12-3

Nurses set priorities fast when they "first look" at patient. As you approach your patient, get in the habit of observing the following:

FIRST LOOK
- Eye contact as you approach
- Speech
- Posture
- Level of consciousness

AIRWAY
- Airway sounds or secretions
- Nasal flare

BREATHING
- Rate, symmetry, and depth
- Positioning
- Retractions

CIRCULATION
- Color

- Flushed
- Cyanotic
- Presence of IV or oxygen
- Pain
- Vital signs (TPR and BP)
- Pulse oximetry
- Cardiac monitor

DRAINAGE
- Urine
- Blood
- Gastric
- Stool
- Sputum

Practice your "first look" the next time you approach a patient. Does this improve your assessment skills?

KEY CONCEPTS

- General time management strategies include having an outcomes orientation, analyzing time cost and use, focusing on priority outcomes, and visualizing the big picture.

- Shift hand-off reports may be given by two different methods: face-to-face meetings or walking rounds.

- The assignment sheet is evaluated at the end of the shift by determining whether priority outcomes have been achieved.

- Time management applies to one's personal life as well as one's job.

- Quality time can be achieved by analyzing time use and setting priorities.

- It is possible to balance work, family, and school.

- Prioritize patient care using the ABC-Safety-Comfort-Teaching Model.

KEY TERMS

activity log
Pareto Principle

time management

REVIEW QUESTIONS

1. The nurse has just finished the change-of-shift hand-off report. Which patient should the nurse assess first?
   A. a postoperative cholecystectomy patient who is complaining of pain but received an IM injection of morphine five minutes ago
   B. a postoperative appendectomy patient who will be discharged in the next few hours
   C. a patient with asthma who had difficulty breathing during the prior shift
   D. an elderly patient with diabetes who is on the bedpan

2. A nurse has been assigned to a medical-surgical unit on a stormy day. Three of the staff can't make it in to work, and no other staff is available. How will the nurse proceed?
   A. Prioritize care so that all patients get safe care.
   B. Provide nursing care only to those patients to whom the nurse is regularly assigned.

   C. Ask selected ambulatory patients if they can help with care of the sickest patients.
   D. Refuse the nursing assignment as the increased number of patients makes it unsafe.

3. Of the following new patients, who should be assessed first by the nurse?
   A. a patient with a diagnosis of alcohol abuse with impending delirium tremens (DTs)
   B. a patient with a newly casted fractured fibula complaining of pain
   C. a patient admitted two hours ago who is scheduled for a nephrectomy in the morning.
   D. a patient diagnosed with appendicitis who has a temperature of 37.8°C (100.2°F) orally

4. A nurse has just come on duty and finished hearing the morning report. Which patient should the nurse see first?

A. the patient who is being discharged in a few hours

B. the patient who requires daily dressing changes

C. the patient who is receiving continuous IV Heparin per pump

D. the patient who is scheduled for an IV Pyelogram this shift

REVIEW ACTIVITIES

1. Make an assignment for a group of patients on your clinical unit using Figure 12-4. Consider all the factors in Table 12-5 in making your assignments.

2. For the next three days, complete an activity log for both your personal time and your work time.

On what activities are you spending the majority of time? When is your energy level the highest? Is your energy level related to food intake? What are your biggest time wasters? How can you schedule your time more productively?

EXPLORING THE WEB

- Web sites offering electronic organizers (e.g., Personal Digital Assistant, Palm Pilot, Casio electronic organizer, Sharp electronic organizer):
  www.casio.com
  www.sharpeusa.com
  www.palm.com

- Web sites offering non-electronic organizers and systems for time management: (e.g., Day-Timer, Franklin Covey):
  www.daytimer.com
  www.covey.com
  www.franklin.com

- Free on-line calendar:
  calendar.yahoo.com

- Mind Tools:
  www.mindtools.com
  Free time management tools and hints.

- Professional organizers:
  www.organizerswebring.com
  Professional time management assistance.

REFERENCES

Covey, S. R., Merrill, A. R., & Merrill, R. R. (2002). *First things first: to love, to learn, to leave a legacy.* New York: Simon & Schuster.

Fitzgerald, M., Pearson, A., Walsh, K., Long, L., & Heinrich, N. (2003). Patterns of nursing: A review of nursing in a large metropolitan hospital. *Journal of Clinical Nursing, 12*(3), 326–332.

Flaherty, M. (1998). The Juggling Act: 10 tips for balancing work, school, and family. *Nurseweek.*

Retrieved on December 7, 2008, from www.nurseweek.com/features/98–5/juggle.html.

Hansten, R. I, Washburn, M.J., & Jackson, M. (2004). *Clinical delegation skills: A handbook for professional practice* (3rd ed.). Sudbury, MA: Jones and Bartlett Publications.

Kirkpatrick, C. (2006). *Safety first: JC's patient safety goals for 2006. Nursing Spectrum.* Retrieved on March 5, 2006, from www2.

nursingspectrum.com/CE/Self-Study_modules/syllabus.html?ID=331.

Maloney, P. (2008). Time management and setting patient care priorities. In P. Kelly (Ed.), *Nursing Leadership & Management* (2nd ed.). Clifton Park, NY: Delmar Cengage Learning.

Marquis, B.L., & Huton, C.J. (2005). *Leadership roles and management functions in nursing: Theory and application.* Hagerstown, MD: Lippincott, Williams & Wilkins.

Maslow, A. H. (1970). (2nd ed.). Motivation and Personality. New York: Harper & Row.

Mind Tools. (1999–2006a). *How to achieve more with your time.* Retrieved February 27, 2006, from www.mindtools.com/tmintro.html.

Mind Tools. (1999–2006b). *How to achieve more with your time.* Retrieved February 27, 2006, from www.mindtools.com/tmgetup.html.

Pareto Principle—The 80–20 Rule—Complete Information. (2008). Available at www.gassner.co.il/pareto/.

Pelletier, D., & Duffield, C. (2003). Work sampling: Valuable methodology to define nursing practice patterns. *Nursing and Health Sciences, 5,* 31–38.

Reed, F. C., & Pettigrew, A. C. (2006). Self-management: stress and time. In P. S. Yoder-Wise (ed.), *Leading and managing in nursing* (4th ed., pp. 413–430). St. Louis: Mosby.

Scharf, L. (1997). Revising nursing documentation to meet patient outcomes. *Nursing Management, 28*(4), 38–39.

Sullivan, E. J., & Decker, P. J. (2004). *Effective leadership and management in nursing.* Lebanon, IN: Pearson.

Upenieks, V. B. (1998). Work sampling: Assessing nursing efficiency. *Nursing Management, 49*(4), 27–29.

Urden, L., & Roode, J. (1997). Work sampling: A decision-making tool for determining resources and work redesign. *Journal of Nursing Administration, 27*(9), 34–41.

Vaccaro, P. J. (2001, April). Five priority-setting traps. *Family Practice Management, 8*(4), 60.

Warren, D., Jarvis, A., Leblanc, L.; the National Triage Task Force members. (2001). Canadian Paediatric Triage and Acuity Scale: implementation guidelines for emergency departments. CJEM;3 (suppl), S1–27.

SUGGESTED READINGS

Cohen, S. (2005). Reclaim your lost time with better organization. *Nursing Management, 36*(10), 11.

Hendry, C., & Walker, A. (2004). Priority setting in clinical practice: Literature review. *Journal of Advanced Nursing, 47*(4), 427–436.

Patterson, E. S., Roth, E. M., Woods, D. D., Chow, R., & Gomes, J. O. (2004). Handoff strategies in settings with high consequences for failure: Lessons for health care operations. *International Journal for Quality in Health Care, 16*(2), 125–132.

Reh, F. J. (2002). *Pareto's principle—The 80–20 rule.* Retrieved February 25, 2006, from management. about.com/cs/generalmanagement/a/Pareto081202.htm

UNIT IV
Quality Improvement of Patient Outcomes

CHAPTER 13

Quality Improvement and Evidence-Based Patient Care

The best outcomes evaluation is likely to come from partnerships of technically proficient analysts and clinicians, each of whom is sensitive to and respectful of the contributions the other can bring.

(Robert L. Kane, Professor of Public Health, University of Minnesota, 1997)

OBJECTIVES

Upon completion of this chapter, the reader should be able to:

1. Articulate major principles of quality improvement, including customer identification; the need for participation at all levels; and a focus on improving the process, not criticizing individual performance.
2. Identify the importance of evidence-based care.
3. Discuss the University of Colorado Model for Evidence-Based Practice.
4. Discuss the Model for Improvement and the FOCUS-PDCA Method.
5. Discuss sentinel events, storyboards, benchmarking, and the use of quality data.
6. Identify how data are utilized for performance and quality improvement (time series data, Pareto charts).
7. Review an organizational structure for quality improvement.

During report, the staff nurse tells you about a 60-year-old woman, Miss Kelly, who was admitted to the unit today with left hip and sciatic pain after a recent fall at home. You immediately begin to think she has a hip fracture. The staff nurse interrupts your thoughts and says, "Wait, there is more. This woman has a new diagnosis of breast cancer and has also developed a pleural effusion, which necessitated the insertion of a chest tube this morning. Her dyspnea has improved since this morning, and her pulse oximetry on 2 liters of oxygen via nasal cannula is 99%."

Miss Kelly has lymphedema of her right hand and arm, and the right breast mass is a very large, open, foul-smelling lesion that bleeds intermittently. She appears anxious and has indicated that she is uncomfortable and afraid to move. She has Tylenol with codeine ordered orally every 4 hours as needed for pain, but has been very reluctant to take the medication because she believes it will alter her ability to think and make decisions regarding her care. Results of a bone scan and CT scan of the abdomen and pelvis indicate that she has further metastatic involvement of the left acetabulum. This could be the cause of her left hip pain—tumor replacing the bone. Although the CT scan does not reveal a fracture, Miss Kelly is at high risk for developing a pathological fracture.

Miss Kelly is single, has no children, and lives with her brother and five cats. She does not smoke or drink. She is a retired clerk for the state Department of Labor. She has been followed by a cardiologist for hypertension for several years. She has often called for prescription refills but canceled her appointments because she feared what the doctor would find or say.

What additional data do you need to develop a protocol of care to improve Miss Kelly's outcomes?

What priorities should be addressed to manage Miss Kelly's care?

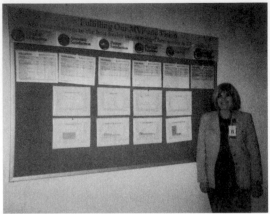

Delmar/Cengage Learning

Quality improvement and evidence-based care (EBC) have been shown to be powerful tools to make health care organizations more effective. Ransom, Joshi, and Nash (2005) stress the importance of management and leadership commitment to the success of quality improvement. The improvement philosophies of quality experts such as Deming (1986) and Crosby (1979) also emphasize the commitment of management, and without that commitment, successful quality improvement is jeopardized.

Nursing leaders and managers are particularly well placed to see that health care institutions have evidence-based care (EBC) and work processes in place that provide professional nurses with support to meet new challenges in the clinical delivery of care. **Evidence-based care** is clinically competent care based on the best scientific evidence available. It incorporates clinical expertise, research, and the patient's preferences. All nurses have responsibility for promoting patient care based on the best scientific evidence available.

This chapter will discuss the importance of Quality Improvement (QI) and EBC to patients and nursing. Nursing uses a scientific process driven by evidence-based standards and practice guidelines while also emphasizing continuing quality improvement.

QUALITY

Quality assurance (QA) emerged in health care in the 1950s, about the same time as hospital-accrediting organizations were founded (AMCQ Series Curriculum, 1998). QA began as an inspection approach to ensure that health care institutions—mainly hospitals—maintained minimum standards of care. QA's methods consisted primarily of chart audits of various patient diagnoses and procedures. The method emphasized "doing it right," and did little to sustain change or proactively identify problems before they occurred. It did, however, encourage monitoring minimum standards of performance and improving performance when standards were not met. QA efforts also began to encourage hospitals to use Donabedian's (1966) structure, process, and outcome framework for looking at quality (See Table 2-2 in Chapter 2).

QUALITY IMPROVEMENT

Quality Improvement (QI) is a management philosophy to improve the organizational structure and the level of performance of key processes in the organization to achieve high quality outcomes. This philosophy states that quality is an organizational issue, that is, that variation in quality is as much due to the way in which care is organized and coordinated as it is to the competence of the individual caregivers (Kimberly & Minvielle, 2003). QI was developed originally by several industrial quality experts and applied successfully in a variety of industries worldwide (Crosby, 1979; Deming, 1986; Juran, 1988). The principles espoused by these experts differ little, but are known by several terms used interchangeably with QI: total quality management (TQM), continuous quality improvement (CQI), and performance improvement (PI). Key philosophical concepts include:

- Productive work involves work processes. Most work implies a chain of processes whereby each worker receives input from suppliers (internal or external to the organization), adds value, and then passes it on to the customer. **Customers** are defined to include everyone internal or external to the organization who receives the product or service of the workers, e.g., patients, nurses, physicians, community, etc.
- The customer is central to every process. Look at improvement of all work processes to meet the customer's needs reliably and efficiently.

- There are two ways to improve quality: eliminate defects in the work process and add features that better meet customers' needs or preferences.
- The main sources of quality defects are problems in the work process. Workers basically want to succeed in carrying out the work process correctly. The problems derive from the work process being wrong.
- Quality defects are costly in terms of internal losses from lowered productivity and efficiency, increased requirements for inspection and monitoring, and dissatisfied customers. Preventing defects in the process by careful planning saves resources.
- Focus first on the most important work processes to improve. Use statistical thinking and tools to identify desired performance levels, measure current performance, interpret it, and take action when necessary.
- Involve every worker in QI and empower them to take action. Use new structures such as teams and quality councils to advise and plan QI strategies. Assure administrative support for QI.
- Set high standards for performance; go for being the best. Emphasize this until it becomes a work habit and part of the organization's daily operations.

QI logic suggests that high quality could lead to a higher volume of use of the organization by patients and providers who have the flexibility to make choices about where they seek health care. Higher volume generally leads to higher profits which, in turn, may be directed toward improving programs and services, thus achieving higher quality, a very positive spiral that can result in the organization's thriving.

Increased quality → Increased volume → Increased profit → Enhanced programs/services → Increased quality

The obverse spiral is more likely when quality is shoddy, a very negative and potentially fatal spiral.

Decreased quality → Decreased volume → Decreased profit → Cutting corners → Decreased quality

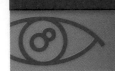

CRITICAL THINKING 13-1

On an orthopedic unit, when the original lengths of stay data by nursing unit were examined, one unit had a much shorter length of stay than the other. At first there was discussion about this variance and the idea emerged of just going to the floor with the longer length of stay and fixing things there. The group members decided that rather than approach the task from this limited perspective, they would study the care delivery process as a whole and determine whether there were steps they could take to improve the process before criticizing the staff on the floor with the longer length of stay. Several excellent opportunities for improvement were identified, for example, the need for preoperative home evaluation, increased physical therapy involvement, and shorter indwelling catheter use. All these areas contributed to the process improvement, and the outcome was that both units ended up reducing their lengths of stay. These opportunities would have been lost had the group members used the data only to say that one unit was doing a bad job. They needed to review the process as a whole to improve the length of stay on both units.

Describe a problem on a patient care unit with which you are familiar. What patient care process could be improved? Who would you ask to work on the improvements with you? Can you suggest ideas for QI to other staff without making them feel that the quality of their care is being criticized?

EVIDENCE-BASED CARE (EBC)

Nursing, medicine, health care institutions, and health policy makers recognize EBC as care based on an approach to collecting, reviewing, interpreting, critiquing, and evaluating research and other relevant literature for direct application to patient care. EBC uses evidence from research; performance data; quality improvement studies such as hospital or nursing report cards, program evaluations, and surveys; national and local consensus recommendations of experts; patient observation; and clinical experience.

The EBC process further involves the integrating of both clinician-observed evidence and research-directed evidence. This then leads to state-of-the-art integration of available knowledge and evidence in a particular area of clinical concern that can be evaluated and measured.

NURSING AND EBC

It was inevitable that nursing would move to EBC. One of the earlier proponents for EBC in nursing was the Joanna Briggs Institute for Evidence Based

Nursing (JBIEBN), established in 1996. Significant work has been done worldwide to implement EBC into Australian, Canadian, and U.K. institutions of care.

In the United States, the Agency for Healthcare Research and Quality (AHRQ) has provided a stimulus for the EBC movement through recognition of a need for evidence to guide practice throughout the health care system. In 1997, the AHRQ launched its initiative establishing twelve evidence-based practice centers. This initiative partnered AHRQ with other private and public organizations in an effort to improve the quality, effectiveness, and appropriateness of care. Several EBC models are used in QI.

THE UNIVERSITY OF COLORADO HOSPITAL MODEL

The University of Colorado Hospital model (Figure 3-1 in Chapter 3) is an example of an evidence-based multidisciplinary practice model (Goode et al., 2000; Goode & Piedalue, 1999). The model depicts nine sources of evidence that can be evaluated and benchmarked.

Benchmarking is defined as the continuous process of measuring products, service, and practices against the toughest competitors or those customers recognized as industry leaders (Camp, 1994). The elements of the University of Colorado's model can be applied to the case of Miss Kelly in the opening scenario of this chapter (Table 13-1).

BENCHMARKING

Benchmarking against the best performers teaches us how to adapt the best practices to achieve breakthrough process improvement and build healthier communities (Gift & Mosel, 1994). Benchmarking focuses on key services or work processes, for example, length of time from the patient entering the emergency department until the time of a treatment PCI procedure. A benchmark study will identify gaps in performance and provide options for selection of processes to improve, ideas for redesign of care delivery, and ideas for better ways to meet customer expectations. There are various types of benchmarking studies, such as clinical, financial, and operational. A clinical benchmark study will review outcomes of patient care, for example, reviewing standards for managing the outcomes of care of patients with diabetes or a stroke. Financial benchmarking studies examine cost/case charges and length of stay. Operational benchmarking studies review systems that support care, for example, the case management system in an organization.

METHODOLOGIES FOR QUALITY IMPROVEMENT

Several models outline methodologies for quality improvement. Two are reviewed here: the Model for Improvement and the FOCUS methodology. Improvement comes from the application of knowledge (Langley, Nolan, Nolan, Norman, & Provost, 1996). Thus, any approach to improvement must be based on building and applying knowledge.

THE MODEL FOR IMPROVEMENT

The Model for Improvement (Langley et al., 1996) (Figure 13-1) begins with these questions:

1. What are we trying to accomplish?
2. How will we know that a change is an improvement?
3. What changes can we make that will result in improvement?

These three questions provide the foundation for the Model for Improvement and will help focus the use of the Plan, Do, Study, Act (PDSA) Cycle to complete the Model for Improvement. We will apply the Model for Improvement to Miss Kelly, the patient in the opening scenario presented at the beginning of this chapter, in relation to pain. This process can also be applied to the patient's pressure ulcers and wound management.

APPLICATION OF THE MODEL FOR IMPROVEMENT TO PAIN MANAGEMENT

Let's apply the Model for Improvement to Miss Kelly, the patient in the opening scenario.

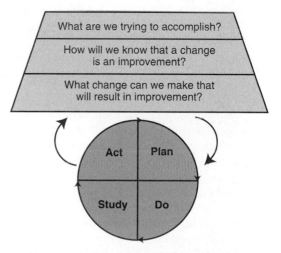

Figure 13-1 The PDSA cycle. (*Source:* From Langley, G. J., Nolan, K. M., Nolan, T. W., Norman, C. L., & Provost, L. P. [1996]. *The improvement guide: A practical approach to enhancing organizational performance.* San Francisco: Jossey-Bass).

TABLE 13-1	**PRACTICE APPLICATION TO ELEMENTS OF THE UNIVERSITY OF COLORADO HOSPITAL MODEL**

Model Element	Application
Benchmarking data	Compare length of stay for Miss Kelly with that of other patients with breast cancer in this hospital and other hospitals nationally. Review the literature.
Cost-effective analysis	Analyze cost-effectiveness of wound care regimens, including nursing time and use of actual products (e.g., hydrogel vs. normal saline dressings). Benchmark with others.
Pathophysiology	Review biopsy results/findings of testing for metastatic disease and implications.
Retrospective/concurrent chart review	Assess changes in condition related to pressure ulcer development using the Braden Pressure Ulcer Risk Assessment Scale.
Quality improvement and risk data	Review and analyze documentation regarding patient progress and risk assessment (e.g., infection, bleeding, pressure ulcer development, and outcomes assessment (e.g., pain rating, falls, and dosage of narcotic administration).
International, national, and local standards	Assess effectiveness of care related to AHRQ guidelines for cancer pain and pressure ulcers.
Infection control data	Review wound culture results and institute appropriate precautions and treatment.
Patient preferences	Discuss, document, and implement patient's wishes regarding advance directives, pain management, and so forth.
Clinical expertise	Consult acute care nurse practitioner and other practitioners for wound, skin, and pain management.

Source: By permission of University of Colorado Hospital Research Council, Denver, CO.

1. *What are we trying to accomplish?* The overall objective is to reduce or alleviate Miss Kelly's pain, which may be related to a variety of physiological, psychosocial, and spiritual issues.

   In conjunction with the other members of the health care team the nurses will identify, implement, and document the best strategies for reducing Miss Kelly's pain.

2. *How will we know that a change is an improvement?* Miss Kelly will state that her pain is decreased or relieved. Behaviors that may indicate decreased pain include her verbal or nonverbal expression of pain relief or improved comfort, her ability to reposition herself, and statements such as "I feel more rested," along with an improved mood.

3. *What changes can we make that will result in improvement?* To standardize pain management for patients like Miss Kelly, the nursing staff will create a protocol that includes a plan to use a trial pain management flow sheet to document the patient's reported pain status and pain interventions at various points in time.

IMPLEMENTATION OF THE PDSA CYCLE   The PDSA Cycle can be individual or system focused. It can be used to solve a specific patient problem or to structure strategies for managing groups of patients with common problems. Based on our answers to the three questions, we will apply the PDSA Cycle as follows:

Planning Phase   Once the three Model for Improvement questions have helped staff identify what should be improved, the multidisciplinary staff (RN, MD, nurse practitioner, pharmacist, and so on) would develop a plan for improvement. The plan would include using the pain management flow sheet and implementing evidence-based unit standards for assessing, managing, evaluating, and documenting patient comfort.

Doing Phase   Nursing staff used the pain management flow sheet to collect data on Miss Kelly during her hospital stay. All nurses assigned to care for Miss Kelly were asked to complete the documentation tool. Data to be collected would include the patient's pain rating, her nonverbal behaviors, level of consciousness, respiratory rate, side effects, activity, nonpharmacological therapies, pharmacological interventions, and patient response to interventions and teaching.

Studying Phase   Data were collected for a period of two weeks. The nurses on the unit met and reviewed the documentation. Several improvements and issues were identified. Documentation of pain assessment and pain parameters had been completed 66% of the time during the two-week period. Staff nurses stated that they referred to the pain management flow sheet when giving reports to the doctor or other nurses about Miss Kelly's pain status. As a result, Miss Kelly's pain management was central in discussions regarding her care, and decisions about changes in her pain medication regimen were made in a timely manner. The nursing and medical practitioners and pharmacists verbalized satisfaction with the flow sheet in terms of being able to see at a glance the amount and type of medication she was getting, how often, and her rating of pain. Within one week, Miss Kelly was reporting that her pain level improved to 2 or 3 on a scale of 0 to 10. She was receiving around-the-clock medication and bolus dosing three to four times a day as necessary. She remained alert and oriented and had no problems with constipation, urinary retention, or other medication side effects. Radiation therapy was started to her left leg in an effort to control her pain.

Acting Phase   After a meeting with the nurse manager, clinical nurse specialist, doctor, pharmacist, staff nurse, and other health care staff to discuss the findings, the staff agreed to continue to test the new pain management interventions and flow sheet for four months on all patients admitted to the oncology unit. This next step in the improvement process reflects the use of additional multiple PDSA cycles (Figure 13-2) to improve not only Miss Kelly's outcomes, but also the total care delivery system.

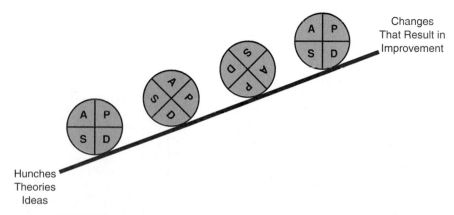

Figure 13-2 Use of multiple PDSE cycle. (*Source:* Langley, G. J., Nolan, K. M., Nolan, T. W., Norman, C. L., & Provost, L. P. [1996]. *The improvement guide: A practical approach to enhancing organizational performance.* San Francisco: Jossey-Bass).

MULTIPLE USES OF THE PDSA CYCLE Multiple PDSA cycles were used to improve care not just for Miss Kelly, but for all patients.

Planning Phase The inpatient oncology staff agreed to collect data for four months using the pain management flow sheet on Miss Kelly and all new patients admitted to the oncology unit. The study also included a plan to orient the staff to the purpose, development, and procedures for using the tool and pain management standards.

Doing Phase All nursing staff working on the inpatient oncology unit attended an inservice reviewing the pain standards and the purpose, development, and procedures for using the pain management flow sheet. Once all the staff had completed the orientation, the data collection period was implemented.

Studying Phase Pain management was reviewed on an ongoing basis and documentation practices were reviewed after four months. Documentation of pain assessment was completed on 78% of all patients' charts on admission to the inpatient unit, 67% were completed 24 hours after admission, and 50% were completed 48 hours after admission. The majority of the unit's nurses agreed that they were using the pain management flow sheet as a basis for their report to the practitioners regarding the patient's pain status. The pharmacist and the practitioners reported that they did review the pain management flow sheet approximately 50% of the time, but they most often relied on the staff to verbally share with them information to improve the patient's pain status.

Acting Phase A protocol for pain assessment, management, evaluation, and documentation was developed and integrated with the pain management flow sheet. Eventually, this process was published in the oncology literature (Jadlos, Kelman, Marra, & Lanoue, 1996). This model for improvement can also be used to focus on other aspects of Miss Kelly's care.

THE FOCUS METHODOLOGY

The FOCUS methodology describes in a stepwise process how to move through the improvement process (Figure 13-3).

F: Focus on an opportunity for improvement. This step asks the question, "What is the problem?" During this phase, an improvement opportunity is articulated and data are obtained to support the hypothesis that an opportunity for improvement exists.

O: Organize a team that knows the process. This means identifying a group of staff members who are direct participants in the process to be examined—the point-of-service staff. A team leader is identified who will appoint team members.

C: Clarify what is happening in the current process. A flow diagram (see Figure 13-4) is very helpful for this.

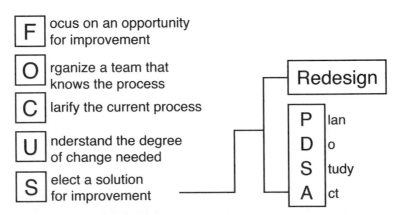

Figure 13-3 FOCUS method. (*Source:* Adapted from Albany Medical Center, Albany, NY).

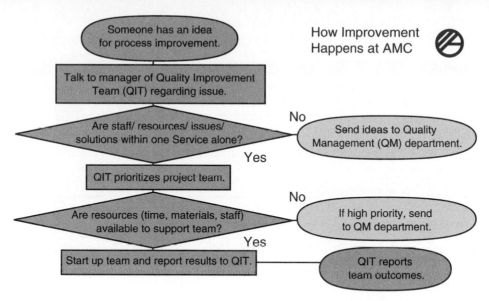

Figure 13-4 Flow diagram—how improvement happens. (*Source:* Courtesy of Albany Medical Center, Albany, NY).

U: Understand the degree of change needed. In this stage, the team reviews what it knows and enhances its knowledge by reviewing the literature, available data, and competitive benchmarks. How are other health care organizations doing the process?

S: Select a solution for improvement. The team can brainstorm and then choose the best solution. It can then use the PDSA Cycle to test this solution. An implementation plan should be used to track progress and the steps required. This implementation plan can be in the form of a work plan or Gantt chart. This is a chart in the form of a table that identifies what activity is to be completed, who is responsible for it, and when it is going to be done. (See sample in Figure 13-5.) It outlines the steps needed to implement the change.

OTHER QUALITY IMPROVEMENT STRATEGIES

Improvement strategies identified at the organizational level involve benchmarking, meeting regulatory requirements, identifying opportunities for

system changes following sentinel event review, using visual measurements, and using a storyboard.

REGULATORY REQUIREMENTS

The Joint Commission (JC) has developed standards to guide critical activities performed by health care organizations. Preparation for an accreditation survey and the survey results will provide a wealth of information and data, which can be utilized as ideas for improvement strategies. In January 2003, the first six National Patient Safety Goals (NPSG) were approved by the JC. Each year, the JC publishes new goals that organizations must have in place to promote specific improvements in care related to patient safety. Recognizing that system design is intrinsic to the delivery of safe, high-quality health care, the goals focus on systemwide solutions wherever possible. The NPSG goals focus on Communication, Patient Identification, Medication Safety, Falls, Correct Surgical Patient Identification and Medication Reconciliation. Specific information regarding the history and ongoing requirements can be found at the JC Web site. (www.jointcommission.org). JC requires that specific data be collected and reported during a survey (ORYX measures). In addition, the Center for Medicare (CMS) requires

Bed Access Improvement Team
Phase 2 Work Plan: Transition to Daily Management and Evaluation

Activity	Responsible Party	8/03	9/03	10/03	11/03	12/03
1.0 Modify the Team						
1.1 Identify Phase 2 tasks to be completed	Team	■				
1.2 Review & Modify Team Composition/membership	Team	■				
1.3 Develop Work Plan	Planning Team	■				
1.4 Review Work Plan with Team	Myers/Nolan		■			
2.0 Review/Modify Ideal Design						
2.1 Identify Modifications/Opportunities for Additional Change	Team			■		
2.2 Revise Ideal Flow Chart	Team			■		
3.0 Modify Structure & Supports: People/Forms Needed						
3.1 Revise Process Management Structure • Modify job descriptions—Triage Manager and Admitting Coordinator	Triage Management Subgroup				■	
3.2 Assess Communication Needed with Nursing Units	Team				■	
4.0 Draft/Standardize Tasks						
4.1 Draft/Standardize Tasks					■	
5.0 Transition to Daily Operations, Develop Data Collection Process, Evaluate, Monitor						
5.1 Evaluate Bed Access Simulation • Review ED & PACU data • Identify accomplishments and opportunities for structure and ideal work process	Team					■
5.2 Develop Plan to Transition Process and Structure to Daily Operations	Planning Team					■
5.3 Develop Data Collection Process	Planning Team					■
5.4 Evaluate Process & Structure (milestone meeting)	Team					■
5.5 Identify Subgroup of Pt Care Delivery System QIT to Monitor Progress	Team					■

Figure 13-5 Gantt chart/work plan. (*Source:* Courtesy of Albany Medical Center, Albany, NY).

reporting on key quality measures, some linked to pay-for-performance. Reporting on quality measures is required in clinical areas such as acute myocardial infarction, congestive heart failure, pneumonia, and surgical infection prevention.

SENTINEL EVENT REVIEW

An adverse **sentinel event** is an unexpected occurrence involving death or serious physical or psychological injury to a patient (Joint Commission 1998).

Events are called sentinel because they require immediate investigation. During analysis of these sentinel events, opportunities for improving the system will arise and should be taken advantage of. Linkage of sentinel event review to the organization's performance improvement system will identify strategies for prevention of future sentinel events. An example of a sentinel event is surgery performed on the wrong extremity of a patient. Reviewing the surgical process and developing a system to mark the appropriate site is an example of a performance improvement to prevent future harmful occurrences.

MEASUREMENTS

To assess and monitor outcomes, heath care organizations collect and report measures at various levels in the organization. The terms *dashboard, balanced scorecard, report cards,* and *clinical value compass* are often used to describe the concept of measuring performance at both a strategic and operational level in the organization. Indicators may be patient clinical or functional status, patient satisfaction measures, cost measures, or organizational performance measures. (Caldwell, 1998) Figure 13-6 illustrates these in the form of a clinical value compass.

Such an approach allows those reviewing data to examine a balanced approach to care (see Figure 13-7). Indicators are selected based on what they have in common, so that if a change occurs in the cost-effectiveness category, it will affect the data in another category. From the control charts on this orthopedic unit, you can see that the total

hip pathway length of stay increased and then decreased. The satisfaction scores remained at around 90%, so even though the length of stay decreased, satisfaction did not deteriorate. The ratio of complications went down; the average number of physical therapy visits varied and then went up. This reporting mechanism offers a balanced view.

The balanced scorecard guides the development of a unit-based performance improvement plan (see Figure 13-8), and provides a tool with which to present the outcomes of performance improvement in the succinct visual format of an executive summary.

STORYBOARD: HOW TO SHARE YOUR STORY

Performance improvement teams share their work with others using a storyboard. The storyboard can be displayed in a high-traffic area of the organization to inform other staff of the QI efforts

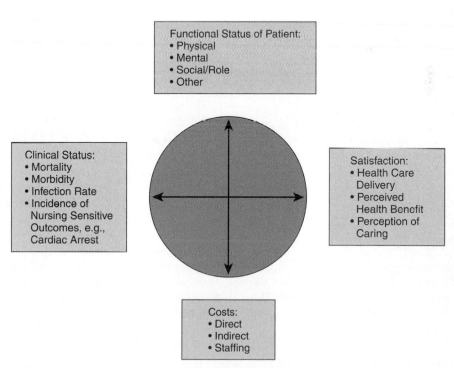

Figure 13-6 Clinical value compass. (*Source:* Developed with information from Albany Medical Center, Albany, NY).

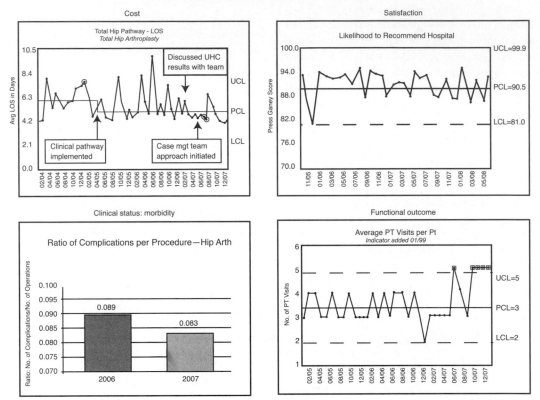

Figure 13-7 Orthopedic balanced scorecard. (*Source:* Courtesy of Albany Medical Center, Albany, NY).

under way. Note the storyboard in the photo at the beginning of this chapter. Storyboarding can be done when an improvement process is complete, or used during the process to communicate information, e.g., clinical outcomes, patient satisfaction, etc.

USING DATA

Several different types of charts are used to examine data in QI efforts. These include time series charts, Pareto charts, histograms, flowcharts, Ishikawa fishbone (root cause) diagrams, pie charts, and check sheets. See Figures 13-9, 13-10 and 13-11.

ORGANIZATIONAL STRUCTURE FOR QI

Figure 13-12 is an organizational chart that shows a structure for quality improvement. Note that it includes staff at the board level to staff on individual quality improvement teams (QITs). Communicating priorities at all levels in the organization is key. Staff members must realize how their day-to-day work influences the accomplishment of strategic goals. Mission, vision, and value statements help accomplish this clarity of focus. This is discussed more in chapter 11.

INPATIENT SURGICAL UNIT

PERFORMANCE IMPROVEMENT PLAN

As part of Bassett's commitment to quality, the Surgical Unit will strive to improve performance through a cycle of planning, process design, performance measurement, assessment and improvement. There will be ongoing assessment of important aspects of care and service and correction of identified problems. Problem identification and solution will be carried out using a systematic intra- and interdepartmental approach organized around patient flow or other key functions, and in concert with the approved visions and strategies of the organization. Priorities for improvement will include high risk, high volume and problem-prone procedures.

The Surgical Unit will:

• promote the Plan-Do-Check-Act methodology for all performance improvement activities
• provide staff education and training on integrated quality and cost improvement
• collect data to support objective assessment of processes and contribute to problem resolution

In identifying important aspects of care and service, the Surgical Unit will select performance measures in the following operational categories:

A. Clinical Quality
1. Patient safety

• Patient falls
• Indicator: # of patient falls per month/# of patient days with upper control limits set by the research department based on statistical deviation

• Medication and IV errors
• Indicator: # of patient IV/medication errors per month/# of patient days with upper control limits set by the research department based on statistical deviation

• Restraint use
• Indicator: % of compliance with policy for use of restraints and overall rate of restraint use

2. Pressure ulcer prevention
• Indicator: Rates of occurrence-quarterly tracking report

3. Surveillance, prevention and control of infection
• Indicator: Infection control statistical report of wound and catheter associated infections
• Indicator: Quarterly monitoring of compliance with standards for Acid Fast Bacilli (AFB) room use, evidence of staff validation in AFB practice

4. Employee safety
• Injuries resulting from
• Back and lifting-related injuries
• Morbidly obese patients
• Orthopedic patients
• Indicators: # of injuries sustained by employees and any resultant workmen's compensation (Human Resources quarterly report)
• 100% competency validation in lifting techniques and back injury prevention
• Respiratory fit testing
• Indicator: competency record of each employee

5. Documentation by exception
Indicators:
• 100% validation of RN/LPN staff
• Monthly chart audit (10% average daily census or 20 charts) meeting compliance with established standards

B. Access:
• Maintenance of the 30 minute standard for bed assignment of ED admissions
• Indicator: Quarterly review of ED tracking record

C. Service:
Patient Satisfaction
Indicator: Patient Satisfaction Survey: 90% or above response to, "Would return", and "Would recommend"

D. Cost:
• Nursing staff productivity will remain at 110% of target of 8.5 worked hours per adjusted patient day within a maximum variance range of 10%

For each of the above performance measures, this performance improvement plan will:

• address the highest priority improvement issues
• require data collection according to the structure, procedure and frequency defined
• document a baseline for performance
• demonstrate internal comparisons trended over time
• demonstrate external benchmark comparisons trended over time
• document areas identified for improvement
• demonstrate that changes have been made to address improvement
• demonstrate evaluation of these changes; document that improvement has occurred or, if not, that a different approach has been taken to address the issue

The Inpatient Surgical Unit will submit biannual status reports to the Bassett Improvement Council (BIC) through the Medical Surgical Quality Improvement Council (MSQIC).
l

Approved by:_____**Date:**_____

(Chief or Vice President)

Figure 13-8 Inpatient surgical unit, performance improvement plan. (*Source:* Courtesy Patricia Roesch, BS, RN, Bassett Healthcare).

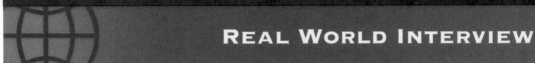

REAL WORLD INTERVIEW

We have developed a nursing practice quality scorecard. The scorecard is a tool to display data on our three organizational priorities: mission, customer orientation, and cost-effectiveness. By looking at measures in all three arenas, we can see how we are doing in these areas. We also can see if changes made in one arena positively or negatively affect the other measures. To look at nursing's mission for nursing practice, we track and trend several of the American Nurses Association national indicators. We track medication errors, patient falls, restraints, nosocomial pressure ulcers, and urinary tract infections. For customer satisfaction, we measure overall satisfaction with nursing care provided and how well patients' pain was controlled. For cost-effectiveness, we track nursing hours per patient day. All of these measures are tracked and trended on control charts every 3 months. The specific data is trended, and measures that are greater than 2 standard deviations of the target are identified as potential points to be reviewed for identification of opportunities for improvement.

Lessons that we have learned in the development of the scorecard is that we needed to set improvement targets earlier in the process to push the search for opportunities for improvement. We also learned that many of these measures are not well defined and therefore benchmarking to other organizations is difficult. We continue to strive for further improvement and utilize the scorecard to measure our success and look for opportunities for improvement. Reviewing nursing outcome data for the entire nursing division has been a powerful tool to ensure that care provided is meeting expected outcomes, and it allows us to benchmark our outcomes to other organizations.

Louann Villani, RN, BSN
Nursing Quality Specialist
Albany, New York

CASE STUDY 13-1

Agroup that was developing a clinical pathway for the care of patients with acute myocardial infarction noted evidence showing that these patients should receive acetylsalicylic acid (ASA) on admission. The research in this area was very clear, and most practitioners believed this was being done. When a chart audit was performed to determine whether this was, in fact, the practice on the unit, it was discovered that only 48% of the patients were receiving ASA within eight hours of admission. The team added administration of ASA to the clinical pathway. After this was implemented, 85% of the patients received ASA within the first eight hours of admission.

What clinical practices do you see on your clinical unit that are based on an evidence-based clinical pathway? How can you participate in improving the care of more patients using evidence-based clinical pathways? Who should be involved in these efforts?

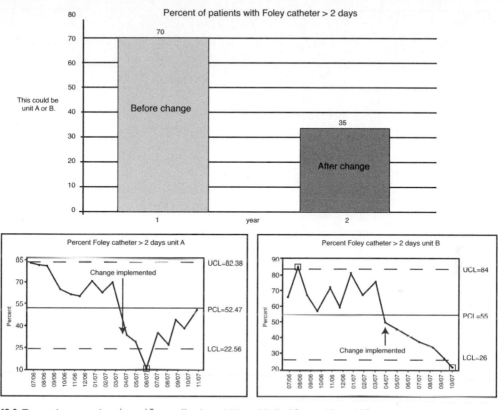

Figure 13-9 Time series versus bar charts. (*Source:* Courtesy of Albany Medical Center, Albany, NY).

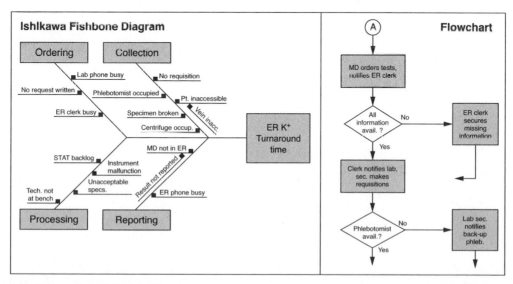

Figure 13-10 Ishikawa fishbone diagram, flowchart, and check sheet. (*Source:* Reprinted with permission from *Clinical Laboratory Management Review*, November/December 1991, 5[6]:448–462. ©Clinical Laboratory Management Association, Inc. All rights reserved).

Check Sheet

Delays in production of Serum K⁺ results from 1/1/91 to 1/7/91

Code/Delay Type		Mon	Tue	Wed	Thur	Fri	Sat	Sun	Total
A	Request not written by physician	I	I			/	I		3
B	Lab phone busy > 2 minutes	I		I		II		I	5
C	Phlebotomists unavailable	III	II	III	III	II	IIII	III	20
D	Requisition not ready	II	I	I	I	I	III	II	11
E	Patient inaccessible	I	I	II	I		II	I	8
F	Vein inaccessible	I		II		I	II		6
G	Centrifuge busy	II		I		I			4
H	Specimen broken	II		I				I	4
I	STAT backlog	III			I		II	I	7
J	Tech. not at bench	II		II		I	II	I	8
K	Unacceptable specimen	I	I		II		I	II	7
L	Lab. sec. unavailable to report	III		I		I	I		6
M	ER phone not answered			I			II		3
N	MD not in ER	II		I		II		I	5
O	MD not answer page	I	I	II		II		II	8
P	Results not reported by ER sec.	II	I	II	I	III	II	II	13

Figure 13-10 *(continued)*

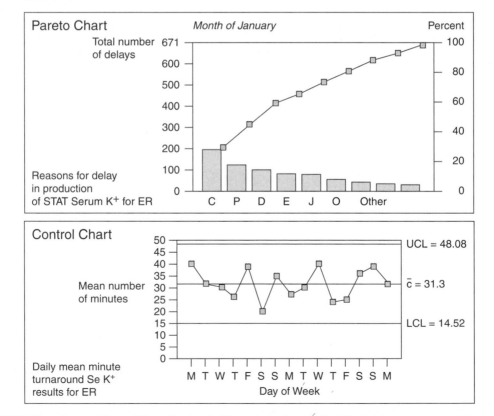

Figure 13-11 Pareto Chart and Control Chart. (Reprinted with permission from *Total quality and the management of laboratories* by K. N. Simpson, A. D. Kaluzny, and C. P. McLaughlin, 1991, Clinical Laboratory Management Review, 5(6), 448–449, 452–453, 456–458. © Clinical Laboratory Management Association, Inc. All rights reserved).

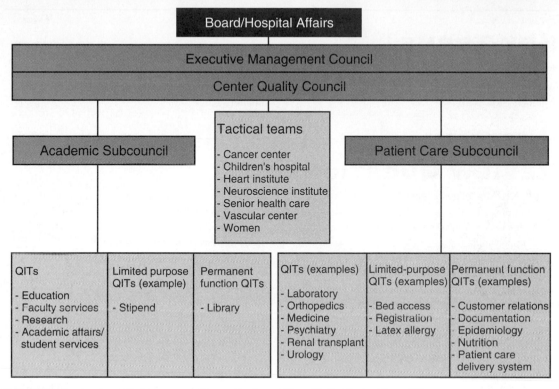

Figure 13-12 Structure for quality improvement. (*Source:* Courtesy of Albany Medical Center, Albany, NY).

KEY CONCEPTS

- Quality improvement is a continuous process focused on maintaining regulatory compliance and improving patient care processes and outcomes.

- Customers of health care are patients, nurses, doctors, the community, and so on.

- Patient care needs should drive improvement opportunities.

- Decisions should be driven by data.

- Improvement initiatives should be linked to the organization's mission, vision, and values.

- Organizational goals and objectives should be communicated up and down the organization.

- There should be a balance in improvement goals focused on patient clinical and functional status, access, cost, and patient satisfaction outcomes.

- A clinical value compass identifies key outcomes that are monitored for quality improvement.

- The University of Colorado Hospital model is an example of a multidisciplinary evidence-based practice model for using different sources of information to change or support your practice.

- The Model for Improvement and FOCUS-PDSA can be applied to a system or an individual.

- Benchmarks are used to monitor quality.

KEY TERMS

benchmarking

customers

evidence-based care

quality assurance

quality improvement

sentinel event

REVIEW QUESTIONS

1. Which of the following describes the benchmarking process?
   A. Reviewing your own unit's data for improvement opportunities
   B. Collecting data on an individual patient
   C. Reviewing data in the literature
   D. Comparing your data to that of other organizations to identify improvement opportunities

2. Identifying opportunities in the health care arena is the responsibility of which group?
   A. Administration
   B. Practitioners
   C. Patients
   D. Everyone

3. Following a sentinel event, which step would be initiated first?
   A. No action
   B. Corrective action of personnel
   C. Reporting to health department/root cause analysis
   D. Immediate investigation

4. To participate effectively in the use of EBC, nurses must
   A. participate in the development, use, and evaluation of practice guidelines.
   B. read and analyze outcomes of research studies.
   C. involve themselves in everyday patient care and nursing practice.
   D. do all of the above.

REVIEW ACTIVITIES

1. Risk management, infection control practitioners, and a benchmark study have revealed that your unit's utilization of indwelling catheters is above average. Brainstorm reasons why this may be occurring. Creating a fishbone (root cause) diagram may help.

2. Think about your last clinical rotation experience. Identify one process that you believe could be improved and describe how you would begin improving the process. Use the FOCUS methodology.

EXPLORING THE WEB

- Visit the University HealthSystem Consortium (UHC) to search for benchmark data: *www.uhc.edu*

- The Institute for Healthcare Improvement (IHI) also includes information on benchmarking: *www.ihi.org*

- These sites are recommended for a team that is looking for evidence-based guidelines or research studies for a particular diagnosis:

  National Guideline Clearinghouse:
  www.guideline.gov
  Cochrane Library:
  www.cochrane.org
  PubMed's home page:
  www.ncbi.nlm.nih.gov
  Evidence-Based Practice Internet Resources:
  www.hsl.lib.mcmaster.ca

- The Web site for the Agency for Healthcare Research and Quality (AHRQ), formerly the Agency for Health Care Policy and Research (AHCPR),

has a clinical information index page that lists evidence reports for topics such as swallowing disorders in stroke patients, evaluation of therapies for stable angina, and access to agency-supported guidelines (e.g., cancer pain, cardiac rehabilitation, and pressure ulcers):
www.ahrq.gov

- Go to:
  www.nursingworld.org
  Search for information about the Nursing Information and Data Set Evaluation Center. Note the ANA Recognized Classification Systems listed.

- Check this source of quality information:
  www.leapfroggroup.org

REFERENCES

AMCQ series curriculum. (1998). Albany, NY: Albany Medical Center, Quality Management Department.

Caldwell, C. (1998). Handbook for managing change in health care. Milwaukee, WI: ASQ Quality Press.

Camp, R. (1994). Benchmarking applied to healthcare. *The Joint Commission on Quality Improvement, 20,* 229–238.

Crosby, P. B. (1979). *Quality is free.* New York: New America Library.

Deming, W. E. (1986). *Out of the crisis.* Cambridge, MA: Center for Advanced Engineering Study.

Donabedian, A. (1966). Evaluating the quality of medical care. *Milbank Memorial Fund Quarterly, 44,* 194–196.

Gift, R. G., & Mosel, D. (1994). *Benchmarking in health care: A collaborative approach.* Chicago: American Hospital Publishing.

Goode, C. J., & Piedalue, F. (1999). Evidence-based clinical practice. *Journal of Nursing Administration, 29,* 15–21.

Goode, C. J., Tanaka, D. J., Krugman, M., O'Connor, P. A., Bailey, C., Deutchman, M., (2000). Outcomes from use of an evidence-based practice guideline. Nursing *Economic$, 18,* 202–207.

Jadlos, M. A., Kelman, G. B., Marra, K., & Lanoue, A. (1996). A pain management documentation tool. *Oncology Nursing Forum, 23,* 1451–1454.

Joint Commission. (JC). (1998). *Comprehensive accreditation manual for hospitals* Oakbrook, IL: Joint Commission.

Juran, J.M. (ed) (1988). *Quality Control Handbook.* (4th ed.). New York, NY: McGraw Hill.

Kane, R. L. (1997). *Understanding health care outcomes research* (1st ed.). Gaithersburg, MD: Aspen.

Kimberly, J. R. & Minvielle, E. (2003) *Quality as an Organizational Problem* (p. 62). In S. S. Mick & M. Wyttenback, M. (Eds.), Advances in Health Care Organization Theory. San Francisco, CA: Jossey-Bass.

Langley, G. J., Nolan, K. M., Nolan, T. W., Norman, C. L., & Provost, L. P. (1996). *The improvement guide: A practical approach to enhancing organizational performance.* San Francisco: Jossey-Bass.

Ransom, S. B., Joshi, M. S., & Nash, D. B. (2005). *The healthcare quality book: Vision, strategy, and tools.* Chicago: Health Administration Press.

Simpson, K. N., Kaluzny, A. D., & McLaughlin, C.P. (1991). Total quality and the management of laboratories. *Clinical laboratory management review, 5(6),* 448–449, 452–453, 456–458.

SUGGESTED READINGS

Allen, D. E., Bockenhauer, B., Egan, C., & Kinnaird, L. S. (2006). Relating outcomes to excellent nursing practice. *The Journal of Nursing Administration (JONA), 36*(3), 140–147.

Arnold, L., Campbell, A., Dubree, M., Fuchs, M. A., Davis, N., Hertzler, B., et al. (2006). Priorities and challenges of health system chief nursing executives: Insights for nursing educators. *Journal of Professional Nursing, 22*(4), 213–220.

Berwick, D. M., Calkins, D. R., McCannon, B. A., & Hackbarth, A. D. (2006). The 100,000 Lives Campaign: Setting a goal and a deadline for improving health care quality. *Journal of the American Medical Association, 295*(3), 324–327.

Cochrane Library at McMaster University. *Using Medline to search for evidence*. Retrieved March, 2000, from www.londonlinks.ac.uk./evidence_strategies/coch_search.htm.

Engelke, M. K., & Marshburn, D. M. (2006). Collaborative strategies to enhance research and evidence-based practice. *The Journal of Nursing Administration (JONA), 36*(3), 131–135.

Guyatt, G. H., Haynes, R. B., Jaeschke, R. Z., Cook, D. J., Green, L., Naylor, C. D., et al. (2000). Users guides to the medical literature: XXV. Evidence-based medicine: Principles for applying the users guides to patient care. *Journal of the American Medical Association, 284,* 1290–1296.

Joanna Briggs Institute for Evidence Based Nursing & Midwifery. Retrieved March 9, 2007, from www.joannabriggs.edu.au/ services/search.php.

Kahn, C. N., Ault, T., Isenstein, H., Potetz, L., & Van Gelder, S. (2006). Snapshot of hospital quality reporting and pay-for-performance under Medicare. *Health Affairs, 25*(1), 148–162.

Ring, N., Coull, A., Howie, C., Murphy-Black, T., & Watterson, A. (2006). Analysis of the impact of a national initiative to promote evidence-based nursing practice. *International Journal of Nursing Practice, 12*(4), 232–240.

CHAPTER 14

Legal Aspects of Health Care

A nurse who concludes that an attending physician has misdiagnosed a condition or has not prescribed the appropriate course of treatment may not modify the course set by the physician simply because the nurse holds a different view . . . However, the nurse is not prohibited from calling on or consulting with nurse supervisors or with other physicians . . . concerning those matters, and when the patient's condition reasonably requires it the nurse has a duty to do those tasks . . .

(Berdyck v. Shinde, 613 N.E.2d 1014, 1024 [Ohio, 1993])

OBJECTIVES

Upon completion of this chapter, the reader should be able to:

1. Discuss the sources of law.
2. Name the most common areas of nursing practice cited in malpractice actions.
3. List some actions a nurse can take to decrease liability.

You are working on a postsurgical unit and have been given an order to discharge a 72-year-old male who has just had a total hip replacement. Per hospital policy, you obtain a set of vital signs before discharging him home and note his temperature to be 100.9°F (38.3°C). Upon assessing the patient, he tells you that he feels a bit "chilled." You notify the practitioner of the elevated temperature and the patient's comments, but you are told to continue with the discharge.

After notifying the practitioner about the elevated temperature, do you need to gather additional information about the patient's condition before you discharge him?

What do you do if the patient appears to be too ill for discharge? Is there anyone else you can contact?

If you discharge the patient and he develops sepsis or a serious illness, are you responsible or is the practitioner responsible?

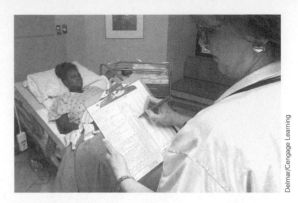

Delmar/Cengage Learning

Law that affects the relationship between individuals is called civil law. Law that specifies the relationship between citizens and the state is called public law. This chapter reviews how various types of law affect nursing practice and actions a nurse can take to minimize risks to her professional practice.

SOURCES OF LAW

The authority to make, implement, and interpret laws is generally granted in a constitution. A **constitution** is a set of basic laws that specifies the powers of the various segments of the government and how these segments relate to each other.

Generally, it is the role of a legislative body, both on the federal and state levels, to enact laws. Agencies under the authority of the administrative branch of the government draft the rules that implement the law. Finally, the judicial branch interprets the law as it rules in court cases. Table 14-1 gives examples of these relationships.

Also, a judicial decision may set a precedent that is used by other courts and, over time, has the force of law. This type of law is referred to as **common law**.

PUBLIC LAW

Public law consists of constitutional law, criminal law, and administrative law and defines a citizen's relationship with government.

CONSTITUTIONAL LAW

Several categories of public law affect the practice of nursing. For example, the nurse accommodates patients' constitutional right to practice their religion every time the nurse calls a patient's clergy as requested, follows a specific religious custom for preparation of meals, or prepares a deceased person's remains for burial.

Nurses may not believe in a right personally and may refuse to work in areas where they would have to assist a patient in exercising a right. Nurses may not, however, interfere with another person's ability to exercise his constitutional right.

CRIMINAL LAW

Criminal law focuses on the actions of individuals that can intentionally do harm to others. Often the victims of such abusive actions are the very young or the very old. These two categories of people generally cannot defend themselves against physical or emotional abuse. The nurse, in caring for patients, may notice that a vulnerable patient has unexplained bruises, fractures, or other injuries. Most states have mandatory statutes that require the nurse to report unexplained or suspicious injuries to the appropriate child or elderly protective agency. Generally, the institution in which the nurse is employed will have clear guidelines

TABLE 14-1	THE THREE BRANCHES OF GOVERNMENT IN THE UNITED STATES		
	Legislative Branch	**Administrative Branch**	**Judicial Branch**
Example at Federal Level	Americans with Disabilities Act (ADA) (1990)	The Equal Employment Commission (EEOC) publishes rules specifying what employers must do to help a disabled employee.	In 1999, the U.S. Supreme Court interpreted the law to require that to be protected by this law, the individual must have an impairment that limits a major life activity and that is not corrected by medicine or appliances (e.g., blood pressure medicine, glasses). (*Sutton v. United Airlines* [1999]; *Murphy v. United Parcel Service, Inc.* [1999]).
Example at State Level	Nurse Practice Act	The state board of nursing develops rules specifying the duties of a registered nurse in that state.	Courts and juries determine whether a nurse's actions comply with the law governing the practice of nursing in a state.

to follow in such a situation. Failure to report the problem as required by law can result in criminal penalties.

Another aspect of criminal law affecting nursing practice is the state and federal requirement that criminal background checks be performed on specified categories of prospective employees who will work with the very young or the elderly in institutions such as schools and nursing homes. Again, this is an attempt to protect the most vulnerable citizens from mistreatment or abuse. Failure to conduct the mandated background checks can result in the institution having to defend itself for any harm done by an employee with a past criminal conviction. One hospital was found negligent for failing to conduct a criminal background check or investigate complaints against an employee who later sexually abused a patient (Fiesta, 1999). However, in another case in which the hospital did investigate such complaints, the appellate court did not find it responsible for the sexual assault on a patient

by an employee (Fiesta, 1999). The rationale for this was that the hospital had done what it was required to do by law in investigating the employee's criminal background and was not liable for these unexpected actions.

The third area in which criminal law concerns affect nursing practice is the prohibition against substance abuse. Both federal and state law requires health care agencies to keep a strict accounting of the use and distribution of regulated drugs. Nurses routinely are expected to keep narcotic records accurate and current.

Nurses' behavior when off duty can also affect their employment status. Abusing alcohol or drugs on one's own time, if discovered, can result in nurses being terminated from employment and their license to practice nursing being restricted or revoked. Frequently, boards of nursing have programs for the nurse with a drug problem, and completion of such a program may be required before the nurse can resume practice. Additionally, health care facilities may do random drug screens

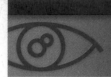

CRITICAL THINKING 14-1

You are new nurse working on the OB unit of your local hospital. Your close friend George Nurse also got a job on this unit. George has a reputation as a smart, likeable, and hard-working nurse, who also knows how to let loose and have a good time outside of work. However, recently George has been coming to work late and appears "out of it." You spoke with George, who told you that he was having a difficult time at home, and had not been as focused at work as he needed to be. He promised that he would try to leave his personal life at home.

For a month after your discussion with George, everything seemed fine. However, in the past two weeks, you have noticed that George has had bloodshot eyes and his speech seems slurred at times. He looks unkempt and unclean, and the narcotic count for Vicodin was off for three separate shifts that he worked. You are concerned that George may be using drugs or alcohol and that it may be impacting his nursing care.

What action do you take? Who can you go to for help in this situation?

on their employees to identify those who may be using illegal substances.

ADMINISTRATIVE LAW

Both the federal government and state governments have administrative laws that affect nursing practice. The laws pertaining to Social Security and, more specifically, Medicare, are interpreted in the *Code of Federal Regulations,* which contains the administrative rules for the federal government. These rules have specific requirements that hospitals, nursing homes, and other health care providers must adhere to if they are to qualify for payment from federal funds. Likewise, state laws are interpreted in administrative rules that specify licensing requirements for health care providers in the state.

FEDERAL LAW **Administrative law** deals with protection of the rights of citizens. It extends some rights and protections beyond those granted in the federal and state constitutions.

As with most federal laws, the agency responsible for implementing the law has a great deal of power to draft specific rules and regulations. For example, the Occupational Safety & Health Administration, an administrative agency, works to establish a safe workplace for employees. This includes enacting regulations concerning storage of hazardous substances, protection of employees from infection, and protection of employees from violence in the workplace. Hospitals are subject to numerous OSHA regulations designed to protect the health and safety of nurses and other health care workers. From the minute the new nurse joins the hospital staff, he or she will come into contact with OSHA-mandated products or programs every day. For example, any unvaccinated nurse joining the staff of a hospital will be offered Hepatitis B vaccination pursuant to OSHA regulations. Additionally, nurses working with patients who may have tuberculosis will be issued special OSHA-approved respirators to prevent the nurse from becoming infected. Every day, nurses will utilize OSHA mandated and approved "sharps" containers that hold used needles and personal protective equipment such as gloves, gowns, and surgical face masks. New nurses should review hospital policies and procedures to ensure they are using these safety devices properly.

STATE LAW An example of a state's administrative law is its nurse practice act. Under nurse practice acts, state boards of nursing are given the authority to define the practice of nursing within certain broad parameters specified by the legislature, mandate the requisite preparation for the practice of nursing, and discipline members of the profession who deviate from the rules governing the practice of nursing. Other professions such as medicine and dentistry have similar practice acts established in state law.

Currently, an issue that is affecting licensure of nursing is the multistate licensure compact, which affords mutual state recognition of nursing licenses.

Multistate Licensure Compact An important issue to nurses is the transferability of their nursing license from one state to another. A license to practice nursing is generally valid only in the state where it is issued. In most cases, a nurse wanting to practice in a state other than where his or her license was issued must apply for a license in that state. For nurses who frequently move from one state to another, this can be a burdensome process. There is an ongoing movement to allow nurses licensed in one state to automatically receive licensure to practice in another state. The Nurse Licensure Compact, a project of the National Council of State Boards of Nursing, is an agreement among states to allow nurses licensed in other states who are parties to the agreement to practice without applying for a new license (Hellquist & Spector, 2004). As of the date of this writing, only 23 states had joined this agreement, meaning that most states still require nurses to apply for a license in the state where they want to practice. You may check the Internet to determine if your state is a member of the compact by pointing your browser to www.ncsbn.org. Of course, nurses should always contact the board of nursing in any state where they intend to practice to determine eligibility and licensure requirements.

CIVIL LAW

Civil law governs how individuals relate to each other in everyday matters. It encompasses both contract and tort law.

CONTRACT LAW

Contract law regulates certain transactions between individuals and/or legal entities such as businesses. It also governs transactions between businesses. An agreement between two or more parties must contain the following elements to be recognized as a legal contract:

- Agreement between two or more legally competent individuals or parties stating what each must or must not do

- Mutual understanding of the terms and obligations that the contract imposes on each party to the contract
- Payment or consideration given for actions taken or not taken pursuant to the agreement

The terms of the contract may be oral or written; however, a written contract may not be legally modified by an oral agreement. Another way this is often expressed is by the phrase "all of the terms of the contract are contained within the four corners of the document"; that is, if it is not written, it is not part of the agreement or contract. A contract may be express or implied. In an express contract, the terms of the contract are specified, usually in writing. In an implied contract, a relationship between parties is recognized, although the terms of the agreement are not clearly defined, such as the expectations one has for services from the dry cleaner or the grocer.

The nurse is usually a party to an employment contract. The employed nurse agrees to do the following:

- Adhere to the policies and procedures of the employing entity
- Fulfill the agreed-upon duties of the employer
- Respect the rights and responsibilities of other health care providers in the workplace

In return, the employer agrees to provide the nurse with the following:

- A specified amount of pay for services rendered
- Adequate assistance in providing care
- The supplies and equipment needed to fulfill the nurse's responsibilities
- A safe environment in which to work
- Reasonable treatment and behavior from the other health care providers with whom the nurse must interact

This contract may be express or implied, depending on the practices of the employing entity. Sometimes, what is determined to be "reasonable" by the employer is not considered "reasonable" by the nurse. For instance, after 20 years of working as a nurse on the orthopedic unit, a nurse may not view it as reasonable to be pulled to the labor and delivery unit for duty as a nurse there. It would be prudent for this nurse to express any misgivings to the supervisor and then to cooperate but take only assignments that are in keeping with the responsibilities the nurse can safely complete. In this instance, it is reasonable to give nursing assistance on the labor and delivery unit that the nurse can competently deliver, although it may not be reasonable to assume total responsibility for these patients without additional education and experience.

TORT LAW

A **tort** is a negligent or intentional civil wrong not arising out of a contract or statute that injures someone in some way, and for which the injured person may sue the wrongdoer for damages (The 'Lectric Law Library's Lexicon On Tort [2008]). A tort can be any of the following:

- The denial of a person's legal right
- The failure to comply with a public duty

- The failure to perform a private duty that results in harm to another

A tort can be unintentional, as occurs in malpractice or neglect, or it can be the intentional infliction of harm, such as assault and battery. In a tort suit, the nurse can be named as a defendant because of something the nurse did incorrectly or because the nurse failed to do something that was required. In either case, the suit is usually classified as a tort suit (Fiesta, 1999). Other tort charges that a nurse may face include false imprisonment, invasion of privacy, defamation, and fraud. See Table 14-2.

NEGLIGENCE AND MALPRACTICE

If a nurse fails to meet the legal expectations for care, usually defined by the state's nurse practice act, the patient, if harmed by this failure, can initiate an action against the nurse for damages. The term

TABLE 14-2	**SELECTED TORTS**

Tort	Definition	Example
Assault	Threat to touch another person in an offensive manner without that person's permission.	Nurse who threatens to give a patient a treatment against his or her will.
Battery	Touching of another person without that person's consent.	Nurse who forces a treatment against a patient's will.
Invasion of privacy	All patients have the right to privacy and may bring charges against any person who violates this right.	Nurse who discloses confidential information about a patient or photographs a patient without consent.
False imprisonment	This occurs when individuals are physically prevented, or incorrectly led to believe they are prevented, from leaving a place.	Nurse who restrains a patient who is of sound mind and is not in danger of injuring self or others.
Defamation, including libel and slander	Intentionally false communication or publication, including written (libel) or verbal (slander) remarks that may cause damage to a person's reputation.	Nurse who makes a statement that could either ruin the patient's reputation or cause the patient to lose his job.

malpractice refers to a professional's wrongful conduct in the discharge of his or her professional duties, or failure to meet standards of care for the profession, which results in harm to another individual entrusted to the professional's care. **Negligence** is the failure to provide the care a reasonable person would ordinarily provide in a similar situation.

Simply proving malpractice or negligence is not sufficient to recover damages. Proof of liability or fault requires proof of the following four elements:

1. A duty or obligation created by law, contract, or standard practice that is owed to the complainant by the professional
2. A breach of this duty, either by omission or commission
3. Harm, which can be physical, emotional, or financial, to the complainant (patient)
4. Proof that the breach of duty caused the harm being complained of

A Louisiana appellate court described the plaintiff's (patient's) specific burden of proof in a negligence or malpractice case against a nurse as follows:

[T]he three requirements which a plaintiff must satisfy to meet plaintiff's burden of proving the negligence of a nurse are (1) the nurse must exercise the degree of skill ordinarily employed, under similar circumstances, by the members of the nursing or health care profession in good standing in the same community or locality; (2) the nurse either lacked this degree of knowledge or skill or failed to use reasonable care and diligence, along with her best judgment in the application of that skill; and (3) as a proximate result of this lack of knowledge or skill or the failure to exercise this degree of care, the plaintiff suffered injuries that would not otherwise have occurred (*Odom v. State Dept. of Health & Hospitals* [1999]).

Once a plaintiff presents his or her case, the defendant nurse must refute the claims either by showing that if a duty was owed, it was fulfilled or by demonstrating that the breach of that duty was not the cause of the plaintiff's harm.

Proving that a duty was owed is not difficult. The person need only show that the nurse was working on the day in question and was responsible for the plaintiff's care. This can usually be accomplished by producing staffing schedules and assignment sheets.

To demonstrate a breach of duty, the courts employ a *reasonable man* standard by asking what a reasonable nurse would do in a like situation. This is accomplished by reviewing the employing institution's policies and procedures and the state's nursing and medical practice acts and hearing testimony from nurses who are accepted as expert witnesses to the standard of nursing practice in the community. Other sources that may be reviewed include evidence-based health care research, nursing and medical literature, standards of professional associations such as the American Nurses Association Standards, equipment manufacturers' manuals, health care accreditation agency criteria, and/or medication books.

The defendant nurse would employ the same methodology to refute the plaintiff's charges. The nurse would present evidence that the institution's policies and procedures were followed and that the care rendered adhered to accepted nursing standards. To present the nurse's case, the nurse's attorney would also use expert witnesses to document that the care given fulfilled the duty owed, was the kind that would be given by a reasonable nurse in such a circumstance, and that it was not the cause of the plaintiff's harm.

It is not sufficient for a patient plaintiff to show a breach of duty to prevail in a tort suit. He must also show that the breach of the duty caused him or her harm. Even if it is proved that a nurse made a medication error, if the error was not the cause of the plaintiff's harm, he or she will not win in recovering damages from the nurse. In a recent malpractice case, a patient with sickle cell anemia died after suffering a cardiopulmonary arrest, attributed to an aspiration that was witnessed by a visitor. The visitor immediately called for and obtained help. Although revived, the patient never regained consciousness and was eventually taken off life support. At trial, the plaintiff was able to prove that the nurse assigned to this patient did not follow the institution's policy of documenting frequent observations, which were mandated because the patient was receiving a blood transfusion at the time of the cardiac arrest. In reviewing the case on appeal, the appellate court noted the following:

[T]he record contains no evidence which suggests what could have been done even if the nurse had been seated at his bedside prior to the arrest. Plaintiff has failed to offer any proof that more immediate assistance would have prevented the catastrophic results of his aspiration.

Based on the evidence in this record, we conclude that more frequent monitoring would have made no difference (*Webb v. Tulane Medical Center Hospital* [1997]).

Thus, even though the plaintiff successfully proved a breach of a duty, the breach was not found to be the cause of the patient's death, and the nurse was not found to be guilty of negligence. Table 14-3 reviews types of nursing

---

TABLE 14-3	**TYPES OF NURSING ACTIONS INVOLVED IN LITIGATION**

Treatment

- Failed to prevent and treat pressure ulcers and malnutrition, resulting in death
- Mishandled shoulder dystocia during delivery, resulting in brachial plexus injury
- Failed to perform intrauterine resuscitation, leading to infant's brain damage
- Failed to properly handle telephone triage calls, resulting in death
- Failed to incorporate patient's emergency room records into patient's hospital chart, resulting in death
- Failed to properly treat pediatric glaucoma, resulting in vision loss
- Burned patient with hair dryer, resulting in third-degree burns
- Failed to accurately count sponges after operation, resulting in retained sponge
- Failed to provide adequate nutrition and implement nursing plan of care, resulting in death
- Injected patient with used needle, leading to emotional distress from possible hepatitis infection
- Failed to properly treat patient's jaundice, resulting in infant's brain damage
- Failed to treat dehydration resulting in death
- Removed internal pacemaker wires improperly, resulting in infection
- Administered suction tube improperly, leading to aspiration and death by suffocation
- Failed to detect arterial blockage after surgery, leading to leg amputation
- Failed to adequately hydrate patient prior to C-section, resulting in maternal hypotension and infant's brain damage
- Failed to administer supplemental oxygen, resulting in vision loss and brain damage

Communication

- Failed to notify physician of
    a. patient burns
    b. bleeding gastric ulcer, resulting in death

(Continues)

TABLE 14-3	TYPES OF NURSING ACTIONS INVOLVED IN LITIGATION (CONTINUED)

    c. increased heart rate, resulting in death

    d. fetal distress, resulting in death, or resulting in brain damage

    e. newborn jaundice, resulting in brain damage

    f. PT level

    g. pain and numbness after spinal surgery, resulting in cauda equina syndrome

    h. vision problems, resulting in vision loss

- Failed to report sexual abuse of patient/resident to police and/or state department of human resources
- Failed to use chain-of-command reporting when medical practitioner refused to come to the hospital promptly

Medication

- Administered insufficient heparin, leading to death by pulmonary embolism
- Administered doses of Dilantin and insulin to a patient in excess of physician's order, leading to patient's disorientation and burns from bedside heater
- Administered excessive dose of IV antibiotics (nafcillin), leading to chemical burn
- Failed to send antibiotics home with patient with meningitis, leading to cerebral palsy
- Failed to recognize dosage error in doctor's order and thereby administered excessive dose of Dilaudid, leading to brain damage

Monitoring/Observing/Supervising

- Failed to monitor premature newborn, leading to death by cardiac arrest
- Failed to detect fetal distress, resulting in death, or resulting in brain damage
- Failed to monitor patient, leading to third-degree burns
- Failed to call a "code blue" in response to patient's respiratory arrest, resulting in death
- Failed to prevent patient falls, leading to death, or leading to quadriplegia, or leading to quadriparesis
- Failed to seek timely medical intervention, leading to death from bleeding ulcer
- Failed to properly monitor heart rate after surgery, resulting in death
- Misidentified and mixed up newborns in nursery
- Failed to monitor respiratory rate after surgery, resulting in death
- Failed to take vital signs of patient in waiting room, resulting in brain damage
- Failed to restrain demented patient, resulting in death
- Failed to properly insert Foley catheter during delivery, resulting in urinary sphincter trauma and incontinence
- Failed to monitor cornea in facial palsy, leading to corneal scarring and vision loss
- Failed to reattach cardiac monitor after x-rays, resulting in death
- Failed to detect brain swelling, resulting in vision loss and diminished IQ

Source: Pozza, R. (2003). Nursing malpractice cases. Unpublished manuscript.

actions involved in litigation reported in the *Professional Negligence Law Reporter*, July 2001 through July 2002 (Pozza, 2003). The clinical settings of these malpractice cases, included hospitals (Medical-Surgical, Maternity, Emergency Room, Pediatrics, Nursery, and Recovery Room units), nursing home, home health care, clinics, and urgent care facilities. Table 14-4 identifies health care facility liabilities other than nursing actions identified in these cases.

When a nurse is listed as a party in a medical malpractice lawsuit, the nurse's liability is reviewed. If state laws mandate that a nurse must have a nursing or medical practitioner's order before doing something, then that practitioner's order must be present. Problems arise when the orders are verbal, and later it is claimed that the nurse misunderstood and acted in error. Another pitfall is illegible writing, which is then misinterpreted and the result causes harm to the patient. Many nurses who have been in practice for a long time have encountered practitioners who write orders that are contrary to accepted practice. In these situations, the nurse must exercise professional judgment and follow the policies and procedures of the institution. Usually these require the nurse to notify the nursing supervisor and the medical director for the area where the nurse works.

The institution's policies and procedures describe the performance expected of nurses in its employ, and a nurse deviating from them can be liable for negligence or malpractice. Failure to adhere to institutional protocol can result in the employer denying the nurse a defense in a lawsuit.

Practicing nurses must also adhere to the standards of practice for the nursing profession in the community. These standards include such things as checking the six "rights" in medication administration or repositioning the bed-bound patient

TABLE 14-4	HEALTH CARE FACILITY LIABILITIES OTHER THAN NURSING ACTIONS

- Failure to provide a safe environment
- Misrepresenting the level of care available
- Failure to adequately train personnel in fall prevention
- Failure to adequately supervise nursing home staff to ensure residents receive proper nutrition, custodial treatment, and medical care at the facility
- Failure to instruct and train personnel regarding the handling of jaundice in newborns
- Failure to adequately train staff on emergency procedures
- Failure to inform medical practitioner of patient burns
- Failure to properly supervise staff
- Failure to provide timely lab services
- Failure to appropriately dispose of used syringes
- Failure to enforce policies to adequately handle emergencies
- Failure to report abuse of nursing home resident
- Allowing unlicensed persons to administer IV medications

Source: Pozza, R. (2003). *Nursing malpractice cases.* Unpublished manuscript.

at regular intervals. It is not uncommon for nurses to encounter conflicts between an employer's expectations and the nursing standards of care, resulting in problems such as having insufficient time or staffing to adhere to the standards taught in nursing school or receiving poor evaluations for taking too long to render care. In all situations, nurses must prioritize and evaluate what standards they must follow to preserve their professional practice, protect patients, and protect themselves from liability.

ASSAULT AND BATTERY   **Assault** is a threat to touch another in an offensive manner without that person's permission. A **battery** is the touching of another person without that person's consent. In the health care arena, lawsuits of this nature usually question whether the individual consented to the treatment administered by the health care professional. Most states have laws that require patients to make informed decisions about their treatment.

Informed consent laws protect the patient's right to practice self-determination. The patient has the right to receive sufficient information to make an informed decision about whether to consent to or refuse a procedure. The individual performing the procedure is responsible for explaining to the patient the nature of the procedure, benefits, alternatives, and the risks and potential complications. The signed consent form is used to document that this was done, and it creates a presumption that the patient had been advised of the appropriate risks.

Often the nurse is asked to witness a patient signing a consent form for treatment. When you witness a patient's signature, you are vouching for two things: that the patient signed the paper and that the patient knows he is signing a consent form (Olsen-Chavarriaga, 2000). For a consent form to be legal, a patient, in most states, must be at least 18 years old; be mentally competent; have the procedures, with their risks and benefits, explained in a manner he can understand; be aware of the available alternatives to the proposed treatment; and consent voluntarily. The nurse must also be familiar with which other people are allowed by state law to consent to medical treatment for another when that person cannot consent for himself. Frequently, these include the person possessing medical power of attorney; a spouse; adult children; or other relatives, if no one is available in one of the other categories listed.

A nurse may also face a charge of battery for failing to honor an advance directive, such as a medical power of attorney, durable power of attorney or living will.

Federal law requires that a hospital ask the patient, upon admission, whether she has a living will; if she does not, the hospital must ask her whether she would like to enact one. A **living will** is a written advance directive voluntarily signed by the patient that specifies the type of care she desires if and when she is in a terminal state and cannot sign a consent form or convey this information verbally. It can be a general statement, such as "no life sustaining measures," or specific, such as "no tube feedings or respirator." Often, the patient's family has difficulty allowing health care personnel to follow the wishes expressed in a living will, and conflicts arise. These should be communicated to the hospital ethics committee, pastoral care department, risk management, or whichever hospital department is responsible for handling such issues. If the patient verbalizes her wishes regarding end-of-life care to the family, such difficult situations can sometimes be avoided, and the patient should be encouraged to do this, if possible.

INVASION OF PRIVACY AND CONFIDENTIALITY   The nurse is required to respect the privacy of all patients. As a health care practitioner, the nurse may be privy to very personal information and must make every effort to keep it confidential. Only authorized individuals can access patient information, although patients have the right to access their own records. Only by obtaining the patient's permission can information be given to others. It is often necessary to monitor conversations with coworkers that have the potential of being overheard by others so that no patient information is accidentally revealed. Sometimes the protection of a patient's privacy conflicts with the state's mandatory reporting laws for the occurrence of specified infectious diseases such as syphilis or human immunodeficiency virus (HIV). The need to protect an individual's privacy may also conflict with the state's mandatory reporting laws on suspected patient abuse, discussed previously. Other information that state or federal law may require to be revealed include a patient's blood alcohol level, incidences of rape, gunshot wounds, and adverse reactions to certain drugs. Failing to strictly follow reporting laws could lead to criminal, civil, or disciplinary action; termination of employment; or all of these. Nurses must consult the institution's policies and confer with its risk management department to ascertain their responsibilities and course of action. The American Nurses Association (ANA) Code of Ethics for Nurses, 2005 states that nurses must protect the patient and the public when incompetence or unethical or illegal practice compromise health care and safety. Many states have adopted this concept in their nurse practice acts, thereby creating a legal obligation to report. If a nurse were to observe unethical behavior in a hospital, he or she should report this as directed in the institution's policies and procedures manual or by the laws of the state.

DEFAMATION   **Defamation** is defined as an intentionally false communication/publication (*Black's Law Dictionary*, 2005). Other similar terms used with this tort are *slander*, which is verbal communication. *Libel* is the term for false written communication.

CASE STUDY 14-1

You are working the night shift. One of your patient's practitioners has ordered a dose of a medication to be given that you know is too high for this patient. You are unable to locate the practitioner to check the order. What would you do to ensure safe care for your patient?

Two essential elements must be proved in a charge of defamation:

1. The information conveyed must be untrue.
2. The false information must be published or communicated to another party.

Note that publication or communication may mean simply telling one other person or writing a friend a letter containing the false information. The nurse may face such an accusation if the nurse communicates inaccurate information to another or if it is claimed that the information charted was untrue. However, several courts have ruled that charting information in a medical record, whether accurate or not, does not constitute publication as required for a charge of defamation.

Following Orders, Including Do Not Attempt Resuscitation (DNAR)   The attending medical practitioner may write a do not attempt resuscitation (DNAR) order on an inpatient, which directs the staff not to perform the usual cardiopulmonary resuscitation (CPR) in the event of a sudden cardiopulmonary arrest. The practitioner may write such an order without evidence of a living will on the medical record, and the nurse should be familiar with the organization's policies and state law regarding when and how a practitioner can write such an order in the absence of a living will. Often, a DNAR order is considered a medical decision that the doctor can make, preferably in consultation with the family, even without a living will executed by the patient.

If the nurse feels that a DNAR order or any order is contrary to the patient's good, the nurse should consult the policies and procedures of the institution. These may include going up the chain of command until the nurse is satisfied with the course of action. See the chain of command figure in the chapter on Delegation. This may entail notifying the nursing supervisor, the medical director, the institution's chief operating officer, the risk manager, the state regulators, and/or the accreditation agency, e.g., the Joint Commission. Often an organization has an ethics committee that examines such issues and makes a determination of the appropriateness of the order. Because of the opportunity for misunderstanding, verbal orders are not encouraged. When a nurse has a problem with a practitioner's order, it is often prudent to discuss it first with the practitioner involved before reporting the problem up the chain of command. Often problems can be resolved at this first step. However, if the problem is not resolved by discussing it with the practitioner, the nurse should report the problem to her supervisor and follow the state law and the agency's polices.

FALSE IMPRISONMENT
False imprisonment occurs when individuals are incorrectly led to believe they cannot leave a place. A claim of false imprisonment may be based on the inappropriate use of physical or chemical restraints. Federal law mandates that health care institutions employ the least restrictive method of ensuring patient safety. Physical or chemical restraints are to be used only if necessary to protect the patient from harm when all other methods have failed. If the nurse uses restraints on a competent person who is refusing to follow the practitioner's orders, the nurse can be charged with false imprisonment or battery. If restraints are used in an emergency situation, the nurse is to contact the practitioner immediately after application to secure an order for the restraints. Also, the nurse must check the institution's policies regarding the type and frequency of assessments required for a patient in restraints and how often it is necessary to secure a reorder for the restraints. These policies ensure the patient's safety and must be consistent with state law.

A charge of false imprisonment may occur because the nurse misinterprets the rights granted to others by legal documents such as powers of attorney and does not allow a patient to leave a facility because the person with the power of attorney (agent) says the patient cannot leave. A **power of attorney** is a legal document executed by an individual (principal) granting another person (agent) the right to perform certain activities in the principal's name. It can be specific, such as "sell my house," or general, such as "make all decisions for me, including health care decisions." In most states, a power of attorney is voluntarily granted by the individual and does not take away his right to exercise his own choices. Thus, if the principal (patient) disagrees with his agent's decisions, the patient's wishes are the ones that prevail.

PROTECTIONS IN NURSING PRACTICE

As discussed earlier in this chapter, nursing practice is guided by state nurse practice acts and agency policies and procedures. Other resources for the nurse include Good Samaritan laws, useful health records, risk management, and professional liability insurance.

GOOD SAMARITAN LAWS

Good Samaritan laws are laws that have been enacted to protect the health care professional from legal liability. The essential elements of commonly enacted Good Samaritan laws are as follows:

- The care is rendered in an emergency situation.
- The health care worker is rendering care without pay.
- The care provided did not recklessly or intentionally cause injury or harm to the injured party.

Note that these laws are intended to protect the volunteer who stops to render care at the scene of an accident. They would not protect a nurse, an emergency medical technician (EMT), or other health care professional rendering care at the scene of an accident as part of her assigned duties and for which she receives pay. In doing their duties, paid emergency personnel are evaluated according to the standards of their professions. (Martin et al., 2008)

USEFUL HEALTH RECORDS

The nurse must communicate accurately and completely verbally, in writing, and electronically. Often a case involving patient care takes several years to come to trial; by that time, the nurse may have no memory of the incident in question and must rely on the record done at the time of the incident. This record is frequently in the courtroom, blown up to billboard size for all to see. All errors are apparent and omissions stand out by their absence, especially if it is data that should have been recorded per organizational policy. The old adage that "if it isn't written, it wasn't done" will be repeated to the jury numerous times.

DOCUMENTATION

Professional responsibility and accountability are two primary reasons why nurses document. Other reasons to document include communication, education, research, meeting legal and practice standards, and reimbursement. Documentation is the professional responsibility of all health care practitioners. Thorough documentation provides:

- accurate data needed to plan the patient's care in order to ensure the continuity of care
- a method of communication among the health care team members responsible for the patient's care
- written evidence of what was done for the patient, the patient's response, and any revisions made in the plan of care
- evidence of compliance with professional practice standards, e.g., American Nurses Association Standards

- compliance with accreditation criteria, e.g., Joint Commission (JC), Healthcare Facilities Accreditation Program (HFAP), etc.
- a resource for review, quality improvement, reimbursement, education, and research
- a documented legal record to protect the patient, organization, and nursing and medical practitioners.

For protection when charting, the nurse should use the FLAT (Factual, Legible, Accurate, and Timely) charting acronym.

ELECTRONIC HEALTH RECORDS

Note that several hospitals have adopted electronic health records (EHR). The EHR eliminates paper record storage, improves access to patient records, controls legibility, and facilitates timely capture of data. The EHR can also be used to gather data about patient care and outcomes, staff activities, and other data for clinical, administrative, and financial decision making.

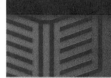

EVIDENCE FROM THE LITERATURE

Citation: Jha, A. K., Doolan, D., Grandt, D., Scott, T., Bates, D. W. (2008). The use of health information technology in seven nations. *International Journal of Medical Informatics*. Jul 24. 254–262.

Discussion: The authors assessed the state of health information technology (HIT) adoption and use in seven industrialized nations. They used a combination of literature review, as well as interviews with experts in individual nations, to determine the use of key information technologies. They examined the rate of electronic health record (EHR) use in ambulatory care and some hospital settings, along with current activities in health information exchange (HIE) in seven countries: the United States (U.S.), Canada, United Kingdom (UK), Germany, The Netherlands, Australia, and New Zealand (NZ). Four nations (the UK, The Netherlands, Australia, and NZ) had nearly universal use of EHRs among general practitioners (each >90%) and Germany also exhibited widespread use (40–80%). The U.S. and Canada had a minority of ambulatory care physicians who used EHRs consistently (10–30%). Although there are no high-quality data for the hospital setting from any of the nations the authors examined, evidence suggests that only a small fraction of hospitals (<10%) in any single country had the key components of an EHR. HIE efforts were a high priority in all seven nations, but early efforts have demonstrated varying degrees of active clinical data exchange.

Implications for Practice: Increased efforts will be needed if interoperable EHRs are soon to become universally available and used in these seven nations. Nurses and other practitioners in these nations must be part of the solution to making the EHR universally used and available.

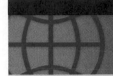

REAL WORLD INTERVIEW

Most nurses are familiar with the phrase, "If it was not documented, it was not done." Insofar as this phrase is used to encourage thorough documentation, it reflects good nursing practice. Timely, accurate, and complete documentation is an excellent way to protect oneself from litigation. However, lawyers who represent plaintiffs in medical malpractice cases are aware of this "rule" and often attempt to use it against nurses in health care liability claims.

Imagine the following scenario: A patient is admitted to the hospital, and Nurse A performs an initial assessment of the patient. Nurse A notes in the patient's chart that the patient has good capillary refill. Nurse A proceeds to take the patient's vital signs, including capillary refill, hourly throughout Nurse A's 8-hour shift. The patient's capillary refill remains reassuring and the nurse makes no further documentation in the chart relating to the patient's capillary refill. After Nurse A's shift, Nurse B takes over the patient's care. One hour into Nurse B's shift, the patient codes and expires. The patient's family sues Nurse A. The plaintiffs' lawyer is cross-examining Nurse A.

Lawyer: "Nurse A, are you familiar with the phrase, 'If it wasn't charted, it wasn't done'?"

Nurse A: "Yes."

Lawyer: "That's a common rule in nursing practice, isn't it?"

Nurse A: "Yes."

Lawyer: "You were taught that in nursing school, weren't you?"

Nurse A: "Yes, I was."

Lawyer: "And after you documented that the patient had good capillary refill upon admission, you did not document anything relating to the patient's capillary refill for the next 8 hours, did you?"

Nurse A: "Well, no."

Lawyer: "So if we use the rule, 'If it wasn't documented, it wasn't done,' we can assume you never checked the patient's capillary refills during your shift after the initial assessment, right?"

Nurse A: "No. I checked, but it hadn't changed, so I didn't chart anything."

Do you see what just happened? Nurse A provided competent nursing care, but the lawyer made it appear as if Nurse A was negligent. A nurse involved in litigation should not blanketly agree with this documentation rule. The rule ignores the concept of charting by exception. You simply cannot document everything noted in an assessment of a patient. Moreover, most nurses would agree that patient care takes priority over charting. This rule ignores that. Bad charting looks bad. Good charting protects you. However, charting by exception does not correlate with providing bad nursing care. Even lapses in charting do not correlate with bad nursing care. Nurses should not lose sight of that when faced with litigation.

Robyn D. Pozza-Dollar, JD
Austin, Texas

The U.S. Department of Veterans Affairs (VA) has the largest EHR, known as the Veterans Health Information System and Technology Architecture (VistA). Health care providers can review and update a patient's EHR at any of the over 1,000 VA organizations nationwide. The EHR has the ability to place orders regarding medications, diet, labs, and, x-rays, etc. The U.S. Indian Health Service has an EHR that is similar to VistA. As of 2005, the United Kingdom implemented its EHR, designed to provide

TABLE 14-5	NURSING CHECKLIST OF ACTIONS TO DECREASE LIABILITY

- Delegate patient care based on patient's needs, staff competency and skill, and the documented education, skill, and experience of licensed and unlicensed personnel. Monitor the outcomes.

- Develop a professional, assertive communication style with nursing and medical practitioners to assist you with meeting patient care goals. Use SBARR as a guide. See Chapter 5.

- Communicate with your patients and keep them informed. Treat them with kindness and respect.

- Acknowledge unfortunate incidents and express concern about these events without either taking the blame, blaming others, or reacting defensively.

- Avoid taking telephone and verbal orders. If necessary to maintain patient safety, however, repeat the order back to the practitioner to assure clarity. Document that you did this, e.g., telephone order repeated back (TORB) or verbal order repeated back (VORB).

- Follow professional standards for education, licensure, and competency in all hiring and promotion decisions, orientation, and ongoing continuing education programs.

- Provide access to professional evidence-based health care standards, policies, procedures, library, and medication information with unit availability and efficient Internet access.

- Have clear policies and procedures for delegation, supervision, and chain-of-command reporting lines for all staff from RN to charge nurse to nurse manager to nurse executive and, as appropriate, to risk management, the hospital ethics committee, the hospital administrator, medical practitioners, the chief of the medical staff, the board of directors, the State Licensing Board for Nursing and Medicine, and the accreditation agency, e.g., The Joint Commission (JC).

- Note that the RN always has an independent responsibility to protect patient safety. Blindly relying on another nursing or medical practitioner is not permissible for the RN.

- Provide standards for regular RN evaluation of NAP and LPN/LVN and reinforce the need for NAP and LPN/LVN accountability to the RN. RNs must delegate and supervise. They cannot abdicate this professional responsibility.

- Develop physical, mental, and verbal "No Abuse" policies to be followed by all professional and nonprofessional health care staff.

- Consider applying for Magnet status for your facility. This status is awarded by the American Nurses Credentialing Center to hospitals that have worked to improve nursing care, including the empowering of nursing delegation and nursing decision making.

- Develop electronic health records and monitor patient outcomes, including nurse-sensitive outcomes, staffing ratios, and other clinical, financial, and organizational quality indicators. Develop ongoing clinical quality improvement practices.

- Maintain ongoing monitoring of incident reports, medication errors, equipment maintenance, patient, family, and staff complaints, and sentinel events, and other elements of risk management and performance improvement of the process and outcome of patient care.

- Attain Joint Commission Patient Safety Goals, 2009.

- Monitor Medicare, "Do Not Pay" list, for example, note that Medicare will not pay for transfusions gone wrong due to human error.

access to 60,000,000 patients' EHRs by 2010. The Canadian province of Alberta began an EHR project in 2005 that is expected to encompass all of Alberta (Electronic Health Record, 2008). Implementation of an EHR has been slowed in the U.S. because of concerns over several legal barriers, e.g., paper era state regulations that may not permit EHRs, Federal Anti-Kickback Statute, Stark anti-referral rules, concerns about malpractice exposure, HIPAA, and anti-trust laws, etc. (Shay, 2005). These concerns are being studied to overcome barriers to implementation of the EHR.

RISK-MANAGEMENT PROGRAMS

Risk-management programs in health care organizations are designed to identify and correct system problems that contribute to errors in patient care or to employee injury. The emphasis in risk management is on quality improvement and protection of the institution from financial liability. Institutions usually have reporting and tracking forms for recording incidents that may lead to financial liability for the institution. Risk management will assist in identifying and correcting the underlying problem that may have led to an incident, such as faulty equipment, staffing concerns, or the need for better orientation for employees. After a system problem is identified, the risk-management department may develop educational programs to address the problem.

The risk-management department may also investigate and record information surrounding a patient or employee incident that may result in a lawsuit. This helps personnel remember critical factors if called to testify at a later time. The nurse should notify the risk-management department of all reportable incidents and complete all risk-management and/or incident report forms as mandated by institutional policies and procedures. Note also that employee complaints of harassment or discrimination can expose the institution to significant liability and should promptly be reported to supervisors and the risk-management department, human resources, or whichever department is specified in the institution's policies. See Table 14-5 for a checklist of actions to decrease the risk of nursing liability.

PROFESSIONAL LIABILITY INSURANCE

Nurses may need to carry their own liability insurance. Nurses often think their actions are adequately covered by the employer's liability insurance, but this is not necessarily so. Although the hospital's insurance company almost always pays malpractice awards, insurance contracts often have provisions that allow them to refuse repayment if the insured intentionally injures another party. Also, if in giving care, the nurse fails to comply with the institution's policies and procedures, the institution may deny the nurse a defense, claiming that because of the nurse's failure to follow institutional policy, or because of the nurse working outside the scope of nursing employment, the nurse was not acting as an employee at that time. Also, nurses are being named individually as defendants in malpractice suits more frequently than in the past. More often, though, hospitals are often a plaintiff's primary target because they typically have deeper pockets than individual practitioners (Pozza, 2003).

It is advantageous for nurses to be assured of a defense independent of that of their employer. Professional liability insurance provides that assurance and pays for an attorney to defend nurses in a malpractice lawsuit. When purchasing malpractice insurance, nurses should clarify whether the insurance covers liability just as long as the premiums are being paid or if the insurance covers a prescribed time period.

Note that in the event that unaffiliated nurses, like agency per diem nurses, are held individually liable for a judgment, their personal insurance carrier will be responsible for paying the verdict rendered against them. Unaffiliated, uninsured nurses could be forced to pay for their own defense and be financially responsible for any judgments rendered against them.

In making the decision of whether to obtain separate insurance, nurses should consider the value of their personal assets. Nurses should also consider the laws of the state where they practice regarding those assets that are exempt from being seized to satisfy civil monetary judgments. Generally, one

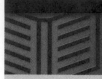

EVIDENCE FROM THE LITERATURE

Citation: Vonfrolio, L. G. (2006). Blow the Whistle? *RN.* October *69*(10), 60.

Discussion: When a nurse "blows the whistle" on an unsafe situation, there are often professional consequences. The nurse may be labeled a "troublemaker," isolated from his or her peers, or, worse yet, fired. Currently, fewer than half of the states in this country offer whistleblower protection. Proceed with caution if you are planning on blowing the whistle. Be sure to:

■ Document the incident(s) and keep a copy for yourself. Send a typed complaint to the Director of Nursing (DON) or anyone in another department with a stake in the case.

■ Avoid being confrontational when discussing the issue with management. Exhaust all internal remedies before taking matters out of house.

■ Keep a personal diary of events after the incident is reported.

■ Seek the support of your colleagues. Nurses must band together to protect patients from incompetent, unethical, or unsafe care.

■ Consider reporting your concerns about quality of care to the Joint Commission Office of Quality Monitoring at: www.jointcommission.org. Click on *Report a Complaint* at the bottom of the home page, or send an e-mail to complaint @ jointcommission.org. If you have concerns about working conditions, try the U.S. Department of Labor (www.dol.gov) or the National Labor Relations Board (www.nlrb.gov).

■ Tell legislators that all nurses in this country need whistleblower protection—now!

Implications for Practice: The decision to become a whistleblower can have far-reaching implications. If you decide to do so, proceed cautiously.

home and one automobile are exempt from seizure (Pozza, 2003).

NURSES INVOLVED IN LITIGATION

Nurses may be sued individually for damages resulting from their negligent acts. However, a plaintiff will often name the nurse's employer as a defendant instead of or in addition to suing the nurse individually. It is a well-established law throughout the United States that "a master is subject to liability for the torts of his servants committed while acting in the scope of employment" (Restatement (second) of the Law of Agency §219 [1958]). This law is called Respondeat Superior. In other words, a hospital, nursing home, clinic, and so on is legally responsible for the damages caused by the negligence of its nurses.

Customarily, plaintiffs in medical malpractice cases name a combination of health care providers as defendants. It is common for some or all of the defendants to settle the cases before they reach the trial phase. However, in the event that a case proceeds to trial, a jury may find that none, some, or all of the defendants were negligent in their care and treatment of the plaintiff. A jury may determine that the nursing care was appropriate, but that the medical treatment was substandard. Likewise, a jury could hold that the medical practitioner rendered appropriate care but that the nurses' conduct fell below the standard of care. Additionally, a new trend in medical malpractice litigation is to name the health maintenance organization (HMO) as a defendant as well. For example, the Illinois Supreme Court recently held that an HMO could be liable under theories of apparent authority, respondeat superior, direct corporate negligence, breach of contract, and breach of warranty (*Jones v. Chicago HMO Ltd. of Ill.*, 2000; Pozza, 2003).

COMMON MONETARY AWARDS

Many malpractice cases are dismissed or settled prior to trial. In those cases that do reach the trial stage, jury verdicts are unpredictable and awards can vary dramatically. For instance, juries awarded the following for the listed injuries:

- Brachial plexus injury ($13.3 million) (Stonieczny v. Gardner, Ill. [2001])
- Wrongful death—pulmonary embolism ($5 million) (*Martinelli v. Lifemark Hospitals of Fla., Inc.* [2001])
- Microcephaly in newborn ($17 million) (*Diver v. Gingo* [2001])
- Vision loss ($8 million) (*Schwab v. Kamat* [2001])
- Arterial impairment ($260,000) (*In re Triss* [2002])

A jury may award the plaintiff both compensatory and punitive damages. Compensatory damages are awarded to compensate the plaintiff for injuries. Compensatory damages include damages for both economic losses (medical expenses, lost wages, lost earning capacity) and noneconomic losses (pain and suffering). Punitive damages are not intended to compensate the plaintiff for any loss. Rather, punitive damages are intended to punish the defendant for acting with "recklessness, malice or deceit" (*Black's Law Dictionary*, 2005). Punitive damage awards are particularly common in cases involving nursing homes. For example, a Texas jury awarded the family of a nursing home resident $90 million in punitive damages for gross negligence that caused the resident to develop pressure ulcers and contractures (*Horizon/CMS Healthcare Corp. V. Auld* [2000]; Pozza [2003]).

MONETARY LIABILITY LIMITS IN SOME STATES. Since 1970, at least 30 states have enacted legislation capping the damages plaintiffs can recover in a lawsuit (Babcock & Pogarsky, 1999). Currently, there exist as many different cap schemes as states that employ them (Pozza, 2003).

A plaintiff may claim that he or she is entitled to damages in excess of the applicable cap. Jurors are customarily not informed of the caps applicable in their states. Therefore, it is common for a jury's award to exceed the state's cap on damages. In the event that a jury awards a plaintiff damages in excess of a statutory cap, the judge will reduce the jury's award to the cap (Pozza, 2003).

OTHER LEGAL RISKS FOR THE NURSE, DOCTOR, OR HOSPITAL

Other than increased insurance premiums, health care providers have plenty at stake when named as defendants in medical malpractice cases. Medical practitioners are required to report adverse verdicts and settlements to the National Practitioner's Data Bank. The National Practitioner's Data Bank was established through the Health Care Quality Improvement Act of 1986. The federal regulations regarding the data bank can be found in 45 CFR Part 60. Significant awards against a practitioner or numerous malpractice payments by a practitioner can affect the practitioner's licensure or ability to gain privileges to practice at certain hospitals and health care entities. Failure to report malpractice payments to the data bank can result in civil monetary penalties. The U.S. Department of Health and Human Services, Office of the Inspector General, may impose a civil money penalty of up to $11,000 for each violation.

Federal and state statutes and regulations prescribe nursing standards of care. See the *Code of Federal Regulations* Title 42—Public Health and Title 45—Public Welfare. Also see the U.S. Code Title 42—Public Health and Welfare. Every jurisdiction that licenses nurses has a Nurse Practice Act. In addition to instructing nurses on the definition of the standard of care for that jurisdiction, the Nurse Practice Act mandates strict rules for reporting and disciplining nurses who violate the standard. Likewise, state boards of nursing and administrative agencies may take action to suspend or revoke the licenses of nurses who it determines have violated the standard of care. Private entities, such as the Joint Commission, and nursing organizations, such as the American Nurses Association, promulgate their own rules of conduct that serve as guidelines for acceptable nursing care (Pozza, 2003).

NURSE/ATTORNEY RELATIONSHIP

Despite the nurse's best intentions, a nurse may be named as a defendant in a lawsuit and need to retain the services of an attorney. LaDuke (2000) made the following suggestions for consulting and collaborating with an attorney:

1. Retain a specialist. Generalists are competent to handle many matters, but professional malpractice, professional disciplinary proceedings, and employment disputes are best handled by specialists in those areas.
2. Be attentive. Read the documents the attorney produces and travel to court proceedings to observe the attorney's performance.
3. Notify your insurance carrier as soon as you are aware of any real or potential liability issue.

Inform your agent about the status of your case every few months, even if it is unchanged.

4. Keep costs sensible. Your attorney should explain initially how the fee will be computed and how you will be billed. The attorney may require you to pay a retainer fee.
5. Keep informed. The attorney should address your questions and concerns promptly. You are entitled to be kept informed about the status of your case. You are entitled to copies of all correspondence, legal briefs, and other documents.
6. Weed through writing. Your attorney needs to explain all facts and options. Examine all relevant documents and do not hesitate to make corrections in the same way you would correct a medical record by drawing a line through the incorrect or misleading information, writing in the correction, and signing your initials after it.
7. Set your own course. Insist on a collaborative relationship with your attorney for the duration of your case.

KEY CONCEPTS

- Nursing practice is governed by civil, public, and administrative laws.

- Nurses need to be familiar with their institution's policies and procedures in giving care and in reporting variances, illegal activities, or unexpected events.

- Nurses must have good oral, written, and electronic communication skills.

- Common torts include negligence and malpractice, assault and battery, false imprisonment, invasion of privacy, and defamation.

- Nurses need to be familiar with their state's nurse practice act.

- The Multistate Licensure Compact allows nurses to practice in more than one state.

- Many sources of evidence are used to identify the standard of care.

- Nursing malpractice examples include treatment problems, communication problems, medication problems, and monitoring/observing/supervising problems.

- Legal protections in nursing practice include Good Samaritan laws, useful health records, risk-management programs, and professional liability insurance.

KEY TERMS

administrative law

assault

battery

civil law

common law

constitution

contract law

criminal law

defamation

false imprisonment

Good Samaritan laws

living will

malpractice

negligence

power of attorney

public law

tort

REVIEW QUESTIONS

1. You are given a written order by a practitioner to administer an unusually large dose of pain medicine to your patient. In this situation, which of the following is an appropriate nursing action?
   A. Administer the medication because it was ordered by a practitioner.
   B. Refuse to administer the medication, and move on to another patient.
   C. Speak with the practitioner about your concerns, and clarify whether the medication dose is accurate.
   D. Select a dose that you feel comfortable with, and administer that dose.

2. A practitioner has issued a Do Not Attempt Resuscitate (DNAR) order for your patient, a fifty-five-year-old man with cancer. You spoke with the patient this morning, and he clearly wishes to be resuscitated in the event that he stops breathing. What is the most appropriate course of action?
   A. Ignore the patient's wishes because the practitioner ordered the DNAR.
   B. Consult your hospital's policies and procedures, speak to the practitioner and your nurse manager, and honor the patient's wishes.

   C. Attempt to talk the patient into agreeing to the DNAR.
   D. Contact the medical licensing board to complain about the practitioner.

3. Which of the following elements is not necessary for a nurse to be found negligent in a court of law?
   A. a duty or obligation for the nurse to act in a particular way
   B. a breach of that duty or obligation
   C. the nurse's intention to be negligent
   D. physical, emotional, or financial harm to the patient

4. Which statement is best to document a patient's behavior in an unbiased way?
   A. "The patient's hostility created difficulties for the nursing staff."
   B. "The patient threw the water pitcher across the room during shift change."
   C. "The patient's rudeness prevented administration of his medications."
   D. "The patient's dressing change was interrupted by his belligerent behavior."

REVIEW ACTIVITIES

1. Identify the various ways in which nurses you observe in your clinical rotations discuss orders and treatments with practitioners and other nurses. How do nurses address incorrect or dangerous

   medication orders? Talk with nurses you encounter about how they handle these situations.

2. Research the various companies that offer nursing malpractice insurance, and determine the cost and

coverage associated with a nursing malpractice policy. Go to an Internet search engine, such as www.google.com. Search for *nursing malpractice insurance.* What did you find? Note the Nursing Service Organization (NSO) Web site at www.nso. com. Recent legal cases are reported there.

3. Discuss how nurses' off-duty behaviors can affect their nursing practice. Note if your state lists any actions in its nurse practice act that you might take

outside of work that might cause your license to practice nursing to be revoked by your state nursing licensure board (e.g., a driving while intoxicated conviction). Check your State's Nurse Practice Act. Go to www.ncsbn.org/
Click on Boards of Nursing. Click on Member Boards, and then click on the map on the state in which you are want to access the State Board information.

EXPLORING THE WEB

■ You have a patient who is to be transferred to a nursing home for recuperation. Where can you tell the family to look to evaluate the local nursing homes regarding their adherence to the federal regulations for nursing homes?
www.medicare.gov
Search for *long term care* and *nursing homes compare.*

■ Where can you find a copy of the ANA Code of Ethics?
www.nursingworld.org
Search for *Code of Ethics.*

■ Check these Internet resources for legal information:

www.findlaw.com
www.lexis.com
www.aslme.com (American Society of Law, Medicine and Ethics)
www.lpig.org (Law and Policy Institutions Guide)
www.law.cornell.edu
www.jointcommission.org
www.cms.hhs.gov
www.nursefriendly.com

■ Note the Medical Liability Monitor at:
www.medicalliabilitymonitor.com

REFERENCES

American Law Institute. (1958). Restatement of the Law of Agency (Second). American Law Institute.

American Nurses Association. (ANA). (2005). Code of Ethics for Nurses. Available at nursingworld.org/ ethics/code/protected_nwcoe813.htm#3.5. Accessed December 28, 2008.

Babcock, L., & Pogarsky, G. (1999). Damages caps and settlement: A behavioral approach. *Journal of Legal Studies, 28,* 341.

Code of Federal Regulations. Available at, www. gpoaccess.gov/CFR/. Accessed October 2, 2008.

Diver v. Gingo, Ohio, No. 305538, Cuyahoga County C. P., Jan. 2001 (16 PNLR 152, Oct. 2001).

Electronic health record. (2008). Available at en.wikepedia.org/wiki/electronic_health_records_ over_paper_records. Accessed October 2, 2008.

Fiesta, J. (1999). Do no harm; When caregivers violate our golden rule, part 1. *Nursing Management, 30*(8), 10–11.

Garner, B. A. (2004). Black's Law Dictionary. (8th ed.). St. Paul, MN: West Group Publishing.

Hellquist, K., & Spector, N. (2004). A primer: The national council of state boards of nursing nurse licensure compact. *Journal of Nursing Administration's Healthcare Law, Ethics, and Regulation, 6*(4), 86–89.

Horizon/CMS Healthcare Corp. v. Auld, 34 S.W.3d 887 (Tex. 2000).

In re Triss, 2002 WL 1271492 (La. App. 4 Cir., 2002).

Jha, A. K., Doolan, D., Grandt, D., Scott, T., Bates, D. W. (2008, July 24). The use of health information technology in seven nations. *International Journal of Medical Informatics.* 254–262.

Jones v. Chicago HMO Ltd. of Illinois, 730 N.E.2d 1119 (Ill. 2000).

LaDuke, S. (2000). What should you expect from your attorney? *Nursing Management, 31*(1), 10.

Martin, J. W., Cain, K., & Priest, C. S. (2008) in Kelly, P. *Nursing Leadership & Management* (2nd ed.), Clifton Park, NY: Delmar Cengage Learning.

Martinelli v. Lifemark Hospitals of Florida, Inc., Fla., No. 99–14491 CA 05, Dade County Cir. Mar. 1, 2001 (16 ATLA PNLR 111, July 2001).

Medicare's Do Not Pay List. (2008). Medicare. Available at www.medicare-medicaid.com. Accessed October 2, 2008.

Murphy v. United Parcel Service, 527 U.S. 516 (1999).

National Practitioner Data Bank. Healthcare Integrity and Protection Data Bank. Available at www.npdb-hipdb.hrsa.gov/. Accessed October 2, 2008.

Nurse Licensure Compact, NCSBN. Available at www.ncsbn.org/158.htm. Accessed October 2, 2008.

Occupational Safety & Health Administration, U.S. Department of Labor, available at www.osha.gov/. Accessed October 2, 2008.

Odom v. State Department of Health & Hospitals, 322 So. 2d 91 (La. 1999).

Olsen-Chavarriaga, D. (2000). Informed consent: Do you know your role? *Nursing 2000, 30*(5), 60–61.

Pozza, R. (2003). *Nursing malpractice cases.* Unpublished manuscript.

Schwab v. Kamat, New York, No. 97–887, Onondaga County Sup. Ct., June 8, 2001 (16 PNLR 154, Oct. 2001).

Shay, E. F. (2005). Legal barriers to electronic health records. *Physician News Digest.* Available at www.physiciansnews.com/law/505.html. Accessed October 2, 2008.

Stonieczny v. Gardner, Illinois, No. 98 L 04578, Cook County Cir. May 29, 2001 (16 PNLR 131, Sept. 2001).

Sutton v. United Airlines, 527 U.S. 471 (1999).

The 'Lectric Law Library's Lexicon On Tort. (2008). Available at www.lectlaw.com/def2/t032.htm. Accessed October 2, 2008.

Vonfrolio, L. G. (2006, Oct.). Blow the Whistle? *RN, 69*(10), 60.

Webb v. Tulane Medical Center Hospital, 700 So. 2d 1142 (La. 1997).

SUGGESTED READINGS

Austin, S. (2006). Ladies and gentlemen of the jury, I present . . . the nursing documentation. *Nursing 36*(1), 56–64.

Austin, S. (2008, Mar.). Seven legal tips for safe nursing practice. *Nursing, 38*(3):34–39; quiz 39–40.

Croke, E. M. (2003). Nurses, negligence, and malpractice. *American Journal of Nursing, 103*(9), 54–64.

Cruzan v. Director, Missouri Department of Health, 110 S. Ct. 2841 (1990).

DeLaune, S. C, & Ladner, P. K. (2006). Fundamentals of Nursing (3rd ed.). Clifton Park, NY: Delmar Cengage Learning.

Green, M. A., & Bowie, M. J. (2005). Essentials of Health Information Management. Clifton Park, NY: Delmar Cengage Learning.

Kay Hall, J. (2004). After Schiavo: Next issue for nursing ethics. *Journal of Nursing Administration's Healthcare Law, Ethics, and Regulation, 7*(3), 94–98.

Marshal v. Methodist Healthcare Jackson Hospital, Mississippi, No. 251–99–000984CIV, Hinds County Cir. Jan. 23, 2001 (16 PNLR 174, Nov. 2001).

National Council of State Boards of Nursing. (NCSBN). Delegation Decision Making Tree. Available at www.ncsbn.org/887.htm?search-text=delegation+decision+making+tree&select=%23. Accessed October 2, 2008.

Priest, C. (2005). Held liable. *Reflections on nursing leadership, 31*(1), 20–22, 36.

Roe v. Wade, 410 U.S. 133 (1973).

Sheehan, J. P. (2000). Protect your staff from workplace violence. *Nursing Management, 31*(3), 24–25.

Sloan, A. J. (1999). Legally speaking: Whistleblowing: There are risks! *RN, 62*(7), 65–68.

The Civil Rights Act of 1964. Available at www.archives. gov/education/lessons/civil-rights-act/. Accessed October 2, 2008.

Toiviainen, L. (2007, Jan.). Nursing Ethics conference on the globalisation of nursing: ethical, legal and political issues. *Nursing Ethics, 14*(1):3–4.

Urgent v. Government of the Virgin Islands, U.S.V.I., No. V.I. Territorial Ct. St. Croix Div. Sept. 13, 2001 (17 PNLR 8, Feb. 2002).

CHAPTER 15

Ethical Aspects of Health Care

Moral excellence comes about as a result of habit, we become just by doing just acts, temperate by doing temperate acts, brave by doing brave acts.

(Aristotle)

OBJECTIVES

Upon completion of this chapter, the reader should be able to:

1. Define ethics.
2. Review the use of ethical theories and principles in professional nursing practice.
3. Discuss a nursing philosophy.
4. Discuss values and values clarification.
5. Identify a guide for ethical decision making.
6. Promote ethical leadership and management in health care organizations.
7. Review ethical codes for nurses.

In a large teaching hospital, a patient you are caring for says he does not want to go on living. He has had cancer for several years and states he is tired of being sick. He has discussed this with his health care practitioner and has been declared Do Not Attempt Resuscitation (DNAR). One of your nursing assistive personnel (NAP) says to you, "I don't know why he is giving up. I think we should call a Code if he arrests." Where are your thoughts on this? Where can you turn for guidance in this situation?

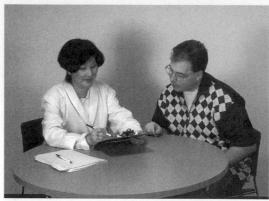

Delmar/Cengage Learning

Throughout its history, nursing has relied on ethical principles to serve as guidelines in determining patient care. Nurses are confronted with ethical dilemmas in all types of practice settings. This chapter provides an overview of ethics and the increased ethical challenges faced by nurses in leadership and management roles in today's health care environment.

ETHICS

Ethics is the branch of philosophy that concerns the distinction of right from wrong on the basis of a body of knowledge, not just on the basis of opinions. **Morality** is behavior in accordance with custom or tradition and usually reflects personal or religious beliefs (DeLaune & Ladner, 2006). Ethics governs professional groups and provides a framework for determining the right course of action in a particular situation. For nurses, the actions they take in practice are primarily governed by the ethical principles of the profession. These principles influence practice, conduct, and relationships that nurses are held accountable for in the delivery of care. An **ethical dilemma** occurs when two or more ethical principles are in conflict and there is no obviously "correct" decision.

Laws, in contrast, are state and federal government rules that govern all of society. Laws mandate behavior. In some health care situations, the distinctions between law and ethics may not be clear. Ethics and law may be similar in some cases. In other cases, ethics and law may differ more dramatically.

MORAL DEVELOPMENT

Lawrence Kohlberg (1971) identified a moral development process that progresses through various levels. At the first level, the Preconventional Level, morals are all about rules imposed by some authority. Moral decisions made at this level are done in response to some threat of punishment. Labels of good and bad or right and wrong have meaning only in reference to a reward and punishment system. People at this Preconventional Level have no concept of the underlying moral code guiding the decision about what is good or bad or right or wrong. They act because an authority tells them to do so.

At the next level, the Conventional Level, people begin to internalize their view of themselves in response to something more meaningful and interpersonal. A desire to be viewed as a good person develops when the person wants to find approval from others. He or she may want to please, help others, be dutiful, and show respect for authority. Conformity to expected social and religious mores and a sense of loyalty often emerge at the Conventional Level. Not all people develop beyond this level.

A morally mature Postconventional Level person is an independent thinker who strives for a moral code beyond that dictated merely by respect for authority. The morally mature Postconventional Level person's actions are based on broader principles of respect for the dignity of all humankind, and not just on principles of respect for authority, duty, or loyalty to others (Kohlberg, 1971).

ETHICAL THEORIES

A standard way of making ethical decisions is to refer to ethical theories. Some of these theories are identified in Table 15-1.

PHILOSOPHY

Philosophy is the rational investigation of the truths and principles of knowledge, reality, and human conduct. Personal philosophies stem from an individual's beliefs and values. These beliefs and values, in turn, develop based upon a person's experiences in life, cultural influences, and education.

PHILOSOPHY OF NURSING

A professional nurse's personal philosophy affects that nurse's philosophy of nursing. Throughout the nursing educational process, students begin forming their philosophy of nursing. This philosophy is influenced significantly by a student's personal philosophy and experiences. One's personal philosophy should be compatible with the philosophy of the nursing department where he or she works.

TABLE 15-1	SELECTED ETHICAL THEORIES
Ethical Theory	**Interpretation**
Deontology	Actions are based on moral rules and unchanging principles, such as, "do unto others as you would have them do unto you." An ethical person must always follow the rules, even if doing so causes a less desirable outcome. This theory states that the motives of the actor determine the goodness or value of the act. Thus, a bad outcome may be acceptable if the intent of the actor was good.
Teleology	A person must take those actions that lead to good outcomes. This theory states that the outcome of an act determines whether the act is good or of value and that achievement of a good outcome justifies using a less desirable means to attain the end.
Virtue ethics	Virtues such as truthfulness and trustworthiness are developed over time. A person's character must be developed so that by nature and habit, the person will be predisposed to behave virtuously. Living a virtuous life contributes both to one's own well-being and to the well-being of society.
Justice and equity	A "veil of ignorance" regarding who is affected by a decision should be used by decision makers because it allows for unbiased decision making. An ethical person chooses the action that is fair to all, including both the advantaged and the disadvantaged groups in society.
Relativism	There are no universal ethical standards, such as "murder is always wrong." Ethical standards are relative to person, place, time, and culture. Whatever a person thinks is right, is right. This theory has been largely rejected.

Memorial's Professional Practice Model
Design for Excellence

Mission--
Professional nurses and nursing teams exist to optimize the health of our patients and communities.

We believe many conditions must work together in order to nurture a professional environment. More specifically, the manner in which Beliefs, Practice, Structure, Relationships, and Operations interact will determine the quality of outcomes for us as well as for those we serve.

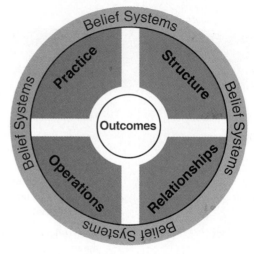

Figure 15-1 Nursing philosophy. (*Source:* Adapted with permission from *Memorial Health System's Professional Practice Philosophy.* Springfield, IL).

This helps the nurse to be an effective leader and practitioner. See Figure 15-1 for a nursing department's philosophy statement. An example of a personal nursing philosophy is:

I believe professional nursing care promotes an optimal level of wellness in body, mind, and spirit to those being served. I believe professional nurses must hold themselves to the highest standards of the profession and honor the profession's code of ethics in all aspects of practice.

VALUES AND VIRTUES

Values are personal beliefs about the truth of ideals, standards, principles, objects, and behaviors that give meaning and direction to life. If you were told that you must pack a bag for a special trip but you may bring only three items from your belongings, what items would you choose? The ones selected are what you value.

It is important to clarify your personal values. Personal values provide a baseline for identifying your professional nursing values. The professional nursing values of altruism, autonomy, human dignity, integrity, and social justice guide the nurse in providing ethical care to patients (American Association of Colleges of Nursing, Essentials of Baccalaureate Education for Professional Nursing Practice, 2008, available at www.aacn.nche.edu/Education/pdf/BaccEssentials08.pdf).

Values Clarification is the process of analyzing one's own values to better understand what is truly

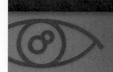

CRITICAL THINKING 15-1

New graduates formulate a philosophy of nursing based on personal beliefs and on values. Reflections on the following questions can assist in the development of a philosophy:

How can nurses influence patient care based on their nursing philosophy? Are compassion, discernment, trustworthiness, and integrity essential both personally and professionally? Do nurses have an ethical responsibility to demonstrate caring and maintain current competency?

important. In their classic work *Values and Teaching*, Raths, Harmin, and Simon (1978) formulated a theory of values clarification and proposed a three-step process for valuing, as follows:

Choosing
1. Analysis of alternative beliefs and their consequences
2. Free choice of your beliefs from alternatives

Prizing
3. Feeling satisfied with your choice
4. Being willing to share your choice with others

Acting
5. Making your choice a part of your behavior
6. Repeating the choice

VIRTUE

Burkhardt and Nathaniel (2006) list four virtues that are more significant than others and that are illustrative of a virtuous person: compassion, discernment, trustworthiness, and integrity. **Compassion** is a deep awareness of the suffering of another along with the desire to relieve it. **Discernment** is possession of acuteness of judgment. **Trustworthiness** is present when trust is well founded or deserving. **Integrity** may be considered to be firm adherence to a code of conduct or an ethical value. These virtues form the foundation for an ethically principled discipline and have been endorsed throughout the nursing profession's history (Burkhardt & Nathaniel, 2006). Nurses who subscribe to these

four virtues are inclined to recall and value that patients also have their own personal values.

ETHICAL PRINCIPLES

In addition to the theories, ethical principles and values provide a basis for nurses to determine the appropriate action when faced with an ethical dilemma in the practice setting. See Table 15-2 for a summary of the major ethical principles and rules.

A GUIDE FOR ETHICAL DECISION MAKING

Burkhardt and Nathaniel (2006) developed a guide for decision making, which new nurses may use when confronted with an ethical decision. See Table 15-3.

AN ETHICS TEST

A practical way of improving ethical decision making is to run decisions that you are considering through an ethics test when any doubt exists. The ethics test presented here was used at the Center for Business Ethics at Bentley College (Bowditch & Buono, 1997) as part of ethical corporate training programs. Decision makers are taught to ask themselves:

- Is it right?
- Is it fair?
- Who gets hurt?
- Would you tell your child or young relative to do it?

TABLE 15-2	ETHICAL PRINCIPLES AND RULES

Ethical Principle/Rules	Definition	Example
Beneficence	The duty to do good to others and to maintain a balance between benefits and harms.	■ Provide all persons, including patients and the terminally ill, with caring attention and information.
Nonmaleficence	The principle of doing no harm.	■ Keep your knowledge and skills up to date.
Justice	The principle of fairness that is served when an individual is given that which he or she is due, owed, deserves, or can legitimately claim.	■ Treat all patients fairly, regardless of economic or social background.
Confidentiality	Ensuring that information is accessible only to those authorized to have access.	■ Become familiar with federal and state laws and facility policies dealing with privacy, e. g., HIPAA legislation.
Fidelity	The principle of promise keeping; the duty to keep one's promise or word.	■ Be sure that you keep your promises.
Autonomy	The right of people to make their own decision; self-determination.	■ Provide all persons with information for decision making. Avoid making paternalistic decisions for others.
Veracity	The obligation to tell the truth.	■ Refuse to participate in any form of fraud. Give an "honest day's work" every day.
Advocacy	The obligation to look out or speak up for the rights of others.	■ Provide patients with high quality, evidence-based care.

- How does it smell? This question is based on a person's intuition and common sense.
- Would you be comfortable if the details of your decision were reported on the front page of your local newspaper or through your hospital's e-mail system?

PATIENT RIGHTS

The American Hospital Association (1992) developed a Patient's Bill of Rights with the expectation that when patients and families participate in treatment decisions, the outcome will be more effective care. The Patient Care Partnership document replaced the Bill of Rights in 2008. See www.aha.org for more information.

ETHICAL LEADERSHIP AND MANAGEMENT

Health care leaders are charged with the responsibility of creating an environment that is ethically principled and that supports upholding the standards of conduct set by the health care professions.

TABLE 15-3	A GUIDE FOR DECISION MAKING

Gather Data and Identify Conflicting Moral Claims

- What makes this situation an ethical problem? Are there conflicting obligations, duties, principles, rights, loyalties, values, or beliefs?
- What are the issues? What facts seem most important?
- What emotions have an impact? What are the gaps in information at this time?

Identify Key Participants

- Who is legitimately empowered to make this decision? Who is affected and how?
- What is the level of competence of the person most affected in relation to the decision to be made?
- What are the rights, duties, authority, context, and capabilities of participants?

Determine Moral Perspective and Phase of Moral Development of Key Participants

- Do participants think in terms of duties or rights?
- Do the parties involved exhibit similar or different moral perspectives?
- Where is the common ground? Differences? What principles are important to each person involved?
- What emotions are evident within the interaction and with each person involved?
- What is the level of moral development of the participants?

Determine Desired Outcomes

- How does each party describe the circumstances of the outcome?
- What are the consequences of the desired outcomes?
- What outcomes are unacceptable to one or all involved?

Identify Options

- What options emerge through the assessment process?
- How do the alternatives fit the lifestyle and values of the person(s) affected?
- What are legal considerations of the various options?
- What alternatives are unacceptable to one or all involved?
- How are alternatives weighed, ranked, and prioritized?

Act on the Choice

- Be empowered to make a difficult decision.
- Give yourself permission to set aside less acceptable alternatives.
- Be attentive to the emotions involved in the process.

Evaluate Outcomes of Action

- Has the ethical dilemma been resolved? Have other dilemmas emerged related to the action?
- How has the process affected those involved? Are further actions required?

Source: Burkhardt, M. A. & Nathaniel, A. K. (2006). *Ethics and Issues in Contemporary Nursing. (2nd ed.).* Clifton Park, NY: Delmar Cengage Learning.

CRITICAL THINKING 15-2

A nurse administered the wrong medication to a patient. The patient then had to be transferred to the Intensive Care Unit and required a longer stay in the hospital. The nurse freely admitted the mistake to her nurse manager. The manager recommended that the two of them go talk with the patient and explain what happened. The administration then heard about the incident and advised the manager against telling the patient immediately about the error. The situation was also referred to the hospital ethics committee. Use the guide for decision making in Table 15-3 and the ethics test discussed earlier in this chapter to decide what should be done.

Research conducted by the Ethics Research Center concluded the following:

- If positive outcomes are desired, an ethical culture is what makes the difference.
- Leadership, especially senior leadership, is the most critical factor in promoting an ethical culture.
- In organizations that are trying to strengthen their culture, formal program elements can help to do that (Harned, 2005).

ORGANIZATIONAL BENEFITS DERIVED FROM ETHICS

Ethical behavior and socially responsible acts are not always free. Investing in work/life programs, granting social leaves of absence, and telling patients the absolute truth about potential problems may not have an immediate return (DuBrin, 2000). Nevertheless, recent evidence suggests that high ethics and social responsibility are related to good financial performance (Positive Leadership, 1998). Profits and social responsibility work two ways. More profitable firms can better afford to invest in social responsibility initiatives, and these initiatives, in turn, lead to more profits. Being ethical also helps avoid the costs of paying huge fines for being unethical, and a big payoff from socially responsible acts is that they often attract and retain socially responsible employees and customers (DuBrin, 2000).

CREATING AN ETHICAL WORKPLACE

Establishing an ethical and socially responsible workplace is not simply a matter of luck and common sense. Nurse managers can develop strategies and programs to enhance ethical and socially responsible attitudes. These may include:

1. Formal mechanisms for monitoring ethics, such as an ethics program or ethics hotline.
2. Written organizational codes of conduct.
3. Widespread communication in the hospital to reinforce ethically and socially responsible behavior.
4. Leadership by example: if people throughout the hospital believe that behaving ethically is "in" and behaving unethically is "out," ethical behavior will prevail.
5. Encouraging confrontation about ethical deviations. Unethical behavior may be minimized if every employee confronts anyone seen behaving unethically.
6. Training programs in ethics and social responsibility, including messages about ethics from executives, classes on ethics at colleges, and exercises in ethics (DuBrin, 2000).
7. Instituting an ethics committee made up of interdisciplinary representatives from

CASE STUDY 15-1

To better relate the study of ethics to yourself, take the self quiz below. Do you agree or disagree with the following statements?

1. I would report a nursing coworker's drug abuse.
2. I see no harm in taking home a few nursing supplies.
3. I would tell the truth to a patient who asked if he was dying.
4. I would tell a patient who asked what narcotic pain medicine he was receiving.
5. It is unacceptable to call in sick to take a day off, even if only done once or twice a year.
6. I would accept a permanent, full-time job even if I knew I wanted the job for only six months.
7. If I received $100 for doing some odd jobs, I would report it on my income tax returns.
8. When applying for a nursing position, I would cover up the fact that I had been fired from a recent job.
9. I would report the family of a child who has findings not consistent with the reported story.
10. I would give ordered drugs on a temporary basis to a drug-addicted patient who is out of narcotics and who presents to the emergency department.

Source: C. S. Faircloth, RN, Personal Communications, March 13, 2003.

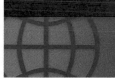

REAL WORLD INTERVIEW

One of my most difficult cases involved a man in his early 40s who was in a coma, ventilator dependent, and declared brain dead. The patient was from a different culture, and when the family arrived six weeks later from abroad, they refused to allow him to be removed from the ventilator. His parents said they were told by the gods that their son would be well several months in the future. After two months in the hospital, the administration began to put pressure on the family to transfer the patient.

Emily Davison, RN
Case Manager
Pleasant Hill, Missouri

nursing, medicine, administration, clergy, consumers, psychiatry, social work, nutritional services, and pharmacy, as well as an ethicist. Additional persons may be invited on an as-needed basis. See Figure 15-2. Ethical dilemmas may be referred to an ethics committee by anyone.

These committees provide guidance to patients and their families, as well as to the health care team.

NURSE-PHYSICIAN ETHICS AND RELATIONSHIPS

Nurses working in organizations often confront ethical dilemmas in working with patients and their families. To resolve these dilemmas, the nurse must often work closely with the medical practitioner. The nurse often finds that medical practitioners hold different beliefs about

values, communication, trust and integrity, role responsibilities, and organizational politics and economics. These beliefs affect their ethical beliefs, which, in turn, affect their decisions

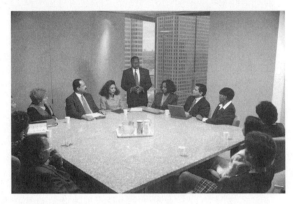

Figure 15-2 Ethics committee at work. (*Source:* Photo courtesy of Photodisc).

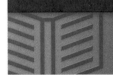

EVIDENCE-BASED PRACTICE

Citation: No abuse zone. (2002, March). *Hospitals and Health Networks, 26,* 28.

Discussion: An astounding number of health care workers, 62% to 96%, say that they experienced or witnessed abusive behavior in the past year from a supervisor, a doctor, or even a patient. For example, a nurse working the night shift gets a medication order she can't read and calls the physician at 2 A.M. for clarification. He yells at her and hangs up without answering the question. The nurse is afraid to call back and gives a fatal dose of the wrong drug.

This article discusses guidelines for a five-stage process to rid health care workplaces of abusive behavior. Deborah Anderson, president of Respond 2, Inc. in St. Paul, Minnesota, is developing the guidelines in conjunction with the Hennepin Medical Society in Minneapolis. Minnesota. The Respond 2, Inc. five-stage process includes: building a team that meets monthly, surveying employees with an assessment tool about their experiences with workplace abuse, devising a plan to deal with workplace abuse, evaluating outcomes with a re-survey, and infusing the workplace with an atmosphere of collegiality by changing policies and procedures that affect culture, hiring, employee orientation, training, reporting processes, performance evaluation, and appropriate patient safety and quality-related initiatives. In developing this five-stage process, it is imperative that strong support be in place from the leaders of the organization.

Implications for Practice: This five-stage process can be very useful in developing a no-abuse workplace. The Joint Commission encourages use of the SBARR communication technique. When this technique is used with the five-stage no-abuse process, the environment for ethical safe practice is enhanced. See chapter 5 in this text for more information on the SBARR Technique. See also the Web site www.chw.org. Search for SBARR.

CASE STUDY 15-2

Select a moderator and an ethical issue of your choice in class, for example, should patients be given placebo medications? The moderator will introduce the issue and be responsible for debate flow and adhering to time requirements.

Divide the group into two subgroups. Ask for one group to give the reasons why patients should be given placebos and one group to give the reasons why patients should not be given placebos.

Instruct your volunteers to consider all pertinent ethical theories and principles, any conflicts between them, any relationships to ethical codes, legal implications, people involved and impacted, and any relevant sociocultural, political, or religious aspects that may influence this ethical issue. Refer to the guide for Decision Making in this chapter.

Each group must state their position and references. They should be familiar with their part so they can "talk it" rather than "read it."

What were the pros identified? What were the cons? Did any of the comments alter your own position on this issue?

Source: Developed with information from Candela, L., Michael, S. R., & Mitchell, S. (2003). Ethical debates: Enhancing critical thinking in nursing students. *Nurse Educator, 28*(1), 37–39.

---

about treatment, which may lead to conflicts between nurses and medical practitioners. These conflicts can be limited with clear ethical guidelines and policies, established by interdisciplinary teams and overseen by an ethical administration. When an ethical issue arises, resolution might be tedious and possibly riddled with resentment if guidelines and policies are not well developed.

The Gallup Organization's 2007 annual poll on professional honesty and ethical standards ranked nurses number one. Of the 22 professions tested, six have high ethical ratings: nurses (83%), pharmacists (71%), medical practitioners (64%), grade school teachers (74%), military officers (65%), and clergy (53%). For more information, see poll.gallup.com. Search for *Ethical Standards.*

ETHICAL CODES

One mark of a profession is the determination of ethical behavior for its members. Several nursing organizations have developed codes for ethical behavior. The International Council of Nurses Code of Ethics for Nurses is available at www.icn.ch/icncode.pdf.

The American Nurses Association has also developed a Code of Ethics for Nurses (2006). See www.nursingworld.org. Click on *Code of Ethics.*

The Canadian Nurses Association (CNA) has also developed a Code of Ethics. The first Code, adopted in 1954, was the International Council of Nursing Code for Nurses. The Code of Ethics for Registered Nurses was adopted in 1997. In 2002, The Code of Ethics for Registered Nurses was expanded and revised. The code may be obtained from the CNA Web site, www.cna-nurses.ca. Search for *Code of Ethics.*

KEY CONCEPTS

- Ethics is the branch of philosophy that concerns the distinction of right from wrong on the basis of a body of knowledge, not just on the basis of opinions.

- A personal philosophy stems from an individual's beliefs and values. This personal philosophy will influence an individual's philosophy of nursing.

- Values clarification is an important step in helping one understand what is truly important.

- Ethical principles include autonomy and confidentiality, beneficence, nonmaleficence, fidelity, autonomy, respect for others, veracity, and advocacy.

- The Burkhardt and Nathaniel guide for decision making is a helpful tool.

- The Patient's Bill of Rights encourages more effective patient care.

- Organizations have a responsibility to society to practice ethically.

- The Ethics test is useful when examining issues.

- Ethics committees provide guidance for decision making about ethical dilemmas that arise in health care settings.

- The International Council of Nurses' Code of Ethics for Nurses influences patient care.

- Various nursing ethical codes influence patient care.

KEY TERMS

advocacy

autonomy

beneficence

bioethics

compassion

discernment

ethical dilemma

ethics

fidelity

integrity

justice

morality

nonmaleficence

philosophy

respect for others

trustworthiness

values

values clarification

veracity

REVIEW QUESTIONS

1. The nurse manager has an ethical responsibility to
   A. the patient.
   B. the organization.
   C. the profession.
   D. the patient, the organization, the profession, and society.

2. The primary role of an ethics committee is to
   A. decide what should be done when ethical dilemmas arise.
   B. prevent the practitioner from making the wrong decision.
   C. provide guidance for the health care team and family of the patient.
   D. prevent ethical dilemmas from occurring.

3. The nurse demonstrates nonmaleficence by doing which of the following? Select all that apply.
   A. observing the six rights of medication administration
   B. reviewing practitioner orders for accuracy and completeness
   C. keeping knowledge and skill up-to-date
   D. dressing professionally with name badge clearly visible

4. When the nurse is obtaining the patient's consent, the patient states that the surgeon did not inform her of the risks of surgery. The nurse should
   A. tell the patient the risks.
   B. report the surgeon to the ethics committee.
   C. report the surgeon to the unit manager.
   D. inform the surgeon that the patient is unaware of the risks.

REVIEW ACTIVITIES

1. An elderly woman, age 88, is admitted to the Emergency Department in acute respiratory distress. She does not have a living will, but her daughter has power of attorney (POA) for health care and is a health care professional. The patient has end-stage renal disease, end-stage Alzheimer's disease, and congestive heart failure. Her condition is grave. The doctors want to intubate her and place her on a ventilator. The sons agree. The daughter states that their mother would not want to be on a machine just to prolong her life.
   Divide into groups. Discuss the ethical theories that can be applied to this situation. Use the class-room debate style from the *Candela evidence-based practice* article identified in Case Study 15-2 to guide you.

2. As a hospice nurse, you are involved with pain control on a regular basis. Many of the medications prescribed for the management of pain also depress respirations.
   Divide into groups and determine a protocol for the use of these medications, keeping in mind that the purpose of hospice is to promote comfort. Support your decision with ethical theories and principles.

EXPLORING THE WEB

- Nursing ethics:
  www.ana.org
  Click on *Code of Ethics*.

- Use the International Council of Nurses Web site to find the ICN Code of Ethics for Nurses:
  www.icn.ch
  Click on the *ICN Code of Ethics*.

- Visit:
  www.aha.org
  Search for *patient care partnership* to view the American Health Association's Patient Care Partnership.

- ANA Center for Ethics and Human Rights:
  www.nursingworld.org/ethic
  Search for *ANA Center for Ethics and Human Rights*.
  Search for *About the Center*. Accessed May 13, 2008.

- National Center for Ethics in Health Care Home:
  www.ethics.va.gov

- The Center for Bioethics and Human Dignity:
  www.cbhd.org

- Nursing ethics network:
  www.bc.edu
  Search for *nursing ethics network*.

REFERENCES

American Association of Colleges of Nursing (AACN). *Essentials of Baccalaureate Education for Professional Nursing Practice, 2008*, available at www.aacn.nche. edu/Education/pdf/BaccEssentials08.pdf.

American Hospital Association (AHA). (1992). *A Patient's Bill of Rights.* Chicago: Author. Available at www.aha.org

American Nurses Association (ANA). (2001). *Code of Ethics for Nurses with interpretive statements.* Washington, DC: American Nurses Publishing.

Bowditch, J. L., & Buono, A. F. (1997). *A primer on organizational behavior.* (4th ed.). New York: Wiley.

Burkhardt, M. A., & Nathaniel, A. K. (2006). *Ethics & Issues in Contemporary Nursing.* (2nd ed.). Clifton Park, NY: Delmar Cengage Learning.

Candela, L., Michael, S. R., & Mitchell, S. (2003). Ethical debates: Enhancing critical thinking in nursing students. *Nurse Educator, 28*(1), 37–39.

Canadian Nurses Association (CNA). (2002). Code of ethics for RN. www.cna-nurses.ca. Search for *code of ethics.*

DeLaune, S. C., & Ladner, P. K. (2006). *Fundamentals of nursing.* (3rd ed.). Clifton Park, NY: Delmar Cengage Learning.

DuBrin, A. J. (2000). *The Active Manager.* Clifton Park, NY: Southwestern College Publishing.

Faircloth, C. S. (2003). Personal communication with Patricia Kelly.

Greene J. (2002). The medical workplace. No abuse zone. *Hospitals and Health Networks.* Mar; 76(3):26, 28.

Harned, P. (2005). National Business Ethics Survey. *Ethics Today Online,* 4(2). Available at www.ethics. org/research/2005-press-release.asp.

International Council of Nurses (ICN). (2006). *Code of Ethics for Nurses.* Geneva: Author.

Kohlberg, L. (1971). Stages of Moral Development as a basis for moral development. In C. M. Beck, B. S. Crittenden, & E. V. Sullivan (Eds.). *Moral Interdisciplinary Approaches.* Paramus, NJ: Newman.

Positive Leadership. (1998). Research reported in sample issue. *Positive Leadership,* 5.

Raths, L. E., Harmin, M., & Simon, S. B. (1978). *Values and teaching* (2nd ed.). Columbus, OH: Merrill Publishing.

SUGGESTED READINGS

Beard, E. L., Jr., Johnson, L. W. (2007, Oct.–Dec.). Conversations in ethics. *JONAS Healthcare Law Ethics Regulation, 9*(4), 117–8.

Lobbyists Debut at Bottom of Honesty and Ethics List – December 10, 2007 by Jeffrey M. Jones. Available at www.gallup.com/poll/1031231lobbyists-debut-bottom-honesty-ethics-list.aspx.

Memorial Health System's Professional Practice Philosophy, Springfield, IL.

Milton, C. L. (2008, Jan.). Boundaries: ethical implications for what it means to be therapeutic in the nurse-person relationship. *Nursing Science Quarterly,* 21(1), 18–21.

Nursing Ethics conference on the globalization of nursing: ethical, legal and political issues. (2007, Jan.) *Nursing Ethics,* 14(1), 3–4.

Pauly, B., Goldstone, I., McCall J., Gold, F., Payne, S. (2007, Oct.). The ethical, legal and social context of harm reduction. *Canadian Nurse, 103*(8), 19–23.

Pendry, P. S. (2007, July–Aug.) Moral distress: recognizing it to retain nurses. *Nursing Economics, 25*(4), 217–21.

Tschudin, V. (2006). How nursing ethics as a subject changes: An analysis of the first eleven years of publication of the journal Nursing Ethics. *Nursing Ethics, 13*(1), 65–85.

Tschudin, V. (2007, Nov.). How is the nursing profession perceived from outside the profession itself…? *Nursing Ethics, 14*(6), 709–10.

CHAPTER 16

Culture, Generational Differences, and Spirituality

If we are to achieve a richer culture, rich in contrasting values, we must recognize the whole gamut of human potentialities, and so weave a less arbitrary social fabric, one in which each diverse human gift will find a fitting place.

(Margaret Mead, 1935)

OBJECTIVES

Upon completion of this chapter, the reader should be able to:

1. Define culture.
2. Discuss cultural competence.
3. Identify key cultural nursing theories.
4. Discuss organizational culture.
5. Review strategies for working with a multicultural team.
6. Discuss generational differences.
7. Integrate understanding of spiritual beliefs into patient care.

Mr. Wu is brought into the Emergency Department with diaphoresis, nausea, and vomiting, and he is clutching his left chest. He is speaking with his wife in Chinese and says he understands only a little English. His wife understands none. Fortunately, Charles Lin, a new nurse, is working this shift and is able to communicate in Chinese with the Wu family. How can Charles most effectively communicate Mr. Wu's concerns to the health care staff? If Charles was not working, how could the other staff communicate with Mr. Wu?

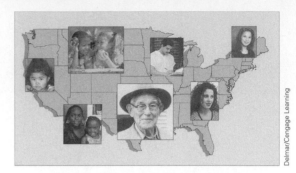

Delmar/Cengage Learning

We live in a global society rich with different and ever-changing cultures, traditions, religions, spiritual beliefs, and generations, all of which influence the delivery of health care. New immigrants arrive daily. Consideration of all of these differences and sensitivity to patient and health care staff diversity is necessary in all nursing roles as situations arise that call for evaluating patient and staff behavior. Though each person is first and foremost an individual, each is also a member of a cultural group. Clues to people's behaviors come from understanding the cultural, generational, and spiritual focus of the individual or group. This chapter will enable the nurse to begin to prepare for cultural, generational, and spiritual aspects of leadership and management with patients and health care staff.

CULTURE

Culture refers to the integrated patterns of human behavior that include the language, thoughts, communication, actions, customs, beliefs, values, and institutions of racial, ethnic, religious, or social groups (Munoz & Luckmann, 2005). Although people from all cultures share most human characteristics, the study of culture highlights both the way individuals differ and are similar to individuals in other cultures. Individuals from different cultures may think, solve problems, and perceive and structure the world differently from individuals of another culture. Cultural beliefs serve as a conscious and unconscious point of reference that guides the outlook and decisions of people. Culture incorporates the experience of the past and

influences the present. It transmits traditions to future members of a culture. Culture influences what we eat, the language we speak, the values we believe in, and the actions we take (Munoz & Luckmann, 2005).

Normally, children learn about their culture while growing up. However, when people emigrate from their native cultures into a new culture, they often experience culture shock. **Culture shock** develops when the values and beliefs upheld by a person's new culture are radically different from the person's native culture. For successful assimilation into a new culture, immigrants may want to learn that culture's important values.

In addition to belonging to a major cultural group, people also belong to a variety of subcultures, or smaller groups within a culture. Each culture has its own value system and related expectations. Subcultures may be based on the following:

- Professional and occupational affiliations (RNs)
- Nationality or race (a shared historical and political past)
- Age groups (adolescents, senior citizens)
- Gender (feminists, men's groups)
- Socioeconomic factors (working class, middle class, upper class)
- Political viewpoints (Democrat, Republican)
- Sexual orientation (gay and lesbian groups)

Upon admission to a hospital, patients also become members of a culture. In this world filled with strange healthcare sights, unfamiliar sounds, and strangers, many patients experience culture shock. This shock intensifies for patients who are recent immigrants or who do not speak English (Munoz & Luckmann, 2005).

RACE AND ETHNICITY

Race describes a geographical or global human population distinguished by genetic traits and physical characteristics such as skin color or facial features. Major U.S. Census classifications of race are American Indian, Asian, Black African, Pacific Islander/Hawaiian, or White, as shown in Figure 16-1 (www.census.gov). Cultural ethnicity identifies a person or group based on a racial, tribal, linguistic, religious, national, or cultural group, for example, Jewish or Irish. In years past, when new immigrants arrived in the United States, they sought to become acculturated to their new country by adopting the conditions, language, and customs of the United States. Acculturation has taken a generation or two in the past and often resulted in the loss of a separate cultural identity. Today's immigrant population is more likely to maintain a strong tradition of valuing their historical cultural identity.

HEALTH CARE DISPARITY

Because of differences in cultural beliefs, there is often the **marginalization** or separation of some cultural groups away from the mainstream. Marginalized groups often suffer from higher rates of morbidity, mortality, and the burden of disease (Keltner, Kelley, & Smith, 2004). These increased rates may be due to a lack of health care access, inadequate financial resources, immigrant resident status, or a lack of knowledge on how to seek help.

According to the U.S. Census Bureau, 30% of Native Americans live below the poverty line, compared with 29.5% of Blacks, 25.3% of Hispanics, 14.1% of Asian/Pacific Islanders, and 9.8% of Whites. Also, Native Americans have the lowest life expectancy of any ethnic group in the United States. Native Americans can expect to live only two-thirds as long as other people in the United States (Wikoff, 2008).

The life expectancy gap between African Americans and Caucasians is 5.6 years, with the average life expectancy being 75.2 years for Caucasians and 69.6 years for African Americans. The infant death rate for African Americans is twice that of Caucasians (Nies & McEwen, 2007).

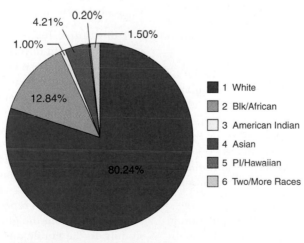

4.21% 0.20%
1.00%   1.50%
12.84%
80.24%

- 1 White
- 2 Blk/African
- 3 American Indian
- 4 Asian
- 5 PI/Hawaiian
- 6 Two/More Races

Hispanics make up 14.1% overall, may be of any race, and are counted under more than one category.

Figure 16-1 2004 estimate of U.S. population by race. (*Source:* U.S. Census Bureau, Census 2000 [www.census.gov]).

Note that concern for quality care must focus not only on ethnic minorities and populations that have a different heritage than Euro-Americans, but also on the needs of other marginalized populations (Hall, Stevens, & Meleis, 1994). Examples of other marginalized populations may include gays and lesbians, older adults, recently arrived immigrants, e.g., from South America or Rwanda, as well as groups that have been in this country for some time, e.g., people from South America and the Middle East. These populations are often less visible than federally defined minorities (Lenburg et al., 1995).

DIVERSITY IN NURSING

While most nurses are Caucasian women, increasing numbers of minority students are graduating from nursing programs. In a survey conducted by the American Association of Colleges of Nursing (AACN) in 2006, minority representation in baccalaureate programs was highest among those identified as Black or African American (12%) and lowest among Native Americans (0.7%). Graduates from Hispanic or Latino groups totaled 5.4%, and Asian, Native Hawaiian, or other Pacific Islanders comprised 0.8% of the undergraduate students who responded to the survey. These totals lag behind the 75.2% reported Caucasian enrollments. The number of men who graduate from basic registered nurse programs is also increasing. In the AACN survey conducted in 2006, 9% of the undergraduates were men.

Of the nurses who indicated their racial or ethnic background in 2004, 88.4% (estimated 2,380,639) were White, non-Hispanic; 4.6% or 122,495 were Black or African American, non-Hispanic; 3.3% or 89,976 were Asian or Pacific Islander, non-Hispanic; 1.8% or 48,009 were Hispanic; 0.4% or 9,453 were American Indian or Alaskan Native; and 1.5% were from two or more racial backgrounds.

Men constituted 5.7% of the RN population in 2004. The initial nursing preparation for many male RNs was an associate's degree. The percentages of male and female RNs completing a baccalaureate or higher degree initial nursing program were similar, 32.7% and 31.5%, respectively.

CULTURAL COMPETENCE

Nurses providing care need to ensure that the cultural needs of their patients are considered. **Culturally competent care** is a complex integration of knowledge, attitudes, and skills that enhances cross-cultural communication and appropriate and effective interactions (American Academy of Nursing, 1992). The goal of culturally competent nursing care is to provide care that is consistent with the patient's cultural needs. The AAN expert panel report (1992) on culturally competent nursing care suggested the following four principles:

- Care is designed for the specific patient.
- Care is based on the uniqueness of the person's culture and includes cultural norms and values.
- Care includes empowerment strategies to facilitate patient decision making in their personal health behavior.
- Care is provided with sensitivity to the cultural uniqueness of the patient.

Since the 1960s, a united effort has been underway to include concepts sensitive to cultural diversity in nursing education. The National League for Nursing (NLN) has made this requirement mandatory for accreditation. Additionally, the Transcultural Nursing Society has been certifying nurses in transcultural nursing since 1988.

A new nurse leader is often asked to work with people from different cultures. To manage and understand these cultures, cultural nursing theories and conceptual models offers direction, i.e., Leininger's Transcultural Nursing (1978, 1997), Purnell's Model for Cultural Competence (2005), Campinha-Bacote's Process of Cultural Competence in the Delivery of Health Care Service (2003), Spector's Cultural Heritage Model (2005), and Giger and Davidhizar's Transcultural Assessment Model (2004). Purnell's Model for Cultural Competence is represented by a circle with rims moving from the global society to the community, to the family, and to the individual. The inner circle has twelve pie slices representing twelve domains of culture, that is, overview/heritage, communication, family roles and organization, workforce issues, biocultural ecology, high-risk

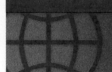

REAL WORLD INTERVIEW

In the southern part of California, we have an underrepresentation of Hispanic nurses in our hospitals. To encourage and promote nursing enrollment, we have brought Hispanic nurses from Mexico to experience our health care system. They are provided with a hospital orientation of key programs in their areas of interest. They also spend time in the clinical area.

At the high school level, we have brought a group of about thirty high school students, the majority Hispanics, to the hospital. We talk to them about health care, nursing opportunities, and the need for Hispanic nursing staff.

As a nursing executive, I feel that it is important to be a role model for minority students. Recently, I participated in mock interviews for high school students. The majority of these students were Hispanic, Black, and Asian. We wanted to mentor and coach them on how to successfully interview for jobs. These are students without role models in their lives. Just by seeing what other people have done creates a high sense of inspiration and desire to do better because they see that it is possible.

Pablo Velez, PhD, RN,
Chief Nursing Officer
Sharp Chula Vista Medical Center
Chula Vista, California

behaviors, nutrition, pregnancy, death rituals, spirituality, health care practices, and health care practitioners. Analyzing the patient belief system in each of the twelve domains gives direction to the nursing process.

These nursing journals will also assist with building your cultural competence:

- *The Journal of Transcultural Nursing*
- *Western Journal of Medicine: Cross Cultural Issues*
- *Journal of Cultural Diversity*
- *Journal of Multicultural Nursing*
- *International Journal of Nursing Studies*
- *International Nursing Review*
- *Journal of Holistic Nursing*

LANGUAGE

As you work with patients, you will encounter a great diversity in both body language and spoken language. For instance, more than 6,000 languages and dialects are spoken today. Mandarin Chinese is spoken by approximately 836 million people.

In the late 1990s, there were nearly as many Spanish speakers, who number 332 million, as there are Hindi speakers, who number 333 million worldwide (Microsoft, 1996). There are 322 million English speakers. If we include individuals who speak English as a second language, which is approximately 418 million speakers, then English is the second most widely spoken language, with Mandarin Chinese being the most widely spoken (Munoz & Luckmann, 2005).

LINGUISTICALLY APPROPRIATE SERVICES Any individual who is seeking health care services and who has limited English proficiency (LEP) has the right, based on Title VI of the Civil Rights Act of 1964, to have an interpreter available to facilitate communication within the health care system. Open and clear communication is essential to develop an appropriate diagnosis and treatment.

Unfortunately, use of family members or friends as interpreters is convenient and continues to be common practice in some health care settings.

CASE STUDY 16-1

Following are different levels of response you might have toward a person.

Levels of Response:

- *Greet:* I feel I can greet this person warmly and welcome him or her sincerely.
- *Accept:* I feel I can honestly accept this person as he or she is and be comfortable enough to listen to his or her problems.
- *Help:* I feel I would genuinely try to help this person with his or her problems as they might be related to or arise from the label or stereotype given to him or her.
- *Background:* I feel I have the background of knowledge and experience to be able to help this person.
- *Advocate:* I feel I could honestly be an advocate for this person.

The following is a list of individuals. Read down the list and place a check mark by anyone you would not Greet or would hesitate to Greet. Then move to response level 2, Accept, and follow the same procedure for all five response levels. Try to respond honestly, not as you think might be socially or professionally desirable. Your answers are only for your personal use in clarifying your initial reactions to different people. How did you do?

Individual	1 Greet	2 Accept	3 Help	4 Background	5 Advocate
1. White Anglo-Saxon American					
2. Hispanic American					
3. Black African American					
4. Native American					
5. Asian American					
6. Filipino American					
7. Chinese American					
8. Pacific Islander American					
9. Jewish American					
10. Iranian American					
11. Muslim American					
12. Amish American					
13. Gay/Lesbian American					
14. Catholic American					
15. Jehovah's Witness American					
16. Protestant American					
17. Male Nurse					
18. Female Nurse					
19. Older Nurse					
20. Young Nurse					
21. Elderly American					
22. American with AIDS					
23. Unmarried expectant teen					
24. Obese American					
25. Alcoholic					

Source: Compiled with information from Munoz, C., & Luckmann, J. (2005). *Transcultural communication.* Clifton Park, NY: Delmar Cengage Learning.

EVIDENCE-BASED PRACTICE

Citation: DeRosa, N., & Kochurka, K. (2006, Oct.). Implement culturally competent healthcare in your workplace. *Nursing Management, 37*(10), 18–26.

Discussion: This article discusses selected verbal and nonverbal communication patterns of culture. Even when two people speak the same language, communication may be hindered by different values or beliefs. Nonverbal differences or ethnic dialects can also block mutual understanding. Communication differences include the following:

■ *Conversational style:* Silence may show respect or acknowledgement. In some cultures, a direct "no" is considered rude, and silence may mean "no." A loud voice or repeating a statement may mean anger or simply emphasis, enthusiasm, or a request for help.

■ *Personal space:* Beliefs about personal space vary. Someone may be viewed as aggressive for standing "too close" or as "distant" for backing off when approached.

■ Eye contact: In some cultures, direct eye contact may be a sign of respect. In other cultures, direct eye contact may be seen as a sign of disrespect.

■ *Subject matter and conversation length:* Even what constitutes an appropriate subject matter, i.e., when it's appropriate to discuss certain ideas, how long the discussion should last, etc. These vary from culture to culture. Some cultures value communication that's subtle and circumspect; forthright discussion is considered rude. In some cultures, it's acceptable to discuss topics such as sexuality and death, whereas in other cultures, these topics are taboo.

The article also discusses elements of a cultural assessment, including nutrition, medications, pain, and psychological and primary language assessment. It also explores how to approach the patient with educational needs.

Implications for Practice: Be aware of these cultural differences when working with patients and staff from other cultures. Remember that not everyone sees things the way that you do.

This practice is discouraged and can be acceptable only when the patient expresses the preference to have a family member or friend be the interpreter. Clearly, situations may arise in which a formally trained interpreter is unavailable and the use of a telephone interpretation service is not practical; family members may then be used with permission from the patient. Although telephone interpreter services are permissible, the use of a face-to-face in-person interpretation is desirable, acceptable, and appropriate.

Health care organizations are expected to make known to all their patients and families the availability of interpreter services at no cost to the patient. Information about available bilingual staff can also help patients access these services. For more information, see the National Standards for Culturally and Linguistically Appropriate Service in Health Care, 2001, available at www.omhrc.gov/assets/pdf/checked/finalreport.pdf.

ORGANIZATIONAL CULTURE

Organizational culture is the system of shared values and beliefs that actively influences the behavior of organization members. The term *shared values* is important because it implies that many people are guided by the same values and that they interpret them in the same way. Values develop over time and reflect an organization's history and traditions. Culture consists of the culture of an organization, such as being helpful and supportive toward new members.

Five dimensions of organizational culture are of major significance in influencing organizational culture (Ott, 1989):

- *Values:* Values are the foundation of any organizational culture. The organization's philosophy is expressed through values, and values guide behavior on a day-to-day basis.
- *Relative diversity:* The existence of an organizational culture assumes some degree of similarity. Nevertheless, organizations differ in how much deviation can be tolerated.
- *Resource allocation and reward:* The allocation of money and other resources has a critical influence on culture. The investment of resources sends a message to people about what is valued in the organization.
- *Degree of change:* A fast-paced, dynamic organization has a culture different from that of a slow-paced, stable one. Top-level managers, by the energy or lethargy of their stance, send messages about how much they welcome innovation.
- *Strength of the culture:* The strength of a culture, or how much influence it exerts, is partially a byproduct of the other dimensions. A strong culture guides employees in many everyday actions. It determines, for example, whether employees will inconvenience themselves to satisfy a patient. If the culture is not so strong, employees are more likely to follow their own whims, that is, they may decide to please patients only when convenient for them.

Each organization will have embedded in its environment the dos and don'ts that are specific to its workplace. When beginning in a new organization, observe and ask questions to learn about the organization and culture and how decisions are made (Table 16-1).

ORGANIZATIONAL SOCIALIZATION

As a new member of a team or workgroup, it is important to be socialized into the organization. Socialization is beneficial to the organization when employees are a good fit, that is, employees have a high commitment to the organization, little intention to leave, high levels of job satisfaction, and little work-related stress. Things to consider when entering

TABLE 16-1	QUESTIONS TO ASK WHEN ASSESSING ORGANIZATIONAL CULTURE

- Are the organization's values consistent with your values?
- What cultures, ages, and genders are represented on the work team? How are members of these cultures similar? How are they different?
- Is the organization or the department centralized or decentralized?
- What is the formal chain of command?
- What is the informal chain of command?
- Do individuals participate in changing policies or procedures?
- What are the rules about how things should be done?
- Where does one take new ideas or suggestions?
- Are risk and change encouraged?
- How are individuals rewarded for quality improvement, or are all rewards oriented primarily toward the total group?
- Does the team work well together?

TABLE 16-2	UNITED STATES ORGANIZATIONAL BEHAVIORAL STYLES

Concepts	Things to Consider
Greetings	■ Americans usually acknowledge each other with a smile, nod of the head, and/or verbal greeting, such as "Hello," or "Hi."
	■ When greeting someone in a business situation, a firm handshake is appropriate, such as when greeting a manager of nursing or a recruiter from human resources.
Titles	■ When introducing yourself, give your first name and your last name, e.g., I am Susan Clover, a Registered Nurse, and I will be caring for you until 7 p.m.
	■ Use the appropriate title the first time you address an individual, such as Mrs., Dr., Ms., or Mr. Wear a badge with your full name and title of RN prominently displayed.
	■ Wait to be directed to call a person by his or her first name. Expect the same respect for yourself.
Time	■ Punctuality is highly respected in nursing. Be on time to interview appointments and work.
Body language	■ Use of direct eye contact is expected in all work situations and when working with patients. However, some people may not respond to direct eye contact, depending on their culture.
	■ In conversation, it is important to keep approximately one arm length's distance from the speaker; closer proximity is considered rude in some cultures.
Dress	■ When in doubt, wear business attire for interviews, that is, a professional suit. For your work environment, ask what the traditional dress is for a particular work area or nursing unit before starting a new job or purchasing new uniforms.
	■ Even in areas where daily dress is more casual, business situations and clinical work settings require professional dress. Avoid uniforms that cover you in cartoons if you expect professional respect.

a new work environment in any culture are the organizational behavior style for greetings, titles, punctuality, body language, and dress (Table 16-2).

Most organizations have a workplace culture that has a strong mission and vision, and members work tirelessly to ensure the organization's success. However, some organizations can only be described as toxic. In these organizations, the staff and/or leadership is dysfunctional. Instead of problem solving, the goal of these organizations is faultfinding and placing blame. This dysfunctional, toxic environment may be a unit within a hospital or the entire organization. Choosing your workplace environment wisely will make your work life more satisfying.

WORKING WITH STAFF FROM DIFFERENT CULTURES

Staff nurses from different cultures may have different perceptions of staff and nursing roles in patient care, a different perception of their own locus of control, a different time orientation, and may speak a different language.

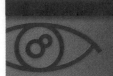

CRITICAL THINKING 16-1

In today's diverse workplace, you will work closely with various nursing and medical practitioners, and ancillary personnel who are from different cultures and who speak English as a second language. How do you feel about working with practitioners who are from foreign countries, or from different racial or ethnic groups? Take a minute to answer the following questions. You do not need to share your answers with anyone, so be honest with yourself. Self awareness is an important step in building cultural competence.

	Agree	Neutral	Disagree
I would rather work with an American nurse than a foreign nurse.			
I find it frustrating to work with medical and nursing practitioners who are not proficient in English.			
If I thought that a medical or nursing practitioner was not fulfilling duties because of cultural or language problems, I would hesitate to report the person for fear that I would be considered prejudiced.			
I enjoy working with a skilled foreign nurse. I feel that I can learn a lot from this person.			
I like to attend classes and informal meetings where I can learn more about how nurses from other countries are educated.			
I do not feel prepared to work with or supervise an nursing assistive worker who has some problems with understanding English.			
Responsible adults prepare for the future and strive to influence events in their lives.			
Intelligent people use their time wisely and are punctual.			
It is disrespectful to address people by their first name unless they give you permission to do so.			
It is rude and intrusive to obtain information by asking direct questions.			

Source: Compiled with information from Munoz, C., & Luckmann, J. (2005). *Transcultural communication*. Clifton Park, NY: Delmar Cengage Learning.

DIFFERENT PERCEPTIONS OF STAFF RESPONSIBILITIES

Cultural values deeply influence whether a person values the rights of the individual more or values the rights of the collective group more. Individualism emphasizes the importance of individual rights and rewards. Collectivism emphasizes the importance of the group's rights and rewards. Staff educated in Western culture may place more value on individualism and independence. These staff may complain to their supervisor if they feel assignments are unfair or involve menial work. Assertive behavior that is consistent with values of equitable work distribution and respect for education and professionalism usually defines the American work style. Staff from other cultures that emphasize collective group rights tend to accept such assignments without complaint. Ensuring harmony, teamwork, and commitment to group loyalty may be more important to these staff.

American staff also want to be individually recognized for their work; for instance, they may want a promotion, or they may dream of being publicly honored for giving outstanding patient care or other accomplishments (Munoz & Luckmann, 2005).

DIFFERENT PERCEPTIONS OF THE NURSE'S ROLE

Nurses from other cultures have different perceptions of the nurse's role and nursing care values, which American nurses may not appreciate. For example, in a study of Philippine American nurses, the most important finding was the theme of obligation to care that prevailed in all aspects of their work (Spangler, 1992). This theme reflected the Philippine American nurses' strong belief that bedside nursing is truly the core of nursing. This value conflicted with the attitude of some American nurses that the physical care of patients is devalued work with low prestige and should therefore be delegated to ancillary personnel (Spangler, 1992).

DIFFERENCES IN LOCUS OF CONTROL

Locus of control refers to the degree of control that individuals feel that they have over events. People who feel in control of their environment have an internal locus of control. People who believe that luck, fate, or chance controls their lives have an external locus of control.

Health care providers who are trained in the United States often have an internal locus of control. American medical and nursing practitioners often feel that it is their duty to diagnose disorders, plan interventions, carry out procedures, and do everything possible to save the patient's life.

Conversely, health care providers from other cultures that promote an external locus of control (some Mexican Americans, Appalachians, and Puerto Ricans) may have a more fatalistic attitude toward their patients and thus feel that they cannot control matters of life and death. For example, when a patient who is expected to die does die on the operating room table, care providers with an external locus of control may be puzzled when hospital administration asks for a quality review of the case (Giger & Davidhizar, 1996). Finally, some American Indians, Chinese Americans, and Japanese Americans believe themselves to be in harmony with nature rather than being controlled by nature or in control of nature (Giger & Davidhizar, 1990).

DIFFERENCES IN TIME ORIENTATION

Cultural groups are either past-, present-, or future oriented. Americans generally value the future over the present. Southern Blacks and Puerto Ricans value the present over the future. Southern Appalachians, traditional Chinese Americans, and Mexican Americans value the present (Munoz & Luckmann, 2005). Many Asian cultures value the past (Munoz, 2009).

The ways in which different cultural groups value time can create challenges in the health care workplace. For example, staff meetings are influenced by the time orientation of staff members. Staff members who are meeting to plan for the future may become annoyed with members who want to spend all of the time on present-day problems and issues.

EDUCATIONAL AND LANGUAGE DIFFERENCES

Foreign nurses are educated differently from American nurses. Generally, nursing education outside of the United States is less theory oriented, focusing primarily on the development of clinical skills. Also, there is less emphasis on meeting the psychosocial needs of patients.

Language differences also raise the potential for serious miscommunications between health care providers and patients. Today, large medical centers in the United States may be primarily staffed by nurses and practitioners for whom English is a second language. For example, in urban medical centers on the East Coast, it is not unusual to hear a Filipino nurse and a Haitian nurse attempting to communicate with a resident practitioner who has been educated in India. Unless these caregivers take the time to clarify their communications, serious errors may result. The potential for miscommunication exists (especially over the telephone) unless words are clarified by a coworker or practitioner (Munoz & Luckmann, 2005).

IMPROVING COMMUNICATION ON THE TEAM

If you are working with a co-worker from a different culture who speaks English as a second language, try these techniques to facilitate communication:

- Recognize that your coworker probably has an educational background in nursing that is very different from your own.
- Acknowledge that the coworker's value system and perception of what constitutes good patient care may differ from your own.
- Clarify your coworker's level of understanding of verbal and written communication.
- Avoid the use of slang terms and regional expressions. For example, Chinese, Japanese, and Filipino nurses may not understand such terms as piggybacking, doing a double, or rigging something to work.

- Provide your coworker with resources, such as written procedures and protocols, that may help to reinforce your verbal communication.
- Remember to praise your coworker's competency in technical skills. Inspiring self-confidence in a foreign nurse will make it easier for that person to ask for assistance when needed.
- Appreciate the knowledge that you can gain by working alongside a skilled nurse from another culture. Observe how foreign nurses relate to patients who are from their culture. If you have an open mind, working with foreign coworkers can increase your knowledge of other cultures, enrich your work as a nurse, and foster personal growth.
- When offering constructive criticism, try to use *I* statements instead of *you* statements. For example: "I think that it's very important to address the patient's emotional state when you chart" is better than "You never seem to chart anything about the patient's emotional state."
- If you feel you cannot achieve effective communication with a coworker, request to work with another person. You do not want to be held accountable for the actions of a nurse with whom you cannot communicate.
- Delegate only appropriate tasks to an unlicensed worker. Match assignments to the worker's level of understanding and skill.
- Do not stop at just delegating an assignment or giving instructions. Instead, make sure that the worker understands your instructions.
- To reduce miscommunication, check for understanding by asking the worker to repeat instructions or do a return demonstration.
- Report to your supervisor if you feel that a nurse or a practitioner is endangering patients because of language difficulties or different cultural values. Record any problems that occur, and keep a copy of the notes you provide to your supervisor (Munoz & Luckmann, 2005).
- Do not take verbal orders, particularly over the telephone. Even when an order is written, take the time to clarify the order with the practitioner. Because patients may also find it difficult to understand a foreign practitioner,

you may need to listen carefully and then explain the practitioner's remarks to the patient.

MANAGERIAL RESPONSIBILITY

Nurse managers may use the following approaches to improve communication:

- Plan informal meetings for nurses to discuss their cultural values. For example, it may benefit Asian nurses to share with American-born nurses their cultural values concerning respect for authority.
- Provide cultural workshops, and ask knowledgeable individuals to present information about the values, behaviors, and communication patterns of the different cultural groups that are represented on staff.
- Provide classes in English as a second language for foreign nurses who do not speak fluent English or who have difficulty pronouncing words.
- Establish a program for orienting foreign nurses to the hospital or agency (Jein & Harris, 1989). The orientation program should be designed to help newcomers adjust to the new work environment. It is helpful to assign each new nurse to a preceptor who is a member of the nurse's cultural group. For maximum benefits, the nurse manager should interview each new nurse every week to find out how that person is adapting to the new hospital culture (Williams & Rodgers, 1993).
- Plan events at which nurses, practitioners, and other staff members can socialize and discuss cultural differences informally, in a relaxed environment. For example, each unit in the hospital might plan one potluck event for each shift on a monthly basis. Potluck meals could be planned around a cultural theme, for instance, a traditional Vietnamese dinner one month and a traditional Costa Rican meal the next month (Burner, Cunningham, & Hattar, 1990).
- Confer with specialists in transcultural communication; also hire experts to identify potential areas of conflict and resolve conflicts

peacefully before they erupt into legal battles (Munoz & Luckmann, 2005).

GENERATIONAL PERCEPTIONS

Different perceptions and values are created as each generation deals with the experiences of their lives as they are altered by the changing times. A **generation** is a group that shares birth years, age, location, and significant life events (Kupperschmidt, 2000). A generation is approximately fifteen to twenty years in length and has a different value system from the preceding generation and later generations. Like culture, we take our generational differences with us into patient care and the work environment. We often assume that those around us are like us and think like us. This is not always true.

Four distinct generations make up the current patient and workforce population. These generations are the Traditional Generation, born before 1940; the Baby Boomers, born between 1940 and 1960; Generation X, born between 1960 and 1980; and the newest generation to hit the workforce, Generation Y (Echo Boomers or Millennials), those born after 1980.

The Traditional Generation came of age after the Great Depression and were raised to be disciplined and obey their elders. They feel obligated to conform and believe that work is one's duty. The Traditional Generation was followed by the Baby Boomers, who came of age during a time of much available education and economic expansion. They work for the challenge of work and career advancement (Calhoun & Strasser, 2005). Baby Boomers have been characterized as workaholic, strong-willed individuals who are working for material gain, promotions, recognition, job security, and corner offices. Baby Boomers are the largest generation. They have had a dramatic financial impact on the present and will continue to impact the future dramatically, as they have begun to retire in 2006.

The Generation Xers are often called latch key kids, as their parents were often away working.

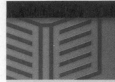

EVIDENCE-BASED PRACTICE

Citation: Grossman, C. L. (2006, Sept. 12). View of God can reveal your values and politics. *USA Today,* 1A.

Discussion: Article reports on the Baylor University religion survey of 1,721 Americans. The survey found that 91.8% of those surveyed say they believe in God, a higher power, or a cosmic force. The other respondents said they were atheists, did not answer, or weren't sure. Respondents had four distinct views of God's personality, that is, Authoritarian, Benevolent, Critical, and Distant. The article discusses how these four views of God affect political issues, such as gay marriage, stem cell research, war, abortion, and federal government involvement in life and world affairs.

Implications for Practice: Many Americans believe in God, a higher power, or a cosmic force and may want assistance with their spiritual needs during times of illness and stress. Nurses can help patients obtain the assistance they need.

They learned to be self-reliant and independent. The Generation Xers are busy looking for career security, not job security. They are willing to change jobs and have little loyalty to their employers. They observed their parents going through multiple changes in their work organizations, such as downsizing and rightsizing. They are not workaholics, and they seek a balance between work and leisure. Generation Xers want a work environment that is technologically current, has competent leadership, and provides a mentor or coach for a boss.

Generation Yers are primarily the children of the Baby Boomers. They grew up with the end of the Cold War, the Internet, and a speak-your-mind philosophy. This generation is just beginning to make its mark on the workforce. What is known is that they are focusing on early retirement. Change is their mantra, and they expect countless options.

In the workplace, these generations all have different goals and needs.

Nursing leadership for this diverse group of workers requires a different management style and increased flexibility. The ACORN Model discussed by Kupperschmidt (2000) illustrates how a new leader can use opportunities to Accommodate employee differences; Create workplace choices; Operate from a theoretically sound, sophisticated management style; and nourish Retention

of Nurses. For example, when creating workplace choices, a nurse leader might devise multiple scheduling options and provide multiple opportunities for cross-training and lateral and upward movement through the organization. Each generation has different needs for orientation, training, and opportunities for advancement and benefits. While meeting these different needs, the nurse manager still needs to bring the groups together and begin to form a team (Hu, Herrick, & Hodgin, 2004). Chapter 5 provides more information on effective team building.

SPIRITUALITY

Spirituality is an important area of assessment during hospitalization. The national health care accrediting body, the Joint Commission, recently focused on the assessment of spirituality, requiring nurses to ask patients some questions regarding their spiritual needs (Hodge, 2001). However, asking the questions, "What is your religion?" or "What religious needs can we meet during your hospitalization?" leaves the nurse with only descriptive labels. To meet the spiritual needs of patients, nurses need to understand more than these labels. Patients may be asked if they would like to see their spiritual leader or advisor, with the understanding that not all patients will want to meet with a clergy member. Nurses can use various resources available for providing spiritual support to patients. Many inpatient facilities have pastoral care departments that conduct formal services, visit and pray with patients and their families, conduct support groups (for example, bereavement), and provide information regarding organ donation, living wills, and other end-of-life services (Duldt, 2002). Kuepfer, as cited in Ray (2004), addresses a shift in the duties of hospital chaplains from focusing mainly on providing religious rites to empowering the hospital staff members to serve the community.

Several research tools are used for measuring spirituality:

- *Spiritual Well-Being:* This tool measures the psychological dimension of spiritual wellness (Ellison & Paloutzain, 1999).
- *JAREL Spiritual Well-Being Scale:* This tool measures harmony as a function of interconnectedness (Hungelmann, Kenkel-Rossi, Klassen, & Stollenwerk, 1989).
- *Spiritual Perspective Scale:* This tool measures the extent to which one holds spiritual views during spirituality-related interactions (Reed, 1986).

For the nurse looking to understand spirituality in an effort to provide comfort to patients during illness or crisis, these tools provide some guidance.

SPIRITUAL DISTRESS

Spiritual distress is a North American Nursing Diagnosis Association (NANDA) term used to identify a condition in which an individual has an impaired ability to integrate meaning and purpose in life through the individual's connectedness with self, others, art, music, literature, nature, or a power greater than oneself (Ackley & Ladwig, 2006). To decrease or eliminate spiritual distress, it is expected that an individual will connect with the elements he or she considers important to arrive at meaning and purpose in life. These elements may include meditation; prayer; participating in religious services or rituals; communing with nature, plants, and animals; sharing of self; and caring for self and others. The Wikoff (2003) Spiritual Focus Questionnaire

(Table 16-3) is designed to ascertain what is spiritually important to the individual. It assesses the concepts of relationships with a Higher Power, Self, Others, Nature, and Religion. Each question can be scored on a 0-4 scale, arriving at a total score for each area of the questionnaire. The tool is not designed to measure the strength or amount of spirituality; rather, the higher score(s) suggest(s) the concepts most important to the patient.

Reviewing the Spiritual Focus Questionnaire helps a nurse develop interventions to help patients. Nursing interventions for spiritual needs could include the nurse requesting a visit from a patient's spiritual leader or helping a patient obtain spiritual or religious tapes or music. The nurse can also offer the patient uninterrupted quiet time to allow him or her time for personal prayer, reading of spiritual and religious material, or meditation.

CHAMPIONING SPIRITUALITY

The nurse leader who champions spirituality for all ensures that this component of holistic nursing is not forgotten or marginalized. Spirituality uses compassion, caring, and nurturing to create an environment that reflects the values and beliefs of the leaders, patients, staff, and organization. For example, an employee may request a Saturday or Sunday off every week to attend religious services. When nurses are needed to work every other weekend, this can pose a problem for the nurse leader. A possible solution is to pair two nurses, where one works every Saturday and the other works every Sunday. Both nurses are then able to meet their spiritual needs without a negative impact on staffing.

Religious holidays or celebrations also have spiritual and cultural significance. An understanding and empathetic approach to vacation requests will help ensure contented staff and minimize turnover. It is also important to consider important markers of life such as weddings, births, and deaths. There are many cultural and spiritual overtones to these life events that need to be respected by nursing leadership practices. Sensitivity to the spiritual practices of the staff will enable the nurse manager to provide compassionate and caring leadership.

TABLE 16-3	WIKOFF SPIRITUAL FOCUS QUESTIONNAIRE

Spiritual Focus Questionnaire Instructions: The following questions assess your expressions of spirituality. Please rate each question by checking the box indicating importance to you as 4=very important, 3=somewhat important, 2=not important, 1=very unimportant, 0=neither important or unimportant.

Question	4	3	2	1	0
1. My strongest relationship is with a Higher Power.					
2. The time I spend in connection with a Higher Power is essential.					
3. In my personal life, I feel close to a Higher Power/Supreme Being.					
4. I spend time daily talking to a Higher Power.					
Higher Power Total Score					
5. I count on myself as my spiritual center.					
6. I feel an internal calmness when I am at peace with myself.					
7. My spirituality comes from within me.					
8. To find spiritual peace, I look inside myself.					
Self Total Score					
9. I renew my spirit with my family/friends.					
10. Special people within my life are my spiritual focus.					
11. When spiritually discouraged, I seek help from my family/ friends.					
12. Others around me help quiet my spirit.					
Others Total Score					
13. I make an effort to spend time in the quiet solitude of nature.					
14. In nature, I reflect on its magnitude and importance to me.					
15. My connection with natural things helps me find inner peace.					
16. When in nature, I feel thankful for my blessings.					
Nature Total Score					
17. Through my religion, I find inner calmness.					
18. My religion gives my life spiritual focus.					
19. The time I spend in religious activities renews my spirit.					
20. My religion helps me keep my life in perspective.					
Religion Total Score					
Overall Total					

Source: Wikoff, K. L. (2003). Development and psychometric evaluation of the Wikoff Spiritual Focus Questionnaire. *Dissertation Abstracts International, 64* (04),1691. (UMI No. AAT 3088678).

KEY CONCEPTS

- Culture affects both the nursing staff and the patient.

- Cultural competence is an important component of nursing.

- Working on a multicultural team requires an understanding of culture.

- Some nursing theorists on culture include Leininger, Giger and Davidhizar, Campinha-Bacote, Purnell, and Spector.

- Organizations that nurses work in have distinct cultures.

- Each generation has different values, goals, and expected outcomes from its work and life experiences.

- Spirituality may include religion and reflects one's values and beliefs.

- Spiritual Assessment is a requisite of holistic nursing.

- Nurses need to be aware of their own spirituality and beliefs to feel comfortable in addressing the spiritual needs of others.

KEY TERMS

culture

culture shock

culturally competent care

generation

marginalization

organizational culture

race

spiritual distress

REVIEW QUESTIONS

1. Which of the following statements must be true for a multicultural team to work together successfully?
   A. Everyone should be focused on the same goals and objectives.
   B. All nurses should be from the same professional background.
   C. Everyone should have the same values about health care.
   D. Everyone in the United States should have the same beliefs because they all are living in the United States.

2. Stephanie, the Gen-X night shift charge nurse, is requesting more time off than any other charge nurse. What reason for this best represents her generation? She
   A. prefers to work the day shift and is hoping for a schedule change.
   B. believes that other nurses are just as capable of performing her role.
   C. wants to increase her leisure time to balance with work.
   D. seeks to be rewarded for time spent at work.

3. During orientation to work on a new unit, the nurse experiences a sense of isolation from his preceptors. Which of the following actions will best increase his socialization into the preceptor group? The nurse should
   A. ask as many questions as he can.
   B. request that his orientation be increased for two more weeks.
   C. study the differences between his values and his preceptor group's values.
   D. arrive late for duty frequently.

4. The Traditional Generation may do which of the following?
   A. value working as one's duty
   B. reflect a speak-your-mind philosophy
   C. value working primarily for the challenge
   D. use the Internet daily as a part of their life

REVIEW ACTIVITIES

1. The hospital where you work is in a predominantly white, non-Hispanic area. Lately, there has been an influx of migrant farmworkers from Mexico because local farms cannot find local workers. What do you perceive as some of the health needs of the migrant farmworkers? How would you facilitate the provision of care for these workers and their families?

2. You are taking care of a trauma patient in the ER. The patient has burns over 70% of his body. The likelihood of the patient's survival is unknown. There is a lot of noise and distraction in the ER, as well as many family members within earshot. The patient asks you to pray for him and his family. How will you respond?

EXPLORING THE WEB

- Language and cultural effects on health care delivery are the focus of this site:
  www.diversityrx.org

- *www.census.gov*
  Search for Statistics. Click on *Latest Race, Ethnic, and Age Estimates,* or click on *Poverty.*

- The International Sigma Theta Tau (nursing honor society) site contains a position paper on diversity. What does the nursing honor society believe about diversity?
  www.nursingsociety.org
  Search for *Diversity.*

- This site contains information about cultural beliefs pertinent to the health care of recent immigrants to the United States:
  www.ethnomed.org
  Click on *Cultural Competency.*

- The U.S. Department of Health and Human Services–Office of Minority Health:
  www.omhrc.gov
  Click on *Cultural Competency.*

- Canadian Nurses Association:
  www.can-nurses.ca

- National Alaska Native American Indian Nurses (NANAINA):
  www.nanainanurses.org

- National Black Nurses Association, Inc.:
  www.nbna.org

- Transcultural Nursing Society:
  www.tcns.org
- Islamic Information Center of American (IICA):
  www.iica.org
- U.S. Citizenship and Immigration Services:
  www.uscis.gov
- American Civil Liberties Union (ACLU):
  www.aclu.org
- American Indian Heritage Foundation:
  www.indians.org
- American Jewish Community:
  www.ajc.org
- Anti-Defamation League:
  www.adl.org

- Asia Society:
  www.asiasociety.org
- National Association for the Advancement of Colored People:
  www.naacp.org
- International Council of Nurses:
  www.icn.ch
- Global Health Council:
  www.globalhealth.org
- World Health Organization:
  www.who.org

REFERENCES

Ackley, B. J., & Ladwig, G. B. (2006). *Nursing diagnosis handbook: A guide to planning care* (7th ed.). St. Louis, MO: Mosby.

American Academy of Nursing (AAN). (1992). AAN expert panel report: Culturally competent health care. *Nursing Outlook, 40*(6), 277–283.

Burner, O. Y., Cunningham, P., & Hattar, H. S. (1990). Managing a multicultural nurse staff in a multicultural environment. *Journal of Nursing Administration, 20*(6), 30–34.

Calhoun, S. K., & Strasser, P. B. (2005). Generations at work. *AAOHN, 53*(11), 469–471.

Campinha-Bacote, J. (2003, Jan. 31). Many faces: Addressing diversity in health care. *Online Journal of Issues in Nursing, 8*(1), manuscript. Retrieved April 18, 2006, from nursingworld.org/ ojin/topic20/tpc20_2.htm.

DeRosa, N., & Kochurka, K. (2006, Oct.). Implement culturally competent healthcare in your workplace. *Nursing Management, 37*(10), 18–26.

Duldt, B. (2002). The spiritual dimension of holistic care. *Journal of Nursing Administration, 32*(1), 20–24.

Ellison, C. W., & Paloutzain, R. F. (1999). *Measures of Religiosity.* Birmingham, AL: Religious Education Press.

Giger, N., & Davidhizar, R. J. (1996). When the operating room has a multicultural team. *Today's Surgical Nurse, 18*(5), 26–32.

Giger, J., & Davidhizar, T. (2004). *Transcultural nursing: Assessment and intervention* (4th ed.). St. Louis, MO: Mosby Year Book.

Grossman, C. L. (2006, Sept. 12). View of God can reveal your values and politics. *USA Today,* 1A.

Hall, J., Stevens, P., & Meleis, A. (1994). Marginalization: a guiding concept for valuing diversity in nursing knowledge development. *Advances in Nursing Science, 16*(4), 23–24.

Hobbs, F., & Stoops, N. (2000). U.S. Census Bureau. Census 2000 special reports. Series CENSR-4. Demographic trends in the 20th Century. U.S. Government Printing Office. Washington, D.C. 2002. Available at www.census.gov/prod/2002pubs/censr-4.pdf

Hodge, D. R. (2001). A template for spiritual assessment: a review of the JCAHO requirements and guidelines for implementation. (Joint Commission on Accreditation of Healthcare Organizations). Social Work. Available at www.accessmylibrary.com/coms2/summary_0286-28917948_ITM

Hu, J., Herrick, C., & Hodgin, K. A. (2004). Managing the multigenerational nursing team. *The Health Care Manager, 23*(4), 334–340.

Hungelmann, J., Kenkel-Rossi, E., Klassen, L., & Stollenwerk, R. (1989). Development of the JAREL Spiritual Well-Being Scale. In R. M. Carroll-Johnson (Ed.), *Classification of nursing diagnoses proceedings of the eighth conference North American nursing diagnosis association* (393–398). Philadelphia: Lipinncott.

Jein, R. F., & Harris, B. L. (1989). Cross-cultural conflict: The American nurse manager and a culturally mixed staff. *Journal of the New York State Nurses Association, 20*(2), 16-19.

Keltner, B., Kelley, F., & Smith, D. (2004). Leadership to reduce health disparities: A model for nursing leadership in American Indian communities. *Nursing Administration Quarterly, 28*(3), 181–190.

Kupperschmidt, B. R. (2000). Multigeneration employees: Strategies for effective management. *Heath Care Management, 19*(1), 65–76.

Lenburg, C., et al. (1995) *Promoting cultural competence in and through nursing education; a critical review and comprehensive plan for action.* Washington, D.C.: American Academy of Nursing.

Leininger, M. (1978). *Transcultural nursing: Concepts, theories and practice.* New York: Wiley.

Leininger, M. (1997). Transcultural nursing research to nursing education and practice: 40 years. *Image Journal of Nursing Scholarship, 29*(4).

Margaret Mead quotation found at www.womenshistory.about.com/cs/quotes/a/qu_margaretmead_3.htm accessed 12–30–08.

Microsoft (1996). Microsoft Encarta 97 Encyclopedia, Microsoft Corporation. Reference for 16–8 H:

Munoz, C. (2009). Personal Communication, January 8, 2009.

Munoz, C., & Luckmann, J. (2005). *Transcultural communication.* Clifton Park, NY: Delmar Cengage Learning.

Nies, M., & McEwen, M. (2007). *Community/public health nursing* (4th ed.). Philadelphia: W. B. Saunders.

Ott, J. (1989). *The organizational culture perspective.* Chicago: Dorsey Press.

Purnell, L. (2005). The Purnell Model for Cultural Competence. *The Journal of Multicultural Nursing and Health, 11*(2), 7–15.

Ray, R. (2004). The faith connection. *NurseWeek, A Nursing Spectrum Publication, 11*(9), 17–20.

Reed, P. G. (1986). Spirituality and well-being in terminally ill hospitalized adults. *Research in Nursing and Health, 35,* 368–374.

Spangler, A. (1992). Transcultural care values and practices of Philippine-American nurses. *Journal of Transcultural Nursing, 4*(2), 28–31.

Spector, R. E. (2004). Cultural diversity in health and illness (6th ed.). Upper Saddle River, NJ: Pearson-Prentice Hall.

Wikoff, K. L. (2003). Development and psychometric evaluation of the Wikoff Spiritual Focus Questionnaire. *Dissertation Abstracts International, 64*(04), 1691. (UMI No. AAT 3088678).

Wikoff, K. L. (2008). Culture, Generational Differences, and Spirituality in Kelly, P. L. (2008). Nursing Leadership & Management. Clifton Park, NY: Delmar Cengage Learning.

Williams, J., & Rodgers, S. (1993). The multicultural workplace: Preparing preceptors. *Journal of Continuing Education in Nursing, 24*(3), 101–104.

Suggested Readings

Buerhaus, P. I., Auerbach, D. I., & Staiger, D. O. (2007, Mar.–Apr.). Recent trends in the registered nurse labor market in the U.S.: Short-run swings on top of long term trends. *Nursing Economics, 25*(2), 59–66; quiz 67.

Casida, J., & Pinto-Zipp, G. (2008, Jan.–Feb.). Leadership–organizational culture relationship in nursing units of acute care hospitals. *Nursing Economics, 26*(1), 7–15; quiz 16.

Christmas, K. (2007, Nov.–Dec.) Workplace abuse: finding solutions. *Nursing Economics, 25*(6), 365–7.

Gaston-Johansson, F., Hill-Briggs, F., Oguntomilade, L., Bradley, V., & Mason, P. (2007, Dec.). Patient perspectives on disparities in health care from African-American, Hispanic, and Native American samples including a secondary analysis of the Institute of Medicine focus group data. *Journal of the National Black Nurses Association, 18*(2), 43–52.

Irwin, W. (2008, Jan 24). Nursing. A reality check for diversity. *Health Services Journal*: 40–1.

NLNAC Accreditation Manual. (2008). National League for Nursing Accrediting Commission, Inc. Available at www.nlnac.org/manuals/NLNACManual 2008.pdf

Racher, F. E., & Annis, R. C. (2007). Respecting culture and honoring diversity in community practice. *Research and Theory of Nursing Practice, 21*(4), 255–70.

Roenkoetter, M. M., & Nardi, D. A. (2007, Oct.). American Academy of Nursing Expert Panel on Global Nursing and Health: white paper on Global Nursing and Health. *Journal of Transcultural Nursing, 18*(4), 305–15.

Scott, D. E. (2008, Jan.–Feb.). The multicultural health care work environment. *American Nurse, 40*(1), 7.

Tracey, C., & Nicholl, H. (2007, Oct.). The multifaceted influence of gender in career progress in nursing. *Nursing Management, 15*(7), 677–82.

CHAPTER 17

NCLEX-RN Preparation and Your First Job

*Luck is a matter of
preparation meeting
opportunity.*

(Oprah Winfrey)

OBJECTIVES

Upon completion of this chapter, the reader should be able to:

1. Discuss preparation for the National Council of State Boards of Nursing Licensure Examination for Registered Nurses (NCLEX-RN)
2. Detail the process of beginning a successful nursing job search.
3. Develop a resume and cover letter.
4. Identify appropriate preparation for a successful job interview.
5. Discuss potential interview questions and identify acceptable answers.
6. Describe typical components of health care orientation.
7. Discuss elements of performance feedback.

Anwar will be graduating from his nursing education program in two months. He plans to focus his current efforts on preparing to take the NCLEX-RN Licensure Examination. He knows that three important areas of examination preparation are having the knowledge, being adept at testing, and controlling test anxiety.

How should he prepare for the examination?

Where should he focus?

How can he decrease his test anxiety?

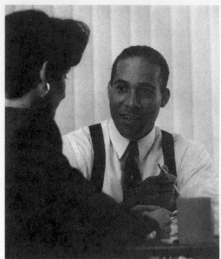

Delmar/Cengage Learning

A new graduate from an educational program that prepares RNs will take the National Council of State Boards of Nursing. Licensure Examination for Registered Nurses (NCLEX-RN). The NCLEX is taken after graduation and prior to practice as an RN. It is wise to schedule the exam date soon after graduation. The examination is given across the United States at professional testing centers. Graduates submit their credentials to the state board of nursing in the state in which licensure is desired. After the state board accepts the graduate's credentials, he or she can schedule the examination. This examination ensures a basic level of safe nursing practice to the public and is essential to working as a professional RN. The examination follows a test plan formulated on four categories of client needs that RNs commonly encounter. Integrated processes include the nursing process; caring; communication and documentation; and teaching/learning. These are integrated throughout the four major categories of client needs (NCSBN, 2007). See Table 17-1. The focus of this chapter is to give new nursing graduates the tools to pass NCLEX and to seek and obtain a nursing position. Included in this chapter are tips on NCLEX preparation, resume writing, sample interview questions and answers, and hints on how and where to search for a job.

PREPARATION FOR NCLEX-RN

Graduates may receive anywhere from 75 to 265 questions on the NCLEX examination during their testing session. Fifteen of the questions are questions that are being piloted to determine their psychometric value and validity for use in future NCLEX examinations. Students cannot determine whether they passed or failed the NCLEX examination from the number of questions they receive during their session.

TEST QUESTION FORMATS AND SAMPLES

Questions are presented in several formats. Multiple-choice questions may be four-option, single-answer items or multiple-option items that require more than one response. Fill-in-the-blank questions or questions that ask the test taker to identify an area on a picture or a graphic may also be included. Some examination questions may require responses to be placed in the correct order. The computer screen displays the questions and their answer choices.

SAMPLE QUESTIONS

The various formats for test questions are illustrated here.

Test Question 1—Fill in the blanks

A man underwent an exploratory laparoscopy yesterday. He is on strict intake and output. Calculate his intake and output for an 8-hour period.

TABLE 17-1	NCLEX TEST PLAN

Client Needs Tested	Percent of Test Questions
Safe and effective care environment:	
Management of care	13–19%
Safety and infection control	8–14%
Physiological integrity:	6–12%
Basic care and comfort	6–12%
Pharmacological and parenteral therapies	13–19%
Reduction of risk potential	13–19%
Physiological adaptation	11–17%
Psychosocial integrity	
Health promotion and maintenance	6–12%

Source: NCLEX-RN Examination. (2007). Test plan for the National Council Licensure Examination for Registered Nurses. Chicago, IL: National Council of State Boards of Nursing. Available at www.ncsbn.org/1287.htm. Accessed October 7, 2008.

Intake	Output
IV-0.9% NS at	Foley urine
125 mL/hr	output-850 mL
PO-1 ounce ice chips	NG tube-200 mL
IVPB-30 mL Q8H	
Intake _____	Output _____

Test Answer 1

Intake = 1,060 mL; Output = 1,050 mL

125 mL/hr (125 mL × 8 hr) is 1,000 mL. 1 ounce of ice chips is 30 mL;

IVPB 30 mL Q8H (30 mL × 1) is 30 mL for a total of 1,060 mL.

Output is 850 mL urine and 200 mL of nasogastric drainage for a total of 1050 mL (Stein, 2005).

Test Question 2—Question that requires more than one response

A woman has been diagnosed with cervical cancer and will be undergoing internal radiation in addition to surgery. The nurse is planning her nursing care. Check all that are appropriate in maintaining a safe environment.

——— Minimizing staff contact with the patient.

——— Utilizing required shielding.

——— Encouraging staff to stay at the foot of the bed or at the entrance to the room.

——— Wearing isolation gowns when entering the room.

Test Answer 2

"Minimizing staff contact with the patient" should be checked. Radiation is cumulative. Limiting the amount of time with the patient limits the nurse's exposure to radiation.

"Utilizing required shielding" should be checked. Shielding made of heavy metal decreases the amount of radiation exposure.

"Encouraging staff to stay at the foot of the bed or at the entrance to the room" should be checked. Exposure decreases with greater distance from the radiation source.

"Wearing isolation gowns when entering the room" should not be checked. Isolation gowns offer no protection against radiation. (Stein, 2005)

Test Question 3—Single answer, multiple-choice question.

The lab results of a 68-year-old male reveal an elevated titer of *Helicobacter pylori*. Which of the following statements, if made by the nurse, indicates an understanding of this data?

1. "Treatment will include Pepto-Bismol and antibiotics."
2. "No treatment is necessary at this time."
3. "This result indicates a gastric cancer caused by the organism."
4. "Surgical treatment is indicated."

Test Answer 3

1. This is the correct choice. *Helicobacter pylori* is the organism believed to cause most peptic ulcers. Treatment with bismuth compounds (Pepto-Bismol), antibiotics, and an acid-suppressing drug (ranitidine [Zantac] or omeprazole [Prilosec]) is indicated to prevent chronic atrophic gastritis (a predisposition to cancer).
2. Treatment with bismuth, antibiotics, and acid-suppressing drugs is indicated when the *H. pylori* titer is elevated
3. An elevated *H. pylori* does not by itself indicate cancer. An untreated infection predisposes to cancer. Cancer is diagnosed with a biopsy. Most people with elevated *H. pylori* do not have gastric cancer.
4. Surgical treatment of an uicer is indicated when medical approaches fail and the client has a bleeding ulcer. (Stein, 2005)

Test Question 4—Fill in the blanks

A medication is ordered to be given at 6 mL/hr. The solution is 20,000 mg/500 mL. How many mg per hour will that deliver to the patient?

Test Answer 4

$$\frac{20{,}000 \text{ mg}}{500 \text{ mL}} = \frac{40 \text{ mg}}{1 \text{ mL}} \text{ mL} = 40 \times 6 = 240 \text{ mg per hour}$$

Test Question 5—Identify the height of the fundus at 22 weeks on this picture. Mark the site with an X.

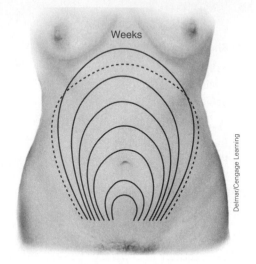

Delmar/Cengage Learning

Test Answer 5

The fundus is located at this site at 22 weeks.

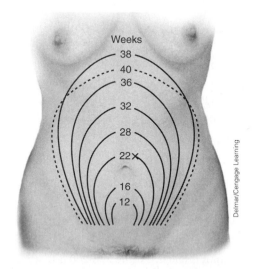

Delmar/Cengage Learning

Test Question 6

Put in correct order

Put these steps in the correct order to insert a Foley catheter.

1. Check integrity of Foley balloon.
2. Attach drainage bag to bed.

3. Send urine specimen to laboratory.
4. Cleanse meatus.
5. Spread the labia.
6. Insert the Foley.

Test Answer 6

1. Check integrity of Foley balloon.
5. Spread the labia.
4. Cleanse meatus.
6. Insert the Foley.
2. Attach drainage bag to bed.
3. Send urine specimen to laboratory.

FACTORS AFFECTING NCLEX-RN PERFORMANCE

Several factors have been identified as being associated with performance on the NCLEX examination. Some of these factors are listed in Table 17-2.

REVIEW BOOKS AND COURSES

In preparing to take the NCLEX, the new graduate may find it useful to focus his or her preparation on three areas: NCLEX knowledge review, NCLEX test question practice, and test anxiety control. Review books often include nursing content, sample test questions, or both. They frequently include computer software disks with test questions. The test questions in the review books and software may be arranged by clinical content area, or they may be presented in one or more comprehensive examinations covering all areas of the NCLEX.

Try to answer as many questions correctly as you can. As you study, be sure to actually practice taking the examinations. Do not jump ahead to the answer section before you have completed an examination. Completing the examinations in this way may improve your performance on the NCLEX.

It is helpful to use several of these books and their computer software when preparing for the NCLEX. Listings of NCLEX review books are available at www.amazon.com.

Prioritize your review by focusing on content in NCLEX-RN in your weak areas.

NCLEX review courses are also available. Brochures advertising these programs are often sent to schools and are available in many sites nationwide. The quality of these programs can vary, and you may want to ask faculty and former nursing graduates for recommendations. You may also find it helpful to note the excellent NCSBN review course and test question of the week at www.learningext.com.

NURSING EXIT EXAMS

Many nursing programs administer an examination to students at the completion of their nursing program, e.g., the HESI Evolve Exit Exam. New graduates who examine their feedback from such an examination have important information regarding their strengths and weaknesses that can help them focus their review for the NCLEX. A strategy for organizing this NCLEX review is outlined in Table 17-3.

TABLE 17-2	FACTORS ASSOCIATED WITH NCLEX-RN PERFORMANCE
■ HESI Exit Exam	■ GPA in science and nursing theory courses
■ Verbal SAT score	■ Competency in American English language
■ ACT score	■ Reasonable family responsibilities or demands
■ High school rank and GPA	■ Absence of emotional distress
■ Undergraduate nursing program GPA	■ Critical-thinking competency

TABLE 17-3	**SELF NEEDS ANALYSIS FOR NCLEX**

Anxiety level (circle)   1   2   3   4   5   6   7   8   9   10

Weak content areas identified on NCLEX Test Plan in Table 17-1, exit exam, or comprehensive exam, etc.:

_____

_____

Nursing courses below a grade of 'B': _____

Factors from Table 17-2: _____

_____

Weak content areas identified in common U.S. patient conditions causes of death:

- Mental Health, for example, schizophrenia, bipolar disorder, anxiety, personality disorders, suicide, eating disorders, abuse, and so on. _____

- Women's Health, for example, antepartum care, intrapartum care, postpartum care, newborn care, and so on. _____

- Adult Health, for example, cancer, myocardial infarction, diabetes, pneumonia, HIV, hepatitis, cholecystectomy, lobectomy, nephrectomy, cardiac arrest, thyroidectomy, shock, appendectomy, and so on. _____

- Children's Health, for example, leukemia, cardiovascular surgery, fractures, cancer, tonsillectomy, asthma, Wilms' tumor, cleft palate, and so on. _____

Weak content areas identified in any of the following areas:

- Therapeutic communication
- Growth and development (developmental milestones and toys)
- Management, delegation, referrals, and priority setting
- Medications
- Defense mechanisms
- Immunization schedules
- Diagnostic tests and laboratory data
- Nutrition

Organize your review. Study when you are fresh. Are you a day person? Are you a night person?

Your study schedule could look like the following, depending on the results of your self-analysis above:

Day 1:   Practice 60 Adult Health test questions. Score the test, analyze your performance, and review test question rationales and content weaknesses. Practice deep breathing, relaxation exercises, and positive thinking.

Day 2:   Practice 60 Women's Health test questions. Repeat above process.

Day 3:   Practice 60 Children's Health test questions. Repeat above process.

Day 4:   Practice 60 Mental Health test questions. Repeat above process.

Day 5:   Continue with content review and test question practice in all weak content areas. Practice deep breathing, relaxation exercises, and positive thinking. Continue this process of practicing 60 test questions daily until you are doing well in all areas and are scheduled to take your NCLEX-RN.

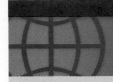

REAL WORLD INTERVIEW

My best advice to anyone preparing for the NCLEX is to take lots of practice tests. I answered close to 1,500 questions in preparation and I feel it did me a world of good. I kept my nursing textbooks handy and when I ran into something I didn't know, I looked it up.

Amanda Meadows, RN, BSN
Huntington, West Virginia

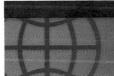

REAL WORLD INTERVIEW

A Dean that I know talks about the fact that she failed what was called in those days "the boards." She tells her students that it was the most traumatic event of her life (or at least *one* of the most traumatic events). When you have given it "your all" to complete a nursing curriculum, you want to be a successful NCLEX candidate. The HESI Exit Exam can help you achieve that goal. Look at your score printout and review any subject area that has a HESI score of less than 85. Remember, HESI scores are NOT percentage scores, but research data indicate that those who have HESI scores of 85 or above have a 94% probability of passing the NCLEX-RN.

Susan Morrison, PhD, RN
President Health Education Systems, Inc. (HESI)
Houston, Texas

KNOWLEDGE, ANXIETY MANAGEMENT, AND TEST-TAKING SKILLS

Successful test performance requires nursing knowledge, anxiety management, and test-taking skills. Knowledge of the test content is the first critical element. Students gain knowledge of nursing as the result of a course of nursing study. Nursing students attend either a two-year associate degree nursing program, a three-year diploma nursing program, or a four-year baccalaureate nursing program to gain the knowledge needed to satisfactorily complete the NCLEX-RN.

Anxiety management through visualization and relaxation techniques before and during the test is the second element of successful test performance. Plan to use any or all of the following to control your anxiety level:

- Positive thinking
- Guided imagery, which requires using your imagination to create a relaxing sensory scene on which to concentrate

- Breathing exercises
- Relaxation exercises
- Relaxation audio tapes (Stein, 2005)

Additional resources for reducing test anxiety include the *Tame Test Anxiety* CD-ROM by Richard Driscoll (2003) and a book: *Taking the Anxiety Out of Taking Tests* by Susan Johnson (2000).

Test-taking skills are the final critical element needed for successful test completion. Strategies to improve test-taking skills include practicing 60 test questions daily from different NCLEX-RN review books, CDs, and online NCLEX review sites, e.g., www.cengage.com/delmar/. Search for NCLEX. Practice until performance is satisfactory in all areas covered by the NCLEX exam. Note that successful students often practice 60 questions

daily in their weak content areas until their performance improves. Sixty questions daily for 30 days exposes students to 1,800 questions (60 × 30 = 1,800). Use the results of an exit exam or comprehensive exam to guide you in your selection of test questions. Practice using the ARKO and ABC-Safe-Comfort methods discussed in the critical thinking exercise later in this chapter as you review the test questions.

TIPS AND MEDICATION GUIDE

Table 17-4 offers some final tips on reviewing for NCLEX. Table 17-5 is a Medication Study Guide Starter to aid you in your NCLEX preparation. Use this guide as a starting point in your medication review for NCLEX.

TABLE 17-4	SELECTED NCLEX TIPS

- Remember Maslow's Hierarchy of Needs. Physical needs are met first, for example, airway, breathing, circulation (ABCs) threats.
  - ❏ Airway threats
    - Altered level of consciousness (LOC)
    - Unconscious
    - Foreign object in airway
  - ❏ Breathing threats
    - Asthma
  - ❏ Circulation threats
    - Cardiac arrest
    - Shock
- Safety needs are met second, for example, safety and infection control threats.
  - ❏ Confusion
  - ❏ Tuberculosis
  - ❏ Isolate noninfectious patients from infectious patients.

- Comfort needs and teaching needs are met after physical and safety needs are met. Don't choose a test question answer that gives the patient comfort or meets teaching needs before his or her ABC and safety needs have been met.
- Remember the nursing process—Assess your patient first; then plan, implement, and evaluate.
- Keep all your patients safe, for example, airway open, side rails up, IV access line in place on unstable patient; monitor vital signs, pulse oximeter, cardiac rhythm, and urine output as needed.
- Know delegation guidelines for RNs, LPNs, and NAPs. Observe the five rights of delegation, that is, the right task, the right circumstance, the right person, the right direction/communication, and the right supervision. See Chapter 8.
  - ❏ The RN assures quality care of all patients, especially complex patients. RNs delegate care of stable patients with predictable outcomes.

(continues)

TABLE 17-4	SELECTED NCLEX TIPS (CONTINUED)

- ❏ The RN uses patient care data such as vital signs, collected either by the nurse or others, to make clinical judgments. The RN continuously monitors and evaluates patient care and delegates care involving standard, unchanging procedures to LPNs and NAPs.

- ❏ The RN makes appropriate referrals to community resources.

- ❏ The RN never delegates patient Assessment, Teaching, Evaluation (ATE), or judgment.

- ❏ Review Chapter 8, especially Tables 8-1 through 8-7 and Figures 8-1 through 8-3, for information on nursing delegation.

- ❏ When delegating care, don't mix the care of a patient with an infection with the care of a patient who has decreased immunity, for example, a patient with AIDS, diabetes, steroids, the very young, the very old, and so on.

- ■ In answering test questions, do the following:

  - ❏ When choosing priorities, select the first action you would take if you were alone and could only do one thing at a time. Don't think that one RN will do one task, and another RN will do another task.

  - ❏ Assume you have the nursing or medical practitioner's order for any possible choices.

  - ❏ Assume you have perfect staffing, plenty of time, and all the necessary equipment for any possible test question choices. Choose the answer that indicates the best nursing care possible.

  - ❏ Assume you are able to give perfect care "by the book." Don't let your personal clinical experience direct you to choose a test answer that is less than high-quality care.

  - ❏ Remember to safeguard the patient ABCs and safety first and then check the equipment.

- ■ Know the most common adult, maternal-child, and psychological health care disorders. For each disorder, know the medications, laboratory and diagnostic tests, procedures, and treatments commonly used.

- ■ Know common medications (see Table 17-5).

- ■ Know common laboratory norms, for example, sodium, potassium, blood sugar, complete blood count, hematocrit, prothrombin time, partial thromboplastin time, international normalized ratio (INR), arterial blood gas (ABG), cardiac enzymes, digoxin level, dilantin level, lithium level, blood urea nitrogen (BUN), creatinine, uric acid, and specific gravity of urine.

- ■ Know communication techniques—look for answers that give patients support and allow them to keep talking and verbalize their concerns and problems. Be their comforting nurse, not their therapist. Avoid giving advice.

- ■ Know common food choices included in special diets, for example, low sodium diet, diabetic diet, and so on.

- ■ Know common food choices for potassium, sodium, vitamin K, calcium replacement, etc.

- ■ Prepare mentally with the following:

  - ❏ Anxiety control and relaxation techniques

  - ❏ Regular exercise

  - ❏ Thinking positively and avoiding negative people

  - ❏ Visualize your name with "RN" next to it on your name badge.

- ■ Remember—you graduated from an accredited nursing program. You can do it!

TABLE 17-5   MEDICATION STUDY GUIDE STARTER

Complete/Add to this as you study for NCLEX*

General Tips

1. Drowsiness and changes in Vital Signs (VS) are side effects of many medications given for their analgesic, antiemetic, antiseizure, tranquilizer, sedative/hypnotic, antihistamine, or antianxiety effects.

2. Drowsiness Guidelines: If drowsiness is listed below, consider the need to monitor the patient's Airway, Level of Consciousness (LOC), Blood Pressure (BP), Pulse (P), Respiration (R), Pulse Oximetry, and Cardiac Monitor. An IV line, side rails, and fall precautions may be necessary to safeguard the patient. He or she may also need to avoid driving and alcohol.

3. Note that if the drug is a cardiac or BP drug, use BP Med Guidelines, i.e., consider the need to monitor LOC, cardiac monitor, BP, P, R, and pulse oximetry. You may also need to monitor postural hypotension and maintain fall precautions.

4. Many meds cause renal, liver, heart, neurological, and bone marrow side effects. Monitor labs that reflect these organs' functions. Check allergies.

5. A Haldol, Ativan, and Cogentin mixture is used PRN for restraints—try psychological and physical non-restrictive approaches first.

Category	Prefix or Suffix	Examples	Patient Implications
Phenothiazine Antiemetic Antipsychotic Antianxiety	Zine	Promethazine (Phenergan); Fluphenazine (Prolixin)-IM	Drowsiness Guidelines Extrapyramidal (EPS) effects, Parkinsonism, Akathisia (restless), Dystonia (jerky movement, spasms, check airway), Tardive Dyskinesia (involuntary movements) Teach patient to report irreversible EPS symptoms early
Benzodiazepines Tranquilizer Hypnotic Antianxiety Antiseizure Anesthetic	Azepam Aze	Diazepam (Valium); Lorazepam (Ativan); Clonazepam (Klonopin); Alprazolam (Xanax); Midazolam (Versed)	Drowsiness Guidelines Check for habituation; taper dose when discontinued Monitor bone marrow, liver, and kidney laboratory tests Versed used for short-term sedation—monitor closely Romazicon (Flumazenil) reverses sedative effect of benzodiazepines

(continues)

TABLE 17-5	MEDICATION STUDY GUIDE STARTER (CONTINUED)

Category	Prefix or Suffix	Examples	Patient Implications
Anticoagulant	Parin	Heparin (antidote is protamine sulfate)	Monitor bleeding, e.g., stool, gums, urine, bruising, etc.
			For Heparin, check ptt level. Give Heparin IV to get ptt level to 1.5–2 times the control time
Anticoagulant		Coumadin (Warfarin)	Monitor bleeding, e.g., stool, gums, urine, bruising, etc.
		(Antidote is Vitamin K)	Check PT/INR (Desirable INR range is 2.0–3.0 for many conditions)
Angiotensin Converting Agent (ACE Inhibitor) Anti-hypertensive	Pril	Lisinopril (Zestril) Enalapril (Vasotec) Ramipril (Altace)	BP Med Guidelines
Angiotensin Receptor Blocking Agents Anti-hypertensive	Sartan	Telmisartan (Micardis) Irbesartan (Avapro) Losartan (Cozaar)	BP Med Guidelines
Beta adrenergic Blockers Anti-hypertensive Antianginal	Olol	Metoprolol (Lopressor) Propranolol (Inderal)	BP Med Guidelines Monitor for bronchospasm, bradycardia
Anti-hypertensive	Pres	Clonidine (Catapres) Hydralazine (Apresoline)	BP Med Guidelines
Calcium channel blockers Anti-hypertensive	Pine	Nifedipine (Procardia) Amlodipine (Norvasc)	BP Med Guidelines
Anti-hyperlipidemic	Vastatin	Lovastatin (Mevacor) Atorvastatin (Lipitor)	Check renal, liver, and cholesterol lab work Severe muscle cramping is side effect
Diuretic	Ide	Lasix (Furosemide)	Monitor intake and output Check potassium

(continues)

TABLE 17-5	MEDICATION STUDY GUIDE STARTER (CONTINUED)		

Category	Prefix or Suffix	Examples	Patient Implications
Potassium		Potassium electrolyte	Give IV slowly—use IV pump for infusions Potassium can kill if given quickly Be sure patient has adequate urine output and normal creatinine level before giving
Anti-Infectives	Mycin Cin	Gentamycin (Garamycin) Vancocin (Vancomycin)	Monitor for ototoxicity, seizures, blood dyscrasias, nephrotoxicity, rash, allergy Monitor peak and trough, BUN, and creatinine
Anti-infective	Ceph Cef	Cephalexin (Keflex) Ceftriaxone (Rocephin)	Check allergy, check liver, and renal lab tests
Antiviral	Vir	Zidovudine (Retrovir) Acyclovir (Zovirax)	Monitor for nausea and vomiting, tremors, confusion Check liver and renal lab tests
NSAID	Cox	Celecoxib (Celebrex)	Tinnitus/GI bleed Check platelets Check renal function, BUN, and creatinine
Steroids Anti-inflammatory Many anti-inflammatory uses for conditions such as CVA, asthma, arthritis, etc.	One	Decadron (Dexamethasone) Prednisone (Deltasone) Methylprednisolone (Solu-Cortef, Depo-Medrol)	Monitor "S's"—sex, sad, stress, sight, susceptibility, sugar, sodium Decreases sex (hormones), stress (inflammatory response), sight (cataracts), and potassium Increases sad (mood), susceptibility (infection, ulcers), sugar (hyperglycemia), sodium (edema), and osteoporosis Wean off steroids to avoid adrenal crisis and shock

(continues)

TABLE 17-5	MEDICATION STUDY GUIDE STARTER (CONTINUED)		

Category	Prefix or Suffix	Examples	Patient Implications
Histamine H2-Receptor Antagonists	Tidine	Ranitidine (Zantac) Famotidine (Pepcid)	Inhibits gastric acid secretion
Proton Pump Inhibitors	Prazole	Esomeprazole (Nexium) Pantoprazole (Protonix) Rabeprazole (Aciphex) Lansoprazole (Prevacid)	Used for erosive gastroesophageal reflux disease
Miotic eye drops		Pilocarpine	Constrict the pupil—reduce intraocular pressure
Mydriatic eye drops		Atropine	Dilate the pupil

Other Medications			
Antipsychotics	Anti-arrhythmics	Antidepressants	Mood Stabilizers
Zyprexa Seroquel Haldol Prolixin Abilify Resperidal (Resperidal M melts in the mouth for patients who are med avoiders)	Amiodarone (Cordarone); Norpace (Disopyramide); Rythmol Propafenone Tambocor (Flecainide); Betapace (Sotalol)	Celexa Cymbalta Lexapro Zoloft Paxil Prozac Remeron (older patient)	Lithium (Know levels) Depakote (Hair loss) Tegretol

*Other important drugs include Atropine, Benadryl, Cogentin, Digoxin, Epinephrine, Insulin, Lasix, Lactulose, Magnesium Sulfate, Morphine, Neurontin, Pitocin, Synthyroid, Isoniazid, Rifampin, Ethambutol, Pyrazinamide, Rhogam, Zyloprim, Activase, etc.

*Use this guide to begin your medication study. Add to it as you study.

Source: Kelly, P., & Hernandez, G. (2010). Medication Study Guide Starter. Unpublished manuscript.

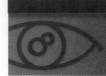

CRITICAL THINKING 17-1

When you are presented with a difficult test question, use these test-taking ARKO Strategies and ABC–Safe–Comfort Tips to help you answer it correctly. Use ARKO Strategies as follows:

- A   Is the question stem asking for you to take Action or take no Action?
- R   Reword the question.
- K   Identify any Key words in the question stem.
- O   Review and eliminate Options.

Apply this ARKO Strategy to the test question below:

What should the nurse do first for a patient with a spinal cord injury who complains of a headache?

A. Insert a new Foley catheter.

B. Assess the patient's pupils.

C. Take the patient's blood pressure.

D. Administer a beta adrenergic blocker.

Apply the ARKO strategy to the question above.

A   Stem asks for the nurse to take Action

R   Reword the question, as follows: What is a priority nursing action for a patient with a spinal cord injury who has a headache?

K   Key words are "first," "spinal cord injury," and "headache"

O   Note the following as you eliminate Options:

Option A may be useful if the patient's blood pressure is elevated, as a plugged catheter can trigger autonomic dysreflexia.

Option B would not give us useful information about this patient.

Option C would be useful to assess blood pressure for autonomic dysreflexia.

Option D would reduce the patient's blood pressure, but the stem does not say his or her blood pressure is elevated.

The correct answer is C.

As you review a test question, it is also helpful to review Maslow's Hierarchy of Needs and use the ABC–Safe–Comfort Tips. Assess your patient's ABCs, then assess his or her Safety, and finally, after these are secured, assess his or her Comfort and then any Teaching needs. Remember this sequence when prioritizing your nursing actions:

A – Airway

B – Breathing

C – Circulation

Safety

Comfort

Teaching

(continues)

CRITICAL THINKING 17-1 (CONTINUED)

Apply these Tips to this test question:

The nurse is unable to obtain a pedal pulse on doppler examination of the cold, painful leg of a patient who has just been admitted with a fractured femur. What is the priority intervention for this patient?

A. Give morphine, as ordered.

B. Teach the patient cast care.

C. Notify the medical practitioner.

D. Comfort the patient and keep the leg elevated.

Apply ABC–Safe–Comfort Tips to the question's options.

A. Comfort can be given with pain medication, but this is an emergency. Call the medical practitioner. Comfort care is done after ABC and Safety are assured.

B. Teaching is done after ABC–Safe–Comfort is assured.

C. Patient has absent pulse on doppler and cold, painful leg—this is an emergency! Patient's arterial circulation cannot be occluded long before there is permanent damage to tissues.

D. Patient is not safe or comforted if there is no arterial circulation to leg. Comfort care is done after ABC and Safety are assured.

The correct answer is C.

Recall that NCLEX often wants you to take all nursing actions before calling the medical practitioner. In an emergency, however, the medical practitioner should be called without hesitation when needed. Always recall that Maslow's Hierarchy of Needs directs us to monitor our patients' ABCs and then keep them Safe. After this is done, we can Comfort and Teach our patients.

BEGINNING A JOB SEARCH

The critical first step in your job search is preparation. Know what clinical area you are interested in and what skills you have that may fit that area.

Consider what type of hospital you want to work in; that is, a large university teaching hospital, a small private community hospital, and so forth.

MAGNET HOSPITALS

In 1993, the American Nurses Credentialing Center (ANCC) established the Magnet Services Recognition Program. A magnet hospital is a health care organization that has met the rigorous nursing excellence requirements of the American Nurses Credentialing Center (ANCC), a division of the American Nurses Association (ANA). As a testament to the increasing recognition given to magnet hospitals, *U.S. News & World Report* recently included magnet designation in its criteria for its annual "100 Best Hospitals of America" list (U.S. News & World Report, 2005).

Of 5,759 hospitals in the United States (AHA, 2006), 202 (or 3.5%) are magnet-designated facilities (ANCC, 2006). This figure is rising daily. Community hospitals, teaching hospitals, and hospital systems, large (more than 1,000 beds) and small (less than 100 beds), in rural and urban settings, have achieved magnet recognition.

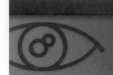

CRITICAL THINKING 17-2

You are responsible for being the nurse you want to be. To do this, set your goals and monitor and evaluate them regularly. Gather data on the following indicators of being a professional nurse and add to the list, as appropriate. What other goals have you added?

- Pass NCLEX-RN.

- Monitor literature so that I am up-to-date on evidence-based care for my patients.

- Monitor data that show that my patients are satisfied, pain-free, and feel cared about.

- Monitor data that show that my patients are complication-free and have no nurse-sensitive outcomes.

- Offer professional nursing service to my patients and my community.

- Give and receive professional respect to and from the health care team.

- Speak up about the important role that nurses play in preventing patient complications.

- Network with other professionals.

- Participate in professional committees at work.

- Communicate assertively with the health care team.

- Receive professional salary and benefits.

- Take good care of myself and strive for professional and personal balance.

- Continue my education, for example, certification, formal education, continuing education, and so on.

- Join my professional organization.

- Dress like a professional.

- Communicate pride in being a nurse.

Not only are nurses in Magnet hospitals more likely to rate their care environment as excellent, but there is also evidence that patient outcomes are better in Magnet hospitals. (Aiken, 2002).

NURSING RESIDENCY PROGRAMS

Consider looking for a one-year nursing residency program like the one currently being implemented through a partnership between the American Association of Colleges of Nursing (AACN) and the University HealthSystem Consortium (UHC). In addition to developing clinical judgment and leadership skills for new nurses, the goal of the residency program is to strengthen the new nurse's commitment to practice in the inpatient setting by making the first critical year a positive working and learning experience. (www.aacn.nche.edu/education/nurseresidency.htm)

MULTISTATE LICENSURE COMPACT

The multistate licensure compact allows a nurse to have one license (in his or her state of residency) and to practice in other states (both physically and electronically), subject to each state's practice law and regulation. Under mutual recognition, a nurse may practice across state lines

Agency and Referral Source	Telephone Number	Contact Name	Resume Sent/Date	Thank-You Letter	Follow-Up

Figure 17-1 Tracker for job leads. (*Source:* Courtesy of Polifko-Harris, K. [2003]. Career Planning. In P. Kelly-Heidenthal, *Nursing Leadership and Management* [2nd ed.]. Clifton Park, NY: Delmar Cengage Learning).

unless otherwise restricted. View guidelines of the multistate licensure compact at *www.ncsbn.org*. Click on *participating states* to view the map.

WHERE TO LOOK

One place many nurses think to begin a job search is the local newspaper. Other places include employment bulletin boards, telephone lines, and job fairs. Many health care employers have an employment bulletin board, telephone line, or Web site that identifies job openings on a weekly basis. It is often helpful to begin a job tracking file. See Figure 17-1. Be sure to look closely at the requirements for the position. If the position requirements state that a skill or education element is a *required* element, recruiters will call first only those candidates who meet the minimum *required* qualifications. If the position requirements state that a skill or education element is a *preferred* element, recruiters will call candidates first who have the *preferred* element.

ELECTRONIC MEDIA AND THE INTERNET

There are several sources of online application for employment. These sources include search engines, job boards, and agency and company

sites such as those for a specific hospital, health care agency, or health care company. Electronic media sites can also include health care journals. Following are some examples of search engines:

- Dogpile (allows you to search multiple search engines at one time; this site is known as a metasearch engine): *www.dogpile.com*
- Excite: *www.excite.com*
- WebCrawler: *www.webcrawler.com*
- Infoseek: *www.infoseek.com*
- Google: *www.google.com*

Some examples of job boards specific to health care include the following:

- *www.healthcareerweb.com*
- *www.medjobs.com*
- *www.rn.com*
- *www.aone.org* (This site requires membership to use.)

A few examples of other sites with job openings include the following:

- *www.rn.com*
- *www.careercity.com*

DEVELOPING A RESUME

Resumes are generally the first opportunity a prospective employer has to see who you are and what your qualifications are for a given position.

A **resume** is a brief summary of your background, training, and experience, as well as your qualifications for a position (see Figure 17-2). It should be viewed as a marketing tool to sell yourself to a prospective employer. Generally, a resume should be no longer than two pages on good quality white or ivory paper. It needs to contain concise information

---

James Mattern
214 Christie Avenue
Gladstone, OH 43523
(604) 775-3424
James123@school.edu

OBJECTIVE:	An entry-level position as an emergency room registered nurse
EDUCATION:	Associate of Science in Nursing, June, 2010 Freedom Community College, Gladstone, OH

          Highlights: *   Maintained 3.66 GPA, Dean's List
                            *   Class President
                            *   Clinical Rotation, Emergency Department, Concordia Hospital, March, 2010.

EXPERIENCE:	Patient Care Assistant, Medical-Surgical Unit St. Mary's Medical Center, Gladstone, OH (August 2008–present)

          Duties: *   Provide basic patient care and monitoring
                           *   Prepare and stock patient rooms

Ambulance Attendant
Mayfair Ambulance Service, Gladstone, OH
(2001–2010)

          Duties: * Answer emergency calls, including mass disasters

CERTIFICATION:	Certified in Advanced Cardiac Life Support, 2001–present Certified in Cardiopulmonary Resuscitation, 2001–present
PROFESSIONAL ORGANIZATIONS:	National Student Nurses Association American Red Cross, Blood Drive Volunteer Gladstone Free Clinic, Registration Volunteer

References available upon request.

Figure 17-2 Resume. (Delmar/Cengage Learning).

that clearly identifies your specific skills, strengths, and experiences. A resume should be honest, neat, easy to read, and have no errors. In companies that are highly desirable to work for, the resume is also often used as a screening tool so that a recruiter's time can best be spent wisely with potential employees who are seen as welcome team members.

There is no one perfect resume style. It is agreed that an effective resume (1) catches the employer's interest; (2) identifies critical areas such as education, work experience, and special qualifications; (3) should be tailored to the employer's needs; (4) creates a favorable first impression about you and your abilities; (5) communicates that you are someone who is a good fit for the position; and (6) is visually appealing. A good resume takes time to prepare. Avoid abbreviations. You should ensure that what is presented on paper is truthful and presents you as a capable person who is able to make immediate and sustained contributions to an organization.

The statement "References available upon request." can be placed on the last line of a resume. You can either provide a listing of references on the application, or bring a separate reference list to a job interview. Include at least three professional references, with names, titles, addresses, and phone numbers—but only after receiving permission from these persons to use them as references. Do not use family, friends, or neighbors as professional references. Notify your references before you interview to let them know they may be contacted.

WRITING A COVER LETTER

A resume should always be accompanied by a letter of introduction, known as the cover letter. This is a one-page letter designed to entice the prospective employer to become interested enough to read the resume. It does not reiterate the entire resume, but presents highlights and a summary of the essential points found on the resume. Figure 17-3 is an example of a cover letter. Your cover letter should highlight your strengths that well suit you to a job opportunity for which the recruiter is actively seeking applicants. Be sure to follow up sending your resume and cover letter with a phone call

to the recruiter. Be professional in your phone call. Consider it part of your interview. If you get the recruiter's answering machine when you call, leave your phone number very slowly twice. Don't abuse the recruiter's time. Don't assume they have your phone number handy even though it is on the resume. Be brief in leaving any phone messages. Don't repeat your whole professional history and goals. The recruiter will see this on your resume.

DEVELOPING AN ELECTRONIC RESUME

Sending cover letters and resumes via the Internet is an acceptable practice. It does require some additional considerations in terms of both safeguards and catching the attention of the reader. It is safest to initially send the e-mail to yourself or to a mentor to determine how it will appear to the reader. Send the resume as an attachment to your cover letter. The human resources personnel or nurse manager can then reproduce it readily and circulate it to other managers or members of the interviewing committee.

Catching the attention of human resources personnel is vital. For example, instead of entering *Resume* in the subject line of your e-mail, enter *Resume for nursing position with 9 years EMT experience,* or *Resume for entry-level RN seeking pediatric nursing position,* as appropriate. Human resources personnel are more likely to read such an e-mail and corresponding resume quickly.

Be specific as to what shift and unit you are seeking. Note that many agencies now scan resumes electronically and search them for key nouns associated with a particular job opening. Those resumes containing the most key word nouns are selected and then ranked. In constructing your resume, be sure to:

- Keep it simple. Use a plain typeface, such as Helvetica for headings and Times Roman for body text, and 10- to 14-point type.
- Avoid fancy highlighting. Use boldface or ALL CAPS for emphasis. Avoid fancy fonts, italics, underlining, slashes, dashes, parentheses, and ruled lines.
- Avoid a two-column format. Multiple columns can be jumbled by scanners that read across the page.

James Mattern
214 Christie Avenue
Gladstone, OH 43523
(604) 775-3424

April 11, 2010

Ms. Eileen Carter, BSN, RN
Director of Human Resources
Concordia Hospital
200 Jones Drive
Austin, OH 43524

Dear Ms. Carter:

I am requesting the opportunity to discuss my career plans with you. I will be graduating on June 30, 2010 from Freedom Community College with an Associate of Science Degree in Nursing. I will take my NCLEX-RN on July 30, 2010.

I have served as an ambulance attendant for nine years. This service provided me with the skills to handle emergency calls, including mass disasters such as airline crashes and hotel and apartment fires. I also performed many tasks of varying priorities within many Fire and Police Departments. I also recently completed a five week clinical rotation in your emergency department. I feel that these skills, combined with my newly acquired nursing skills, will be an asset to your Emergency Department.

I would appreciate the opportunity to discuss my career plans with you. I will call you next week to schedule an appointment to discuss employment possibilities. In the meantime, I can be contacted at (604) 775-3424 or at James123@school.edu. I am willing to rotate shifts.

Thank you for your time and consideration of my resume.

Sincerely,

James Mattern

James Mattern

Figure 17-3 Cover letter. (Delmar/Cengage Learning).

One way to assure that your resume can be read by any computer is to create an ASCII version or "text file." Select "Save as Text only" from your desktop menu, and reformat your ASCII page as needed. (Lannon, 2000).

A SUCCESSFUL INTERVIEW

In preparation for an interview, learn more about the agency and the possible questions you may be asked or that you should ask (Hart, 2006). You would be wise to obtain a copy of the job description beforehand. Familiarize yourself with it, as this will further demonstrate your interest in the position. It will also give you an opportunity to prepare appropriate interview questions. For example, if the job description requires the nurse to demonstrate the use of computer equipment, you can clarify what type of computer equipment is used in the unit. Go online and find the agency's Web site. Review what you find there. Search for the agency by name and location by using a search engine, for example, www.google.com.

Arrive shortly before the interview to demonstrate your time management skills. The interviewer will note this. Prepare a folder that contains a description of the organization and its services, extra copies of your resume, questions you have researched and are prepared to ask, and blank paper as well as a pen and any other documents that may be helpful. The nurse manager or representatives of the Human Resources department will verify your license, assess your competency, review your employment references, and complete background and criminal checks, as appropriate. They will assess your ability to meet any health requirements or any other job requirements of a nursing position. Your ability to fit in with the agency's culture as well as the patient care unit's culture will be assessed. Your communication skills, maturity, dependability, and learning and nursing skills, as well as your ability to delegate, take initiative, use judgment, and be loyal and dedicated to your work are all items that may be assessed. The nursing representatives and the human resources representatives will often offer you a competitive salary or hourly rate within approved budget guidelines, and they will assure the completion of any required organizational and governmental paperwork. Some organizations may require a group interview with multiple persons interviewing you to assess such things as your ability to work on a team, and so on. For entry-level position interviews, it is customary to have only the nursing manager or the nurse manager and a nurse recruiter or human resources person present during the interview. In some situations, other staff nurses are included in interviews for new unit staff.

You will also want to assess such items as whether the organization offers a nurse internship program for new graduates, what the program consists of, who serves as preceptors for the program, their backgrounds, and the salary during the internship. Note that internship programs may vary from organization to organization in content, length, preceptor requirements, salary, and so on.

Rehearse an interview scenario with a trusted colleague or by video. Types of interviews can vary from one-to-one interviews, panel interviews, telephone interviews, and follow-up interviews with varying types of questions involving hypothetical case scenarios. You are applying for an entry-level position, and therefore the questions will be directed at your nursing care knowledge. For example, if you are applying for a nursing position on a general medical unit, be ready to give the nursing interventions for a patient experiencing chest pain or hypoglycemia. You may also be asked to recall a difficult nursing situation and describe your behavior in that situation. For example, you may be asked, "If you are faced with a demanding patient who has been waiting for a long time to have his dressing changed, what would you do?" To respond, use the STAR acronym and include each component. Describe Specifically (S) what happened; the Task (T), problem, or issue; the Action (A) you took; and the Result (R) of the action. The interviewer is looking for what you learned from the situation and how you would handle a similar situation in the future (Table 17-6).

Interviews that ask about your behavior are designed to provide the employer with information about how you have handled both negative and positive experiences in the past. Employers are seeking employees who are able to reflect on their past performance and learn from the experience. In this information age, nursing employers are recognizing the need to transform work sites into learning sites (Holden, 2006).

During the introductory phase of the interview, the employer should outline the job and the conditions of employment. If the job and conditions do not reflect your understanding of the position, be sure to clarify by asking questions at this time. The employer is looking for the traits that successful registered nurses demonstrate, such as flexibility and a willingness to work in various areas, organizational skills and the ability to complete work assignments, and the ability to remain calm and collected during times of crisis.

The employer may ask, "Tell me about a time when you had to work in an area of the hospital in which you had very little orientation." Or "Tell me about a time when you had to complete an unusually large amount of work." Or "Tell me about a time when you had to deal with a stressful crisis at work."

TABLE 17-6	STAR INTERVIEWS
Specifics	A patient was overdue for his dressing change. He became angry and demanded that I come now to change his dressing.
Task	I was busy with other high-priority patients. I was having trouble getting to this dressing change.
Action	I called my charge nurse and asked for help. The charge nurse was able to change the patient's dressing, talk with him, and help him to relax. I stopped in to tell the patient I was sorry for the delay.
Result	I asked the charge nurse to review assignments for future care of this type of patient who has extensive dressing change needs. I also resolved to examine the way I prioritize my patients at the beginning of a shift to determine the best way to meet patient care needs. I resolved to change my future patients' dressings early in the shift before it gets busy.

The employer may ask you to job shadow. This job shadow is in effect a second interview. Often, the prospective employee will show a very different side of his or her personality while shadowing. Input from current employees who spent time with the prospective employee during the job shadow will likely be sought. Valuable information about the prospective employee's personality fit with the department may be gained (Olmstead, 2007).

The next phase of the interview will begin with the employer asking you questions about your cover letter and resume. All the questions during the interview will reflect the job description. Familiarize yourself with the legal and illegal questions that may be asked. See the Web site www.hospitalsoup.com. Legally acceptable questions include your reason for applying, your career goals, any problems you foresee, and your strengths and weaknesses. Illegal questions include asking if you are a citizen of the country, your age, cultural heritage, membership in social organizations, family characteristics, and medical history (Tetterton, 2006).

Rather than refusing to answer an illegal question, which may be seen as being uncooperative or confrontational, respond as if it is a legally acceptable question. For example, should the interviewer ask how many children you are caring for at home, respond by indicating that you are able to handle the demands and hours of the job for which you are applying. Responding in this manner may signal to the interviewer your ability to serve as a team player without compromising the legal or ethical issues of the job requirements.

Highlight specific personal and professional accomplishments that reflect your ability; however, be careful not to inflate them as this can raise doubts concerning your truthfulness and accuracy. If you give the interviewers reason to question your veracity, you may lose the job opportunity. Respond in a calm, problem-solving fashion to all questions. See Table 17-7 for other interview questions you may be asked.

Avoid any discussion of how bad your last employer or faculty was or how incompetent you think that your coworkers or classmates are. Keep the entire interview process as positive as possible. Avoid any discussions of any personal problems. If an employer has a choice between you and the person who lost their last job because they kept calling in sick over child care or personal problems, they're going to pick you every time.

TABLE 17-7	INTERVIEW QUESTIONS

Question	Potential Response
Tell me about yourself.	Do not go into a long list, but offer two to three traits that are solid (for example, "I am a positive person and look for new learning experiences.").
Why do you want to work here?	Describe several attributes of the work environment, the staff, or the patients (for example, "I enjoyed my rotation on 5 West—the staff worked as a team and I am looking for that type of support in my first position.") Comment on any attractive organizational strengths you saw on the organization's Web site, such as Magnet status.
What do you want to be doing in five years?	Identify a long-term goal and your plan to achieve it with progressive responsibilities and achievements.
What are your qualifications?	Discuss experiences that you have had that qualify you for the new position.
What are your strengths?	This is a favorite question. Look at the job description. What qualities do you have that are required? Are you able to work under stress, are you organized, are you eager to learn new skills, do you enjoy new challenges?
What would your references say?	You may want to ask your references this question. Would they say you are easily distracted or focused? A team player or solo player? A problem solver or one who ignores problems?
Are you interested in more schooling?	Most people who have just graduated may want to say no, but an employer wants someone who is interested in lifelong learning, especially in the nursing profession.
What has been your biggest success?	Think of a success ahead of time that may fit with the organization. It does not have to be in nursing.
What has been your greatest failure?	Again, think ahead, but this time, make sure you can state what you learned from the negative experience. After all, to fail is to learn, so state what you would do differently next time and why.
Why do you want to leave your current job?	For an RN, you can say that you are seeking new responsibilities, experiences, and challenges. Give an example of a new experience you are looking for.

Source: Compiled with information from Polifko-Harris, K. (2003). Career Planning. In P. Kelly-Heidenthal, *Nursing Leadership and Management* (2nd ed.). Clifton Park, NY: Delmar Cengage Learning.

DRESSING FOR THE INTERVIEW

Dress appropriately for the position by wearing professionally acceptable, comfortable, and neatly pressed clothing. For women, this may be a solid-color conservative suit with a coordinated blouse, medium-heeled polished shoes, limited jewelry, neat professional hairstyle, and neutral hosiery. Skirt length should be long enough so you can sit down comfortably. Choose a soft color that complements your skin tone and hair color such as brown, tan, beige, black, blue, navy, or gray. Use light makeup and perfume and have neat, manicured nails.

For men, appropriate dress may be a solid-color dark blue, gray, muted pinstripe, or very muted brown conservative suit with a white long-sleeved shirt and conservative tie. Wear a conservative stripe or paisley tie that complements your suit, in silk or good quality blends only. Wear dark socks with professional polished leather dress shoes, brown, cordovan, or black only. Wear limited or no jewelry and have a neat professional hairstyle. Limit aftershave and have neatly trimmed nails. Both women and men should avoid body piercing jewelry and cover tattoos. Don't chew gum, eat, or use a cell phone or iPod during the interview. Use a breath mint before you enter the building for the interview.

TERMINATION

Terminating an interview is important. The employer will close an interview by asking if you have any questions (Table 17-8).

Expect to be quite exhausted by the end of the interview. However, take time to review your notes, seek clarification regarding any concerns, and conclude the interview by asking when you can expect to hear from the employer. Asking this indicates that you are actively seeking employment and suggests that if the employer is serious about hiring you, he may want to offer you a position. Many sources recommend waiting to ask questions such as the following until after a position has been offered: What is the salary? When do raises occur? Is there a shift differential? Is there a differential for advanced nursing degrees? What type of health, dental, retirement, vacation, holiday time, sick time, continuing education, and educational reimbursement benefits are offered? Note the regular salary surveys done by many nursing journals, for example, *RN* (October 2005), *Nursing* (October 2006), *AORN* (December 2005), and so on.

WRITING A THANK-YOU LETTER

Within 24 hours after your interview, you should send a thank-you letter to the interviewer. Many people do not take the time to write a personal

TABLE 17-8	**SAMPLE QUESTIONS TO ASK DURING AN INTERVIEW**

1. How can I prepare myself to work on this unit and do a good job?

2. May I have a copy of the job description (Figure 17-4) and performance appraisal form? How often will I be evaluated?

3. Is there a clinical ladder program that identifies clinical, managerial, and educational levels for promotion?

4. Who is my preceptor?

5. What shift will I be scheduled to work? Will I rotate shifts? Are special requests for time off honored?

6. What holidays and weekends am I scheduled to work?

7. What type of benefits are offered with this position? (Health, dental, retirement, holiday time, sick time, continuing education opportunities, educational reimbursement)

8. What type of orientation or nursing residency program will I receive? How long is it? Does it address how to work well with other practitioners?

9. What is the salary? When do raises occur? Is there a shift differential? Is there a differential for advanced nursing degrees?

10. Is this a Magnet hospital? Do you monitor nurse-sensitive outcomes?

ALBANY MEDICAL CENTER HOSPITAL PATIENT CARE SERVICES
Job Description—REGISTERED PROFESSIONAL NURSE

SUMMARY: The Registered Professional Nurse utilizes the nursing process to diagnose and treat human responses to actual or potential health problems. The New York State Nurse Practice Act and A.N.A. Code for Nurses with Interpretive Statements guide the practice of the Registered Professional Nurse. The primary responsibilities of the Registered Professional Nurse as leader of the Patient Care Team is coordination of patient care through the continuum, education, and advocacy.

ESSENTIAL DUTIES AND RESPONSIBILITIES include the following. Other duties may be assigned.

— Performs an onGoing and systematic assessment, focusing on physiologic, psychologic, and cognitive status.
— Develops a goal-directed plan of care which is standards based. Involves patient and/or significant other (S.O.) and health care team members in patient care planning.
— Implements care through utilization and adherence to established standards which define the structure, process, and desired patient outcomes of the nursing process.
— Evaluates effectiveness of care in progressing patients toward desired outcomes. Revises plan of care based on evaluation of outcomes.
— Demonstrates competency in knowledge base, skill level, and psychomotor skills.
— Documents the nursing process in a timely, accurate, and complete manner, following established guidelines.
— Participates in unit and service quality management activities.
— Demonstrates responsibility and accountability for professional standards and for own professional practice.
— Supports research and its implications for practice.
— Establishes and maintains direct, honest, and open professional relationships with all health care team members, patients, and significant others.
— Seeks guidance and direction for successful performance of self and team, to meet patient care outcomes.

QUALIFICATION REQUIREMENTS: To perform this job successfully, an individual must be able to perform each essential duty satisfactorily. The requirements listed below are representative of the knowledge, skill, and/or ability required. Reasonable accommodations may be made to enable individuals with disabilities to perform the essential functions.

EDUCATION and/or EXPERIENCE: Graduate of an approved program in professional nursing. Must hold current New York State registration or possess a limited permit to practice in the State of New York.

LANGUAGE SKILLS: Ability to read and interpret documents such as safety rules and procedure manuals. Ability to document patient care on established forms. Ability to speak effectively to patients, family members, and other employees of organization.

MATHEMATICAL SKILLS: Ability to add, subtract, multiply, and divide in all units of measure, using whole numbers, common fractions, and decimals. Ability to compute rate, ratio, and percent.

REASONING ABILITY: Ability to identify problems, collect data, establish facts, and draw valid conclusions.

PHYSICAL DEMANDS: While performing the duties of this job, the employee is regularly required to stand; walk; use hands to probe, handle, or feel objects, tools, or controls; reach with hands and arms; and speak or hear. The employee is occasionally required to sit or stoop, kneel, or crouch.

The employee must regularly lift and/or move up to 100 pounds and frequently lift and/or move more than 100 pounds. Specific vision abilities required by this job include close vision, distance vision, peripheral vision, depth perception, and the ability to adjust focus.

WORK ENVIRONMENT: While performing the duties of this job, the employee is regularly exposed to bloodborne pathogens.

The noise level in the work environment is usually moderate.

Figure 17-4 Albany Medical Center hospital patient care services job description for registered professional nurses, excerpt. (*Source:* Courtesy of Albany Medical Center, Albany NY).

note, but doing so may set you apart from other potential employees as someone who is professional and sincerely interested in joining the organization. Figure 17-5 illustrates a thank-you letter as a follow-up to an interview. Be sure to call your recruiter as you have indicated in your follow-up letter. Have your resume in front of you when you call her. Be professional and call from a landline that will have enough minutes or, if calling from a cell phone, call from a place with an adequate signal that will allow you to concentrate on any recruiter questions. Do not call when you are driving, cooking, or doing something else.

Focus on the recruiter and her questions and respect her time.

ORIENTATION TO YOUR NEW JOB

Many health care organizations divide nursing orientation into general and unit-specific sections. Once hired, new nurses receive a general orientation including information and skills that all nurses new to the facility need, regardless of their eventual unit assignment. Figure 17-6 is a sample

---

James Mattern
214 Christie Avenue
Gladstone, OH 43523
(604) 775-3424

April 26, 2010

Ms. Eileen Carter, BSN, RN
Director of Human Resources
Concordia Hospital
200 Jones Drive
Austin, OH 43524

Dear Ms. Carter:

     Thank you for the time you spent with me as I interviewed for a position as a registered nurse at Concordia Hospital. I enjoyed meeting the emergency department nurse manager and several of the staff nurses yesterday and was especially impressed with the sense of professionalism among the staff.

     I have requested that my transcripts be sent directly to your office, and I will have three of my instructors complete the reference forms you gave me. I look forward to hearing from you soon about my second interview and will contact you in two weeks as directed.

                   Sincerely,

                   James Mattern

                   James Mattern

Figure 17-5 Follow-up to interview letter. (Delmar/Cengage Learning).

RN Orientation Template
Week One

Monday Perdiems/Weekend Staff attend May 21	Tuesday Perdiems/Weekend attend May 22 0745 meet in main lobby	Wednesday Perciems/Weekend attend May 23	Thursday Perdiems/Weekend attend May 24	Friday May 25
Human Resource/Safety Education *Remember to sign in on your unit if you want to get paid for the days you attend orientation.	8:00–11:30 Intro/Tour Nursing at AMC Education Opportunities 11:30–12:00 Tina Raggio-Project Learn 12:00–1:00 Lunch 1:00–2:00 Delegation/Assigning *Donna Harat* 2:00–4:30 Modules *some orientees may need to attend the SMS Computer class in the P building from 11:30–2:30-check with Education**	08:00–11:00 Documentation Standards of Care, protocols, I/O, graphic, Clinical Pathways Unit Day Prep *(ED exempt: modules)* 11:00–11:30 Restraints 11:30–12:00 Back Video Nurse Scheduling 12:00–1:00 Lunch 1:00–4:30 Skills Lab Afternoon Emergency Care and Mock Code (ACLS or PALS exempt and does rot apply to NICU). IV/ Phlebotomy Skills, Accucheck, PCA Pump	08:00–09:30 Modules 09:30–11:00 Epidemiology *Carolyn Scott* 11:00–11:30 Lunch 11:30–2:30 SMS Computer Class 3:00–4:00 Math Calculation Class (**optional-check with Educator**) 4:00–4:30 Planning for next week/ core orientation/orientee assessment forms	07:30–10:30 SMS Computer/ P Building-If needed 10:30–12:00 Independent Activities on Unit of Hire or Modules 12:00–1:00 Meet with Director Main 4 Office Lunch Provided 1:00–2:00 Pastoral Care Room U477 2:00–4:00 Modules

Required Modules:

Age Specific ☐	IV Therapy ☐	Blood and Blood Products ☐	RN Medication ☐	Patient Rights ☐
Peds or Adult Emergency Care ☐	Latex Allergy ☐	Patient Classification ☐		
Order Transcription (not for ED, PACU) ☐	Pain Management ☐	Documentation ☐		CPR: (see handout) ☐

Dept of Education- #262–3705

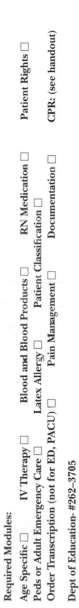

Figure 17-6 Registered professional nurse general orientation schedule template—Week One. (*Source:* Courtesy of Albany Medical Center, Albany, NY).

schedule for the first week of general orientation at one medical center.

General orientations are usually outcome based, requiring the orientee to demonstrate competency, perhaps by written medication or knowledge tests or skills measurement. Information about the Joint Commission, the hospital accrediting body, and National Patient Safety Goals is also often given at general orientation.

Unit-based orientation, whether it follows the general orientation or is interspersed throughout, focuses on the specific competencies a new nurse needs to care for the diagnoses and ages of patients typical to the assigned unit. Many organizations have developed unit- specific competency tools that list those skills orientees need to demonstrate. These lists provide a useful road map with which to plan a learner-specific orientation. Figure 17-7 is an excerpt from an Emergency Department's unit-based orientation tool. It is also useful to identify your personal learning needs and set your own learning goals to prepare yourself to deliver quality patient care and to meet your responsibilities in a professional style. See Table 17-9.

PRECEPTORS

Preceptors can play a key role in introducing the new nurse to coworkers and other members of the health team. The orientee needs to be introduced to the specific functions and roles of those people who interact daily with the nurses on the unit. This helps the new nurse identify relationships within the unit and between the unit and the larger health care organization.

A good preceptor is clinically experienced, enjoys teaching, and is committed to the role. If you find it difficult to work with your assigned preceptor, make this known early in the orientation process. The nursing manager or educator should be notified and the situation discussed and resolved. Good preceptors are familiar with the organization's policies and procedures, willing to share knowledge with their orientees, and model behaviors for their orientees.

REALITY SHOCK

In 1974, Kramer described "reality shock" and discussed the difficulties some new graduates have in adjusting to the work environment. Kramer identified a conflict between new graduates' expectations and the reality of their first nursing position. A skilled preceptor can assist new nurses through this transition by offering them opportunities to validate their impressions. The support of other new nurses in a similar situation, such as those participating in the same core orientation, is particularly helpful. Note that all nurses may experience reality shock throughout their career whenever they enter a new career area (Brunt, 2005).

MENTORS

Developing a mentoring relationship with a more experienced, successful nurse is another strategy for professional growth and help in setting long-term goals. A mentor coaches a novice nurse and helps him develop skills and career direction. A mentor may introduce the new nurse to professional networking opportunities and assist him in workplace problems.

To find a mentor, a new nurse needs to communicate a willingness to learn and grow. A newer nurse usually needs to seek out a prospective mentor rather than wait to be approached by one. An ideal mentor is an experienced nurse who is willing to support and counsel other nurses when asked. This may lead to a formal structured relationship or a more informal role-modeling association.

PERFORMANCE FEEDBACK

Everyone needs feedback about his or her performance, particularly when in a new position. Some preceptors and managers recognize new employees for their progress, but in many cases, the new nurse needs to solicit their feedback. A concrete mechanism to measure one's own performance is

Name:	Preceptor:	Unit/Dept.:	Emergency Dept:	Date:

At the completion of orientation, the RN will perform technical nursing skills specific to the age and characteristics of the patients served, consistent with the Standards of Nursing Practice.

Self-Evaluation Scale 1 2 3	RN Technical Skill Checklist	Method of Validation/ Code	Date Met/ Initials

	1. Cardiovascular
	 A. Initiate IV therapy
	  1. Adult, non-trauma
	  2. Trauma patient
	  3. Pediatric
	  4. Newborn
	  5. Phlebotomy percutaneous approach
	
	 B. Blood sampling:
	  1. arterial line
	  2. blood sampling: port-a-cath
	  3. Triple lumen/trauma cath/central line
	
	 C. Central venous line management: securing/dressing/caps/tubing
	  1. Trauma catheter/triple lumen
	  2. Implanted device external access (i.e., Hickman)
	  3. PICC line
	  4. Port-a-cath
	
	 D. Infusion pumps
	  1. IV pumps
	  2. Syringe pumps
	  3. Programmable pediatric pump
	  4. Patient Controlled Analgesia
	
	 E. Spacelab bedside and central monitors
	  1. Cardiac rhythm interpretation
	
	 F. Defibrillator operation
	  1. Zoll
	  2. Physiocontrol 10 and 9
	
	 G. External transcutaneous pacer–Zoll
	
	 H. Transvenous pacer pack: Emergent
	
	 I. Transvenous pacer pack: Urgent
	  1. Pulse generator
	  2. Ushkow's lead
	
	 J. Blood products administration
	
	 K. Level I blood warmer and rapid infuser
	
	 L. Spun Hct
	
	 M. Utilization of doppler for vascular assessment
	2. Gastrointestinal		

Figure 17-7 Emergency department competency-based orientation tool sample page, excerpt. (*Source:* Courtesy of Albany Medical Center, Albany, NY).

TABLE 17-9   DEVELOPING A PROFESSIONAL STYLE

1. Assess your current education and experience.
2. As you start your new nursing role, review the following on your unit:
   - Most common medical diagnoses
   - Most common nursing diagnoses
   - Most common medications and IV solutions
   - Most common diagnostic tests
   - Most common laboratory tests
   - Most common nursing and medical interventions and treatments
3. Set goals for any additional education and experience that you may need.
4. Review your own job description and the roles and job descriptions of nursing and other health care and medical staff you work with.
5. Identify the names and contact information of all nursing, medical, and health care staff you work with.
6. Discuss delegation with your preceptor, and observe how the preceptor delegates to others.
7. Observe the impact of delegation on both the delegate and the person delegated to.
8. Remember the golden rule: do unto others as you would want them to do unto you.
9. Recognize that, under the law, the RN holds the responsibility and accountability for nursing care.
10. Practice assertiveness and work at being direct, open, and honest in your new role.
11. Exercise your power with kindness to all.
12. Hold others accountable for their responsibilities as spelled out in their job description.
13. Be open to performance improvement feedback about your personal delegation style.
14. Modify your communication approach to fit the needs of patients, staff, and yourself.
15. Take action to assure your patients receive high-quality, safe care.

through the objective learning materials, job descriptions, and competency-based orientation tools provided by nurse educators. New nurses must successfully pass the written and technical parts of orientation. While in orientation, and at least annually thereafter, new graduates should meet at regular intervals with their preceptor and manager to review progress.

At each of these sessions, it is important for the new nurse to solicit feedback. Ask, "How do you think I'm doing? Am I at the level you would expect? What should I focus on next?" Answers to questions such as these allow the orientee to measure progress and set goals for the future.

A sample performance goals outline might look like the following:

By the next scheduled performance assessment, nurse Joanne Johnson will do the following:

- Successfully complete the advanced pediatric assessment course.
- Assume the primary nurse role for patients with an anticipated length of stay greater than three days.

- Become an active participant on a unit-based or hospital-wide committee.
- Attend a pediatric nursing conference.

360-DEGREE FEEDBACK

Some health care organizations have moved to an evaluation program known as **360-degree feedback**. In the 360-degree feedback system, an individual is assessed by a variety of people in order to provide a broader perspective. For example, a nurse may complete a self-assessment and submit a portfolio that documents competency, critical thinking, values, beliefs, and skills (O'Malley, 2008). The portfolio may include elements of nursing orientation, nursing practice, leadership, teamwork, scholarly activity, documentation, and committee work. The portfolio also documents peer reviews, evaluation by the nurse's immediate supervisor, and patient interviews.

CORRECTIVE ACTION PROGRAMS

Sometimes, performance evaluation indicates the need for significant improvement. Most health care organizations have a prescribed corrective action program. One of the first steps in helping employees improve their performance is identifying whether poor performance is developmental or related to a failure to follow policies or procedures. For example, a nurse may be having difficulty completing assignments in an appropriate time frame. The manager needs to coach the nurse, assisting with whatever support will help him or her improve. Another category of corrective action is disciplinary corrective action. Most organizations have a series of progressive steps for corrective action in cases in which employee performance does not improve. For example, a manager may begin by providing a verbal warning to an employee whose attendance is minimally

---

CASE STUDY 17-1

Maria Diaz is a senior nursing student working as a patient care assistant on an oncology floor in a small community hospital. Maria is well liked by the staff of the floor and is offered a full-time registered nurse position upon graduation. While Maria is flattered and relieved that she has an offer, she feels that she should at least interview at another hospital, including a nearby teaching hospital, for comparison.

How would maria begin her job search at other hospitals? What are the key elements to securing an interview at other hospitals? Once maria has an interview, what type of questions should she be prepared to answer from the interviewer? What type of questions should maria be prepared to ask?

---

acceptable. If the nurse's attendance problem continues, he or she may receive a written warning. Without improvement, this could proceed to a suspension, final warning, and eventually termination. In a union environment, the employee may have the right to union representation after a verbal reprimand.

Nurses who receive a verbal warning from their manager should immediately demonstrate a commitment to and plan for improvement in order to avoid any progression toward corrective action. It is useful, although not always easy, to avoid taking the corrective action personally and look on the feedback as an opportunity for improvement.

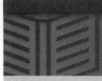

EVIDENCE FROM THE LITERATURE

Citation: Snodgrass, S. G. (2001, June 10). Wish you were a star? Become one! *Chicago Tribune,* D1.

Discussion: The most logical way to predict your future is to create it, so if you want to be a star, start by becoming a top performer now. Companies are drawn to those who use up-to-date skills and leadership to produce measurable results. Organizations seek such people out. Surprisingly, few people understand this. You can begin to position yourself now with exceptional performance.

Start by delivering more than you promise and consistently outperform yourself. Exceed expectations on a regular basis, seek more responsibility, value teamwork and diversity, provide leadership, and always go beyond the call of duty. Communicate effectively and know how to network with others. Be resourceful, comfortable with ambiguity, and open to saying, "I don't know, but I'll find out." In addition, take initiative and persevere until you reach quantifiable results. Finally, assume some personal risk by thinking outside the box and exploring bold, new solutions to challenges. Provide yourself with a margin of confidence through lifelong learning. Be open, flexible, and adapt to new ideas. Spend time with those who challenge your thinking.

You should also be creative, seek innovative solutions, and supplement your past experience with a fresh perspective. Learn how to put your ideas into action and be persistent because achieving results takes time. In addition, do your homework. Understand the business agenda and close any gaps between what you are and what you could be. In other words, define your goals, then create and implement a personal development plan. Finally, demonstrate respect for others, and apply the golden rule. Achieving great results with great behavior enables your star to rise. You can begin the process right now with these specific steps:

- See the big picture. Know why your job was created, how it relates to your organization, and what opportunities it contains. You can positively influence outcomes through performance and achievement.

- Invest in your organization; make decisions as if you owned the company. Determine which actions promise the most significant impact, and then pursue them with zeal.

- Push your comfort zone by seeking challenges, finding the positive in negative situations, taking action, and learning from the past.

- Make time for people; understand the culture, values, and beliefs of the organization; keep things in perspective; and have fun.

- Inspire those around you to exceed expectations; also, convey a sense of urgency, and consistently drive issues to closure.

After you do all this, how do you ensure that you will be noticed? Ask how your company identifies and rewards top performers. Inquire as to whether there is a high-potential category. You should pursue an environment in which the best are recognized and valued. It should be an organization that provides career growth, lifelong learning, and development opportunities. You also want meaningful work, an opportunity to contribute, and an environment that prizes new ideas and fresh perspectives. In addition, you deserve honest feedback and the opportunity to provide the same in return. Finally, seek an organization that energizes and empowers you, encourages your good health, respects your point of view, and honors your performance. Many such organizations abound.

Implications for Practice: Though a business professional wrote this article, the advice rings true for nurses as well. Take the steps to stardom identified above and help your career grow.

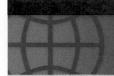

REAL WORLD INTERVIEW

Here are a few lessons I learned as a new graduate:

1. You will manage to get every single type of body fluid on you at one time or another (blood, trach gunk, fistula juice, stomach residual, stool, urine). Bring a pair of backup scrubs to work.

2. You learn from your mistakes. I was taking care of a patient on an insulin drip during the night shift. She was up all night long and her daughter didn't think too highly of the care she was getting. When the patient and her daughter finally fell asleep, I skipped her 3 A.M. Accucheck. Her 4 a.m. Accucheck was 27. Needless to say, I have never skipped an Accucheck since.

3. If a preceptor shows you something, don't say that he or she is doing it wrong and then pull out a policy book. Your preceptor will hate you for life.

4. Never pass up an opportunity to learn something, even if you think you have seen it before. Maybe someone will teach you a new and better way to do it.

5. You will think you are ready for your first really sick patient, but you are not. The senior staff will help you through it. I still replay my first really sick patient in my head and think back to all the things I wish I had done differently. Luckily, no one else dwells on it. I am my worst critic!

6. Find a person besides your preceptor whom you admire, maybe for their nursing skill, their personality, or their way of making everything look easy. Ask if he or she will mentor you. It doesn't need to be a super-serious conversation. I made mine a joke and asked a nurse if she would be my Nighttime Sensei. She accepted and to this day she has my back when things got crazy.

7. Always do the little things. I was a patient care tech before I was a nurse. I always make sure my rooms are stocked, everything is put away, my patient is clean, the patient's meds are in the drawer, etc. Little things like this can really help out your next coworker. There is nothing worse than walking into a patient's room and it looks like a bomb went off.

8. Always help out your coworkers. I work in an ICU, and there is a real sense of teamwork. As a new graduate, I always felt like I never had enough time to do my work, but I always made time to help the other nurses turn their patients, do a bath, move them to a chair, etc. That stuff doesn't take that long and your coworkers really appreciate it. Plus, next time you need help with something, easy or not, they will be there for you.

9. I think my first month off of orientation, I cried in the shower at least once a week. Some of it was about the patients I took care of, some was about working with not nice people, some of it was just because I needed to cry. I always tried to keep my emotions out of my workplace. Some people are very emotional at work, and it makes others uncomfortable. I am not saying that you can never cry at work or with a patient's family, but if you are crying during every shift, your coworkers will start to think that you can't handle your job.

10. I live by the mottos, "never show fear" and "do it right." Always walk into the patient's room with confidence. If you are doing something for the first time, run through it with someone experienced before going into the patient's room. You are taking care of someone's mom, dad, or child, and they are trusting you with their lives. Don't give them a reason to lose that trust.

Erin Mahoney, BSN, RN
Loyola University Hospital
Maywood, Illinois

KEY CONCEPTS

- The NCLEX-RN Test Plan reviews patient needs in the following areas: safe, effective care environment; physiologic integrity; psychosocial integrity; and health promotion and maintenance.

- The NCLEX-RN contains several new types of questions.

- Multiple factors are associated with NCLEX-RN performance as identified in Table 17-2.

- It is useful to have a plan to review any NCLEX-RN weaknesses.

- Organizational orientation is both general and unit based. Orientation is a time for developing strong relationships with preceptors and members of other disciplines, as well as for mastering competencies needed for safe patient care.

- Nurses receive performance feedback both informally and as part of periodic evaluations.

This input is valuable in developing personal goals.

- Newspapers, electronic media and the Internet, job fairs, and employment hot lines are all possible avenues for job opportunities.

- An effective resume will (1) get the employer's interest; (2) identify critical areas such as education, work experience, and special qualifications; (3) be tailored to the employer's needs; (4) create a favorable first impression about you and your abilities; (5) communicate that you are someone who is a good fit for the position; and (6) be visually appealing.

- When preparing for an interview, practice answering potential interview questions with a colleague, friend, or family member before the actual interview so that you have practiced answers to difficult questions.

KEY TERMS

feedback

resume

360-degree

REVIEW QUESTIONS

1. Which of the following is the best response to the interview question "What are your strengths?"
   A. "I have many. Where do you want me to begin?"
   B. "I have strong communication skills, both written and verbal, and I am someone who values completing a task."
   C. "I think I am well liked and get along with everyone."
   D. "Well, I am just a new nurse without many strengths right now, but I will be learning with this new job."

2. What is the primary function of a cover letter?
   A. to entice the prospective employer to become interested enough to read the resume
   B. to have a letter to include with your resume
   C. to include references that are not listed on a resume
   D. to reiterate all that is on your resume

3. A 16-year-old presents to the emergency department. The triage nurse finds that the teenager is legally married and signed the consent for

treatment form. What would be the appropriate INITIAL action by the nurse?

A. Refuse to see the patient until a parent or legal guardian can be contacted.

B. Withhold treatment until telephone consent can be obtained from the spouse.

C. Refer the patient to a community pediatric hospital emergency room.

D. Assess and treat in the same manner as any adult patient.

4. A patient had 20 mg of Lasix (furosemide) PO at 10 AM. Which would be essential for the nurse to include in the change-of-shift report?

A. The patient lost two pounds.

B. The patient's potassium level is 4 mEq/liter.

C. The patient's urine output was 1500 cc in five hours.

D. The patient is to receive another dose of Lasix at 10 PM.

REVIEW ACTIVITIES

1. Set up a group to study for the NCLEX with several of your friends. Have each member of the group buy an NCLEX review book from a different publisher. Practice answering questions for one to two hours daily separately. Don't mark your answers in the review book. Share your study schedule and your review books with each other to encourage each other and increase your exposure to various authors' test questions.

2. You are graduating in two months from a nursing program. Develop a resume using the format in this chapter.

3. You are a new nurse who has been asked to interview for a position on the orthopedic floor. Develop a cover letter expressing interest in the position. Make a list of possible interview questions.

EXPLORING THE WEB

- There are many Web sites specific to nursing employment opportunities. Try some of these:
  www.americanmobile.com
  www.rnwanted.com
  www.healthcareerbuilder.com
  www.healthcarerecruitment.com
  www.healthcaretraveler.com

- Look up several of these nursing sites:
  Association of Pediatric Oncology Nurses:
  www.apon.org
  Association of Rehabilitation Nurses:
  www.rehabnurse.org
  Association of Women's Health, Obstetric and Neonatal Nurses:
  www.awhonn.org
  Trauma Nursing:
  www.trauma.com

- Check this site for job opportunities:
  healthcare.monster.com

- Check this site:
  National Student Nurses' Association:
  www.nsna.org

- Go to:
  www.learningext.com.
  Note: NCSBN's Review for the NCLEX is offered through this NCSBN learning extension. This self-paced, online review features NCLEX-style questions, interactive exercises, topic-specific course exams, and a diagnostic pretest that can help you develop a personal study plan. Visit this site every Monday to see its new NCLEX-RN test question samples.

- Visit:
  www.nursecredentialing.org
  Click on *find a facility.*

- Check this guide to education in nursing:
  www.allnursingschools.com

REFERENCES

Aiken, L. (2002). Superior outcomes for magnet hospitals: The evidence base. In M. L. McClure & A. S. Hinshaw (Eds.), *Magnet hospitals revisited: Attraction and retention of professional nurses* (pp. 61–81). Washington, DC: American Nurses Publishing.

Albany Medical Center. (2001). Emergency department competency-based orientation tool sample page excerpt. Albany, NY: Author.

Albany Medical Center. (2001). Registered professional nurse general orientation schedule template—week one. Albany, NY: Author.

American Hospital Association. (AHA). (2006). *Statistics and studies: Fast facts on U.S. hospitals.* Retrieved May 6, 2006, from www.aha.org/ahresource-center.

American Nurses Credentialing Center. (ANCC). (2006). *Benefits of becoming a magnet-designated facility.* Retrieved May 6, 2006, from nursingworld.org/ancc/magnet/benes.html

Bacon, D. (2005, Dec.). Results of the 2005 AORN salary survey—trends for perioperative nursing. www.ncbi.nlm.nih.gov/pubmed/16478080?ordinalpos=1&itool=EntrezSystem2.PEntrez.Pubmed.Pubmed_ResultsPanel.Pubmed_DefaultReportPanel.Pubmed_RVDocSum AORN J. 82(6):965-72.

Bauer, J. (2005, Oct.). 2005 earnings survey: how does your pay stack up? www.ncbi.nlm.nih.gov/pubmed/16259186?ordinalpos=2&itool=EntrezSystem2.PEntrez.Pubmed.Pubmed_ResultsPanel.Pubmed_DefaultReportPanel.Pubmed_RVDocSum RN. 68(10):46-52.

Brunt B.A. (2005, Nov.–Dec.). Models, measurement, and strategies in developing critical-thinking skills. www.ncbi.nlm.nih.gov/pubmed/16372714?ordinalpos=4&itool=EntrezSystem2.PEntrez.Pubmed.Pubmed_ResultsPanel.Pubmed_DefaultReportPanel.Pubmed_RVDocSum Contin Educ Nurs. 36(6):255-62. Review.

Driscoll, R. (2003). Tame test anxiety: Powerful stress reduction means more gain with less pain. CD-ROM. Westside Publishing.

Hart, K. (2006). Student extra: The employment interview: Tips for success selecting an employer for the perfect fit. *American Journal of Nursing, 106*(4), 72AAA–72CCC.

Holden, J. (2006). How can we improve the nursing work environment? *The American Journal of Maternal/Child Nursing, 31*(1), 34–38.

Johnson, S. (2000). *Taking the Anxiety out of Taking Tests.* Barnes & Noble.

Kramer, M. (1974). *Reality shock: Why nurses leave nursing.* St. Louis, MO: Mosby.

Kelly, P., & Hernandez, G. (2010). Medication Study Guide Starter. Unpublished manuscript.

Lannon, J. M. (2000). *Technical Communication.* (8th ed.). Upper Saddle River, NJ: Addison-Wesley.

Mee, C. L. (2006, Oct.). Nursing 2006 salary survey. www.ncbi.nlm.nih.gov/pubmed/17019347?ordinalpos=1&itool=EntrezSystem2.PEntrez.Pubmed.Pubmed_ResultsPanel.Pubmed_DefaultReportPanel.Pubmed_RVDocSum Nursing. 36(10):46-51.

National Council of State Boards of Nursing (2007) NCLEX-RN Examination. Available at www.ncsbn.oprg/RN_test_plan_2007_web_.pdf accessed 12-03-08.

NCLEX-RN Examination. (2007). Test plan for the National Council Licensure Examination for Registered Nurses. Chicago, IL: National Council of State Boards of Nursing. Available at www.ncsbn.org/1287.htm. Accessed October 7, 2008.

Olmstead, J. (2007, Mar.). Predict future success with structured interviews. *Nursing Management, 38*(3), 52–53.

O'Malley, P. A. (2008, June). Profile of a professional. *Nursing Management, 39*(6), 24–27.

Polifko-Harris, K. (2003). Career Planning. In P. Kelly-Heidenthal, *Nursing Leadership and Management* (2nd ed.). Clifton Park, NY: Delmar Cengage Learning.

Snodgrass, S. G. (2001, June 10). Wish you were a star? Become one! *Chicago Tribune,* D1.

Stein, A. M. (2005). NCLEX-RN Review (5th ed.). Clifton Park, NY: Delmar Cengage Learning.

Tetterton, S. K. (2006). Interviewing potential staff. Retrieved January 4, 2006, from www.libsci.sc.edu/boclass/clis724/SpecialLibrariesHandbook/tetterton.htm

U.S. News & World Report. (2005). *America's best hospitals: 2005 methodology.* Retrieved May 9, 2006, from www.usnews.com.

SUGGESTED READINGS

Aucoin, J. W., & Treas, L. (2005). Assumptions and realities of the NCLEX-RN. *Nursing Education Perspective, 26*(5), 268–271.

Beeman, P. B., & Waterhouse, J. K. (2003). Post-graduation factors predicting NCLEX-RN success. *Nurse Educator, 28*(6), 257–260.

Bondmass, M. D., Moonie, S., & Kowalski, S. (2008, Apr.1). Comparing NET and ERI standardized exam scores between baccalaureate graduates who pass or fail the NCLEX-RN. *Int J Nurs Educ Scholarsh., 5,* Article16. Epub.

Bonis, S., Taft, L., & Wendler, M. C. (2007, Mar.–Apr.). Strategies to promote success on the NCLEX-RN: An evidence-based approach using the ACE Star Model of Knowledge Transformation. *Nurs Educ Perspect., 28*(2), 82–7.

Crow, C. S., Handley, M., Morrison, R. S., & Shelton, M. M. (2004). Requirements and interventions used by BSN programs to promote and predict NCLEX-RN success: A national study. *Journal of Professional Nursing, 20*(3), 174–186.

Cunningham, H., Stacciarini, J. M., & Towle, S. (2004). Strategies to promote success on the NCLEX-RN for students with English as a second language. *Nurse Educator, 29*(1), 15–19.

Daley, L. K., Kirkpatrick, B. L., Frazier, S. K., Chung, M. L., & Moser, D. K. (2003). Predictors of NCLEX-RN success in a baccalaureate nursing program as a foundation for remediation. *Journal of Nursing Education, 42*(9), 390–398.

Davenport, N. C. (2007, Jan.-Feb.). A comprehensive approach to NCLEX-RN success. *Nurs Educ Perspect., 28*(1), 30–3.

DiBartolo, M. C., & Seldomridge, L. A. (2008, Sept.–Oct.). A review of intervention studies to promote NCLEX-RN success of baccalaureate students. *Comput Inform Nurs., 26*(5 Suppl), 78–83S.

Downey, T. A. (2003). Predictive NCLEX success with the HESI exit examination: Fourth annual validity study. *Computer, Informatics, Nursing, 21*(6), 296–297; author reply 297–299.

Downey, T. A., & Nibert, A. T. (2003). Indicia: Letters to the editor and reply. *Computers, Informatics, Nursing, 21*(6), 296–299.

Downey, T. A. (2008, Sept.-Oct.). Predictive NCLEX success with the HESI Exit Examination: Fourth annual validity study. *Comput Inform Nurs., 26*(5 Suppl), 35S–36S; author reply 36S–38S.

English, J. B., & Gordon, D. K. (2004). Successful student remediation following repeated failures on the HESI exam. *Nurse Educator, 29*(6), 266–268.

Frith, K. H., Sewell, J. P., Clark, D. J. (2008, Sept.–Oct.,). Best practices in NCLEX-RN readiness preparation for baccalaureate student success. *Comput Inform Nurs., 26*(5 Suppl), 46S–53S.

Giddens, J., & Gloeckner, G. W. (2005). The relationship of critical thinking to performance on the NCLEX-RN. *Journal of Nursing Education, 44*(2), 85–90.

Griffiths, M. J., Papastral, K., Czekanski, K., & Hagan, K. (2004). The lived experience of NCLEX failure. *Journal of Nursing Education, 43*(7), 322–325.

Higgins, B. (2005). Strategies for lowering attrition rates and raising NCLEX-RN pass rates. *Journal of Nursing Education, 44*(12), 541–547.

Impollonia, M. (2004). How to impress nursing recruiters to get the job you want. *Imprint, 51*(1), 11–15.

Lewis, C. (2005). *Predictive accuracy of the HESI Exit Exam on NCLEX-RN pass rates and effects of progression policies on nursing student Exit Exam scores.* Unpublished doctoral dissertation, Texas Woman's University, Denton, TX.

Lyons, E. M. (2008, June 5). Examining the effects of problem-based learning and NCLEX-RN scores on the critical thinking skills of associate degree nursing students in a Southeastern Community College. *Int J Nurs Educ Scholarsh., 5,* Article 21. Epub.

McDowell, B. M. (2008, Apr.). KATTS: A framework for maximizing NCLEX-RN performance. *J Nurs Educ., 47*(4), 183–6.

Miller, J. C. (2003). Twelve frequently asked questions about the NCLEX-RN. *Imprint, 50*(1), 73–75.

Miller, J. C. (2004). Tips on passing the NCLEX-RN. *Imprint, 51*(1), 61–62.

Miller, J. C. (2005). Tips on taking the NCLEX-RN. *Imprint, 52*(1), 28–32.

Morton, A. M. (2008, Sep.–Oct.). Improving NCLEX scores with structured learning assistance. *Comput Inform Nurs., 26*(5 Suppl), 89S–91S.

Morrison, S., Adamson, C., Nibert, A. T., & Hsia, S. (2004). HESI exams: An overview of reliability and validity. *Computers, Informatics, Nursing, 22*(4), 220–226.

NCLEX practice questions. (2005). *Nursing, 35*(8), 68–70.

Nibert, A., Young, A., & Adamson, C. (2002). A fourth validity study of the HESI Exit Exam. *Computer Information for Nursing, 20*(6), 261–267.

Nibert, A. (2005). Benchmarking for progression: Implications for students, faculty, and administrators. In L. Caputi (Ed.), *Teaching nursing: The art and science* (Vol. 3, pp. 314–335). Chicago: College of DuPage Press.

Nibert, A., Young, A., & Britt, R. (2003). The HESI Exit Exam: Progression benchmark and remediation guide. *Nurse Educator, 28*(3), 141–145.

Nibert, A. T., Young, A., & Adamson, C. (2008, Sept.–Oct.). Predicting NCLEX success with the HESI Exit Exam: fourth annual validity study. *Comput Inform Nurs., 26*(5 Suppl), 28S–34S.

Nibert, A. T., Young, A. (2008, Sept.-Oct.). A third study on predicting NCLEX success with the HESI exit exam. *Comput Inform Nurs., 26*(5 Suppl), 21S–27S.

O'Neill, T. R., Marks, C. M., & Reynolds, M. (2005). Reevaluating the NCLEX-RN passing standard. *Journal of Nursing Measures, 13*(2), 147–165.

Poorman, S. G., & Mastorovich, M. L. (2004). A clinical strategy to help students with leadership/management NCLEX questions. *Nurse Educator, 29*(4), 142–143.

Poster, E. C. (2004). Psychiatric nursing at risk: The new NCLEX-RN test plan. *Perspective Psychiatric Care, 40*(2), 43–44.

Reising, D. L. (2003). The relationship between computer testing during a nursing program and NCLEX performance. *Computers, Informatics, Nursing, 21*(6), 326–329.

Schwarz, K. A. (2005). Making the grade: Help staff pass the NCLEX-RN. *Nursing Management, 36*(3), 38–44.

Seldomridge, L. A., & Dibartolo, M. C. (2004). Can success and failure be predicted for baccalaureate graduates on the computerized NCLEX-RN? *Journal of Professional Nursing, 20*(6), 361–368.

Sifford, S., McDaniel, D. M. (2007, Jan.–Feb.). Results of a remediation program for students at risk for failure on the NCLEX exam. *Nurs Educ Perspect., 28*(1), 34–6.

Sitzman, K. L. (2007, Jul.). Diversity and the NCLEX-RN: A double-loop approach. *J Transcult Nurs., 18*(3), 271–6. Review.

Spector, N., & Sheets, V. (2004). NCLEX results to disclose or not disclose. *JONAS Health Law Ethics Regulations, 6*(2), 38–39.

Spurlock, D. R., Jr., & Hanks, C. (2004). Establishing progression policies with the HESI Exit Examination: A review of the evidence. *Journal of Nursing Education, 43*(12), 539–545.

Spurlock, D. R., Jr., Hunt, L. A. (2008, Apr.). A study of the usefulness of the HESI Exit Exam in predicting NCLEX-RN failure. *J Nurs Educ., 47*(4), 157–66.

Sutherland, J. A., Hamilton, M. J., & Goodman, N. (2007, Aug.). Affirming At-Risk Minorities for Success (ARMS): Retention, graduation, and success on the NCLEX-RN. *J Nurs Educ., 46*(8), 347–53.

Uyehara, J., Magnussen, L., Itano, J., Zhang S. (2007, Jan.–Mar.). Facilitating program and NCLEX-RN success in a generic BSN program. *Nurs Forum, 42*(1), 31–8.

Waterhouse, J. K., & Beeman, P. B. (2003). Predicting NCLEX-RN success: Can it be simplified? *Nursing Education Perspective, 24*(1), 35–39.

Wood, R. M. (2005). Student computer competence and the NCLEX-RN examination: Strategies for success. *Computer, Informatics, Nursing, 23*(5), 241–243.

Yin, T., & Burger, C. (2003). Predictors of NCLEX-RN success of associate degree nursing graduates. *Nurse Educator, 28*(5), 232–236.

CHAPTER 18

Career Planning and Achieving Balance

To Nurse
To Care
To Solace
To Touch
To Feel
To Hurt
To Need
To Heal others,
As well as ourselves.

(Carol Battaglia, 1996)

OBJECTIVES

Upon completion of this chapter, the reader should be able to:

1. Identify strategies for professional growth.
2. Discuss certification and clinical ladders.
3. Define health.
4. Identify the six concepts of health, i.e., physical, intellectual, emotional, professional, social, and spiritual health.
5. Describe selected strategies to maintain physical, intellectual, emotional, professional, social, and spiritual health.

You have just started in your new nursing position. You are excited and want to do a good job, as well as plan for the future. You want to continue to grow professionally and yet have a life outside nursing also. You are thinking about many questions. Where do you see yourself 1, 5, or 10 years from now? What opportunities exist for certification and additional education? How can you ensure some balance and less stress in your life both inside and outside nursing?

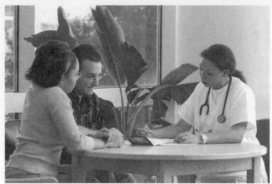

Delmar/Cengage Learning

At the turn of the twenty-first century, the nursing demand far exceeded the supply of registered professional nurses. As of 2005, one in ten nursing jobs were unfilled, and according to the Bureau of Labor and Statistics, the nursing shortage will reach one million by 2012 (Erickson et al., 2005).

Statistical data from 2004 showed that the average age of nurses was 46.8 years; the average age at graduation for recent RN graduates was 29.6 years; and the number of RNs who are advanced practice nurses is 240,461 or 8.3% of the total RN population. In December 2005, the NLN (National League for Nursing) released statistics indicating that while there was a significant increase of almost 20% in enrollment for all types of nursing programs, the number of qualified instructors/professors continued to decline (www.nln.org). Nursing programs rejected 32,617 qualified applicants due to lack of qualified nurse educators available to teach these future generations of RNs, according to preliminary survey data released by the American Association of Colleges of Nursing (AACN) (www.aacn.nche.edu).

An issue confronting nursing has been identifying what the appropriate entry-level educational degree should be, and what a nurse really is because of the many levels of educational preparation. In December 1965, the American Nurses Association (ANA) House of Delegates (HOD) adopted a motion that the ANA continue to work toward baccalaureate education as the educational foundation for professional nursing practice. By 1985, the ANA HOD agreed to urge State Nursing Associations to establish the BS degree with a major in nursing as the minimum educational requirement for licensure and to retain the title of registered nurse (RN) (American Nurses Association [ANA], 2000). To date, there are still a variety of paths an individual can take to become an RN. These include a two-year associate degree, a three-year diploma, and a four-year baccalaureate degree.

A major advancement within nursing has been the emergence of several areas of advanced nursing practice, i.e., the certified registered nurse anesthetist (CRNA), the clinical nurse specialist (CNS), the nurse practitioner (NP), and the certified nurse-midwife (CNM). The profession has also significantly upgraded its educational, clinical, research, and managerial focus. This chapter will examine career planning and maintaining balance in your nursing and non-nursing life.

CAREER PLANNING

Career planning is an ongoing process that involves personal and professional self-assessment, setting goals, and regular self-evaluation.

Determining your goals using a common SMART acronym for goal setting is useful. SMART stands for Specific (S), Measurable (M), Achievable (A), Realistic (R), and Timely (T) goal setting. Being SMART will help you describe specifically what you want to accomplish with your strategic planning for your career. For example, when you are

TABLE 18-1	SMART CAREER PLANNING GOALS
Specific	Employment as an RN in an Emergency Department (ED)
Measurable	Function independently full-time
Achievable	Employment at hospital that allows recently graduated RNs to work in ED
Realistic	Presence of other new graduates that were able to achieve goal
Timely	Achieve goal within two years

planning your career, you may want to work in a specialty patient care unit after graduation. Your SMART career planning goals may be as follows in Table 18-1. You may want to also include goals for continuing your education. Visit www.allnursingschools.com and search "All Programs," for listings of bachelor, masters, nurse practitioner, and doctoral nursing programs. Career planners suggest setting short-term goals for one to three years, intermediate goals for three to five years, and long-term goals for six to twenty years.

CERTIFICATION

Certification in nursing represents an example of professional credentialing and is a voluntary process undertaken by practicing nurses. It is a marker of the knowledge and experience of a professional RN and is more than just a symbolic title. The American Board of Nursing Specialists (ABNS) defines the certification process as the formal recognition of the specialized knowledge, skills, and experience demonstrated by the achievement of standards identified by a nursing specialty to promote optimal health outcomes (Stromberg et al., 2005). Basic eligibility requirements for specialty nursing certification are available at www.nursecredentialing.org.

Professional certification, through a wide variety of organizations, is also monitored by the American Board of Nursing Specialties (www.abns.org) and includes the clinical component of nursing (bedside nurses, advance practice nurses, and so on) as well as nursing administration. Several of the larger certifying organizations include the ANA; American Association of Nurse Anesthetists (AANA); National Association of Pediatric Nurse Associates and Practitioners (NAPNAP); Association of Women's Health, Obstetric and Neonatal Nurses (AWHONN); and The Association of Critical Care Nurses (ACCN).

COMPETENCE

Professional growth and practice require competent staff. **Competency** is defined as possession of a required skill, knowledge, qualification, or capacity (Merriam-Webster, 2005) and is best determined in practice by a group of one's peers. Competency of professional staff can be ensured through credentialing processes developed either at an agency or through certification by a national nursing organization. See Table 18-2.

CLINICAL LADDER

A clinical or career ladder may be in place in an agency. Although the criteria may vary, most programs have three or four distinct levels. **Clinical ladders** offer the nurse the opportunity to seek promotion in a specific track, within a clinical, educational, research, or managerial focus. For example, to be promoted from a new Graduate Level I to a Level II RN, the nurse may be required to complete a specialty course such as Advanced Cardiac Life Support (ACLS) or EKG interpretation, join a unit- or hospital-based committee, and finish

TABLE 18-2	CERTIFICATIONS AVAILABLE FROM AMERICAN NURSES ASSOCIATION

Advanced Practice
Nurse Practitioners

- Acute Care
- Adult
- Adult Psychiatric/Mental Health
- Advanced Diabetes Management
- Family
- Family Psychiatric/Mental Health
- Gerontological
- Pediatric

Clinical Nurse Specialists

- Advanced Diabetes Management
- Adult Health (*formerly known as Medical-Surgical*)
- Adult Psychiatric/Mental Health
- Child/Adolescent Psychiatric/Mental Health
- Gerontological
- Pediatric
- Public/Community Health

Other Advanced-Level Exams

- Advanced Diabetes Management—Dietician
- Advanced Diabetes Management—Pharmacist
- Nursing Administration, Advanced

BS in Nursing or Higher Degree

- Cardiac/Vascular Nurse
- Gerontological Nurse
- Informatics Nurse
- Medical-Surgical Nurse
- Nursing Administration
- Nursing Professional Development
- Pediatric Nurse
- Perinatal Nurse
- Psychiatric/Mental Health Nurse
- Public/Community Health Nurse

Associate Degree or Diploma in Nursing

- Cardiac/Vascular Nurse
- Gerontological Nurse
- Medical-Surgical Nurse
- Pediatric Nurse
- Perinatal Nurse
- Psychiatric Mental Health Nurse

Diploma, Associate, Baccalaureate or higher degree in Nursing

- Ambulatory Care Nurse
- Nursing Case Management
- Pain Management

Source: Certification. American Nurses Credentialing Center, 2009. Available at www.nursecredentialing.org/Certification.aspx.

the preceptor course. Clinical ladders offer an objective way to measure a nurse's achievements.

The Colorado Differentiated Practice Model (Figure 18-1) builds on the work of Benner (1984) regarding career ladder stages. Stage I is characterized as the entry/learning stage. Stage II is characterized by the individual who competently demonstrates acceptable performance adapting to time and resource constraints. Stage III is characterized by the individual who is proficient. And Stage IV is characterized by the individual who is an expert. The stages in this model are specifically defined by behaviors that are consistently exhibited or practiced over a defined period of time.

Colorado Differentiated Practice Model

The Colorado Differentiated Practice Model for Nursing has a separate clinical ladder for the six preparatory backgrounds depicted on the conceptual model (Diagram 1). The framework for each educational ladder has four weighted components as follows:
- Competency Statements 60%
- Skills 10%
- Institutional Goals 15%
- Professional Activities 15%

Conceptual model

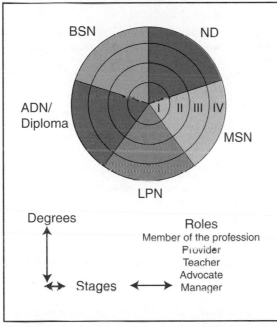

Sample ladder

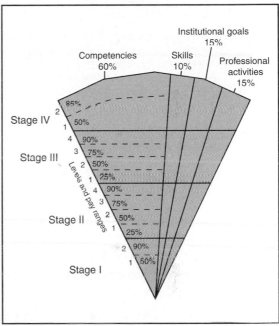

Diagram 1

Diagram 2

Figure 18-1 Colorado differentiated practice model. (*Source:* Courtesy Marie E. Miller, Colorado Nursing Task Force, 2001).

HEALTHY LIVING– ACHIEVING BALANCE

Nursing is a caring profession. Nurses spend their days helping others, many times at the expense of themselves. But, if there is nothing left for nurses, they will not be able to maintain the strength to care for their patients. Florence Nightingale described health as "being well and using every power the individual possesses to the fullest extent" (Nightingale, 1969 [1860], p. 334). The World Health Organization

(2006) describes **health** as a "state of complete physical, social, and mental well-being, and not merely the absence of disease or infirmity. Health is a resource for everyday life, not the object of living."

GOALS FOR HEALTHY PEOPLE 2010

In January 2000, more than 1,500 individuals, health professionals, and organizations convened in Washington, D.C. to discuss goals for health promotion and disease prevention for the United States population (U.S. Department of Health and Human Services, 2001). Healthy People 2010 has

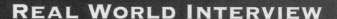

REAL WORLD INTERVIEW

There are five levels of our clinical ladder, which is similar to Benner's novice to expert model. The RN Is or novices are new graduates in orientation. The experts are the clinical specialists. A lot of them have also become nurse practitioners so that the organization can receive some reimbursement for their patient care services. This is a good thing because otherwise I'm afraid we wouldn't have these expert nurses anymore. They are the true mentors for nursing staff, especially when you are working with a very complex or difficult patient situation.

Staff nurses also mentor each other. During orientation, your preceptor guides you along the path from RN I to RN II. When you decide you'd like to advance to RN III, you can choose another mentor. RN IIIs provide much more clinical leadership for staff and for the overall unit. I decided I was ready to be promoted to that level when other staff consistently were coming to me for clinical guidance and with patient care questions. Now, as an RN III, I am the chairperson of our unit-credentialing committee, which is part of the quality council of our shared governance model.

Our clinical ladder uses a portfolio as the main tool to evaluate the nurse's readiness to advance. When you are an RN I in orientation, you are first introduced to the idea of a portfolio and how to put it together. It is difficult at first, as people do not know what is expected. However, after that first time when you are promoted from an RN I to an RN II, it becomes easier. You just build on what is already in the portfolio.

A portfolio should include the following:

Licenses	Examples of participation in development of
Your resume	the team plan of care
Letters of reference	Exemplars
Evaluations	CEU certificates
Clinical documentation of patient care	Presentations
Validations for competencies related to technical skills (medication administration, IV therapy)	Publications

The portfolio tells the story of your practice. When a group of people are ready for promotion, the members of the credentialing committee meet. We review the portfolios and make recommendations related to advancement. The nurse manager is a member of this committee. She always reviews the portfolio and gives us her feedback even if she is unable to attend the credentialing meeting. I enjoy reading the exemplars the most. Exemplars are mini-stories that paint the pictures of each nurse's practice, and they are all so different.

Stacey Conley,
RN, BS, Staff Nurse
Cooperstown, New York

developed ten leading health indicators which will be used to measure the overall goals for the nation. The indicators are physical activity, responsible sexual behavior, environmental quality, overweight and obesity, mental health, immunization, tobacco use, injury and violence, access to health care, and substance abuse (www.healthypeople.gov).

AREAS OF HEALTH

Health is a complex and dynamic state of being. A healthy person must balance various aspects in life to achieve and maintain good health. When one area of life is affected, other areas of health are also affected. There is overlap among each area, but for purposes of discussion in this chapter, health has been divided into the following six elements: physical health, intellectual health, emotional health, professional health, social health, and spiritual health. The tool in Table 18-3 will assist you in identifying your health trends in each of the six areas of health.

PHYSICAL HEALTH

Physical health, the first element of health, encompasses nutrition as well as exercise, coupled with a balanced amount of sleep. Physical health also includes health promotion and disease prevention behaviors such as avoiding smoking, maintaining a healthy

TABLE 18-3	HEALTH ASSESSMENT TOOL		
Physical Health		**Yes**	**No**
1. I exercise at least 30 minutes daily.			
2. My BMI meets the optimal health guidelines.			
3. I sleep eight hours a night.			
4. My immunizations are up-to-date.			
5. I avoid risky behaviors, e.g., smoking, drugs, tanning booths, unprotected sex.			
6. I have regular health screenings, dental cleanings, Pap tests, mammograms, and do monthly testicular or breast self-examinations.			
Intellectual Health			
7. I plan to purchase a home soon.			
8. I read at least one book a month and practice critical thinking.			
9. I have a 401K or 403b savings plan for retirement.			
10. I know how much money I have invested in Social Security.			
11. I have invested in diversified mutual stock and bond funds.			
12. I save 10% of my income for the future.			
13. I have a hobby I enjoy.			
Emotional Health			
14. I have developed strategies to deal with my own anger.			
15. I have developed strategies to deal with the anger of others.			
16. I work well with others.			
17. I practice stress management techniques.			
18. I try to be empathetic and sense what others are feeling.			

(continues)

TABLE 18-3	HEALTH ASSESSMENT TOOL (CONTINUED)

	Yes	No
Emotional Health		
19. I try to find a reason to laugh daily.		
20. I avoid thought distortions.		
Professional Health		
21. I have professional goals including certification and additional nursing education.		
22. I have a mentor.		
23. I have attended at least three workshops in the past year.		
24. I subscribe to three nursing journals.		
25. I belong to at least one professional organization.		
26. I use appropriate personal protective equipment.		
27. I never recap a needle.		
28. I follow safe patient handling policies when moving patients.		
29. I follow standards of care when handling gaseous waste, disinfectants, and chemotherapy.		
30. I follow standards of care in dealing with lasers, radiation equipment, and environmental hazards.		
31. I avoid workplace violence.		
Social Health		
32. I go out with my friends at least once a week.		
33. I see my family regularly.		
34. I have at least one friend I can confide in.		
35. I have a wide diversity of professional, family, neighborhood, and church friends.		
36. Not all my friends are nurses.		
37. I do volunteer work.		
Spiritual Health		
38. I pray or meditate every day.		
39. I believe in a higher power.		
40. I attend meetings at a place of worship regularly.		
41. I read spiritual books or spend time in quiet meditation daily.		
42. I maintain a daily journal.		
43. I seek help from professional counselors as needed.		

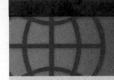

REAL WORLD INTERVIEW

As NPs face the new millennium, it is advisable to listen to the wisdom of the famous author on China, Pearl Buck, who said, "To understand today, you have to search yesterday." Further, to envision the future, think "outside the box" creatively, constructively, and globally. Unfortunately, most people hate change; so do professionals. By their very nature, professionals can become myopic, territorial, and conservative. Some that are so resistant to change become arrogant, self-important, and greedy. Nursing must face the future differently. Tomorrow's practitioners will face globalization, not only of economics but of every field of human endeavor. Demographics, technological advances, transportation, and communication will expand beyond imagination and at lightning speed. Health information will no longer belong exclusively to the health professions. The Internet will see to that. The challenge for NPs is to be proactive rather than reactive in creating a social, cultural, political, and physical environment in which to successfully live, work, and thrive as a responsible member of the new society and as an advocate for our patients and their families. So, thoroughly examine the past, keep the enduring human values of caring, compassion, and courage in nursing, listen to your best teachers—the patients—and create your own future accordingly.

Loretta Ford,
EdD, RN, FAAN Founder, Nurse Practitioner Program
Rochester, New York

body mass index with healthy nutrition and exercise, and having annual Pap smears and other screening procedures that detect health problems early.

BODY MASS INDEX CALCULATION

You can assess your body weight in relation to your height by calculating your body mass index (BMI). You can calculate this at *www.nhlbi.nih.gov;* search for Body Mass Index. The National Institutes of Health has established the following guidelines for interpretation of the BMI:

- 30 and above is obese
- 25 to 29.9 is overweight
- 18.5 to 24.9 is optimal health
- Below 18.5 is considered underweight

SLEEP

Sleep is another component of physical health. It is not uncommon for nurses to sleep less than 8 hours per night. Nurses who work nights may find it especially difficult to sleep for an uninterrupted

block of time. Nurses who are constantly changing shifts are more susceptible to sleep deprivation. It is estimated that it can take from 4 to 6 weeks to change sleeping patterns. In spite of this, nurses may work various shifts within a week. If it is necessary to swing to a different shift, it is best to rotate from days to evenings to nights. People generally adapt better if shift rotation is done clockwise (Frank 2005; Hughes & Rogers, 2004).

Sleep-deprived individuals become petulant and find it difficult to remember or concentrate on the simplest tasks. Nurses who work more than 12 hours a day or commit to more than 60 hours per week are at the greatest risk of making errors that can impact patient safety (Institute of Medicine, 2004). Patient safety is the utmost concern. The drive home after work for a nurse can be equally as dangerous. For each extra shift worked during one month, there is a 9.1% increased risk of a motor vehicle accident during the commute home from work. Nurses who work rotating shifts are at the greatest risk of fatigue compared to those committed to one shift. Nurses who rotate to evenings or nights are almost twice as likely to nod off while driving home (Frank, 2005). A period of twenty-four hours of wakefulness is equivalent to a blood alcohol level of 0.10% (Dawson & Reid, 1997).

How do you know if you are sleep deprived? Assess your sleepiness index by answering eight simple questions using the Epworth Sleepiness Scale at the following Web site: provigil.com. Adapted from Johns MW. A new method for measuring daytime sleepiness: the Epworth Sleepiness Scale. *Sleep.* 1991;14(6):540-545. Test your

knowledge regarding sleep deprivation with the tools and quizzes at the National Sleep Foundation Web site, www.sleepfoundation.org. Search for Tools and Quizzes.

INTELLECTUAL HEALTH

Intellectual health is the second element of health and encompasses those activities that maintain intellectual curiosity. Intellectually healthy people are able to think critically and make sound decisions. They read, have hobbies, learn from experience, and are flexible and remain open to new ideas. For

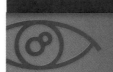

CRITICAL THINKING 18-1

Consider the ten Healthy People 2010 Indicators at www.healthypeople.gov. How is your personal behavior related to each of the indicators? How can you do better? How can you help your family, friends, and community do better? Keep a diary for one week on how you are doing on five or more of the indicators. The other Healthy People 2010 Indicators are substance abuse, injury and violence, environmental quality, immunization, and access to health care. See Figure 18-2 for a sample diary. At the end of the week, assess to see how well you have taken care of yourself. Is this a typical week? Do you need to make any changes? Were there any surprises? You can also record for several weeks and compare the outcomes.

	Physical Activity	Overweight and Obesity	Tobacco Use	Responsible Sexual Behavior	Mental Health	Other
Monday						
Tuesday						
Wednesday						
Thursday						
Friday						
Saturday						
Sunday						

Figure 18-2 Healthy People 2010 diary. *Source:* Leading health indicators. Healthy people 2010. (2010). available at www.healthypeople.gov

purposes of this chapter, the term *intellectual health* also includes doing personal financial planning.

PERSONAL FINANCIAL PLANNING

The first step in personal financial planning is to identify your annual salary. The average nursing salary for RNs is $58,600. For nurses with five or fewer years experience, the mean annual income is $43,500 (Mee, 2005).

Next, begin to think about the percentage of your salary you want to save; most experts recommend 10% to 15%. There is no better time than now to invest in your future. Now is the time to begin saving for such things as a home, your children's education, and retirement. A nurse who invests $2,000 yearly at an 8% annual rate of return beginning at age 20 will earn over $850,000 by age 65 versus a nurse who makes the same yearly investment but begins at age 30. The latter nurse will earn only about $350,000 by age 65.

Note also that a nurse who is making $50,000 annually will make $1,800,000 in a thirty-year working career. If this nurse invests $200 per month at 12% interest for the next 30 years, the nurse will have more than $1,000,000 in a retirement account at age sixty-five.

Savings for retirement are three-pronged: (1) Social Security funds, (2) employee retirement funds, and (3) additional personal savings. You should annually check the accuracy of your Social Security account by reviewing the information sent to you by the Social Security Administration, available at *www.ssa.gov*.

EMPLOYEE RETIREMENT FUNDS

The most common retirement funds are the 401K or 403b plans. The only difference between the two is that the 403b is a plan offered by a nonprofit organization and the 401K is offered by a for-profit organization. Otherwise, the two plans are exactly alike. For purposes of this discussion, the term *401K* will be used.

Both the employee and employer contribute retirement money to a **401K**. This is a great way to save because some health care institutions may match the funds that you contribute. Once your money is put into the fund, it is tax sheltered, meaning you do not pay any taxes on the amount contributed until it is withdrawn. For example, if you earn $58,000 per year and contribute $5,800 to the 401K, you will be taxed on only $52,200 of income. If the money is withdrawn before you reach the age of 59½, you will pay a 10% federal penalty. This is an incentive to keep the money in the account until retirement; the plan should be considered a long-term investment.

Once the money is in the fund, you must decide how the company administering the plan will invest it for you. You have two basic choices: bond mutual funds and stock mutual funds. Each of these investment opportunities has risks and benefits. Many financial advisors recommend diversifying and including a mix of these funds in your planning depending on your age. Several reliable information sources rank mutual funds for quality. These include the annual ratings by *Consumer Reports* and the Morningstar ratings available through the Internet. (See "Exploring the Web" at the end of this chapter.)

Individual Retirement Account (IRA). Another type of retirement fund is the individual retirement account (IRA). This account is an option for anyone with sufficient employment income. Contributions could not exceed $5,000 per year (for 2008). This fund may or may not be tax deductible, depending on what other retirement accounts you held and which type of IRA you opened. There are two kinds of IRAs: the traditional IRA and the Roth. The **Roth IRA** was first introduced in 1998. A Roth IRA is taxed prior to the investment but grows tax-free and there is no penalty for early withdrawal.

PERSONAL SAVINGS AND REAL ESTATE

After investing in retirement funds, you also have a few more options for investment. You can open a **money market account**, checking account, and/or a savings account.

You also have the option to invest in stock or bond mutual funds or individual stocks or bonds outside of your retirement account. You can start your research by reviewing Valueline at your local library (see "Exploring the Web" at the end of this chapter).

The key to successful investment is to diversify, meaning to spread your money around in many different types of investment options, stocks, bonds, mutual funds, and so on.

Owning your own home is a smart investment (Silbiger, 2005). When purchasing a home, obtain as much information as possible. Research properties in the area you want to buy. Investigate the school system, tax base, typical list price, and average time of homes on the market. Drive by and examine the neighborhood. Is this where you would want to live? Next, plan how to finance the property. Work with a real estate agent.

How to Educate Yourself

There are many ways to learn more about investments. Brokerage firms offer classes periodically. Try taking a course on personal finance at a local college. You can also go to the Internet (see "Exploring the Web" at the end of this chapter).

Another option is to hire a financial planner, but that can become expensive. Check their fees first and educate yourself by reading financial books.

Suze Orman (2008) is an author who many find easy to understand and very relevant. Subscriptions to *Money, Barron's,* and *Kiplinger Magazine* can also be educational. Complete your net worth yearly. This can be done by making a list of all your financial assets and deficits. See Table 18-4. Your goal is to see an increase in your assets when you complete this document each year.

Emotional Health

Emotional health is the third element of health. Our emotions express how we are feeling about an event. Emotions can be intense and evoke a strong response. Our challenge as human beings is to acknowledge the emotion and then respond appropriately. Truly, emotions are one of our greatest gifts and add spice to our lives (Dossey, Keegan, & Guzzetta, 2005). Note the discussion of Emotional Intelligence in Chapter One.

Anger

Anger is a universal, strong feeling of displeasure that is often precipitated by a situation that frustrates or prevents a person from attaining

TABLE 18-4	NET WORTH—YEAR 1 AND 2		
Year-I **Assets**		**Deficits**	
Car	$5,000	School Loan	$2,000
Assets − Deficits = Net Worth		Car Loan	$2,000
$5,000 − $4,000 = $1,000 Net Worth − Year 1			$4,000
Year-II **Assets**		**Deficits**	
Home	$75,000	Home Mortgage	$59,000
Car	$ 5,000	School Loan	$ 1,500
Savings	$ 500	Credit Cards	$ 200
	$80,500	Car Loan	$ 1,500
			$62,200
$80,500 − $62,200 = $18,300 Net Worth − Year 2			

a goal or getting what is wanted from life. Anger is influenced by one's beliefs. Ellis (1997) describes anger as an irrational response that arises from one of four irrational ideas: (1) that the treatment one received was awful (awfulizing), (2) feeling that one can't stand having been treated so irresponsibly and unfairly (can't stand-it-itis), (3) believing that one should not, must not behave as he did (shoulding and musting), and (4) believing that because one acted in a terrible manner, he is a terrible person (undeservingness and damnation). Ellis maintains that beliefs remain rational as long as the evaluation of the action does not involve an evaluation of the person. Rational and appropriate responses are feelings of disappointment. Anger, on the other hand, can be unmanageable and self-defeating. Ellis believes that we all have the ability to choose our response to anger.

WAYS TO COPE WITH ANGER.   Thomas (2003) recommends numerous ways nurses can learn to cope with anger at work. Make a commitment to be supportive and honest with co-workers. Reach out to colleagues, and don't be afraid to disclose your honest opinion and utilize self-disclosure. Don't get caught up in workplace gossip. Discuss difficult situations with a confidant. Obtain skills in conflict resolution by taking classes in assertiveness training, bargaining, and negotiating. You may need to seek counseling if your anger is intense or sustained.

Sometimes anger and frustration are caused by sensory overload or overcommitment. It is important to have time for yourself. If nurses are to be effective caretakers, they first must care for themselves. Saying no, be it to a supervisor, friend, or family member, may at times be necessary. Learn to say no.

HUMOR AND STRESS MANAGEMENT

Laughter is the best medicine. Laughter has many benefits such as helping to boost the immune system, promoting relaxation, and decreasing blood pressure, heart rate, and respiratory rate

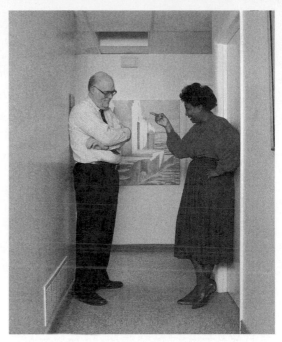

Figure 18-3 Laughter is an effective stress reliever. (Delmar/ Cengage Learning).

(Holistic Online, 2006). But best of all, laughter is contagious and it is free. Laughter is a critical stress management technique (Figure 18-3) (Table 18-5). Visit "Ivy Push," the acting name of Hob Osterlund MS, RN, CHTP, who has created DVDs of comical nursing situations. You can obtain more information about her shows at www.ivypush.com.

AVOIDING THOUGHT DISTORTIONS

Research on thinking processes has shown that people sometimes make mistakes in the way they perceive information and think about the world around them. When people are depressed, their automatic thoughts are loaded with distorted thinking. If one can recognize this distorted thinking (Table 18-6), one can begin to turn his or her life in a more positive direction.

TABLE 18-5	STRESS MANAGEMENT TECHNIQUES	
Meditate.	Do relaxation exercises.	Be polite to all.
Think peaceful thoughts.	Do something different for lunch.	Take a walk.
See things as others might.	Give yourself a pat on the back.	Read.
Forgive your mistakes.	Join a support group.	Join a club.
Do not procrastinate.	Talk about your worries.	Sing a song.
Set realistic goals.	Be affectionate.	Forgive and forget.
Do a good deed.	View problems as a challenge.	Listen to music.
Vary your routine.	Get/give a massage.	Take a hot bath.
Appreciate what you have.	Say a prayer.	Call an old friend.
Focus on the positive.	Expect to be successful.	Let go of the need to be perfect.

PROFESSIONAL HEALTH

Professional health is the fourth element of health. A person is professionally healthy when he is satisfied with his career choice and thinks that there is continual opportunity for growth. The professionally healthy individual is goal directed and seeks every opportunity to obtain knowledge and new learning experiences. This may include going back to school for more education, becoming certified in his or her clinical practice area, and avoiding occupational hazards.

OCCUPATIONAL HAZARDS COMMON AMONG NURSES

An important aspect of professional health is avoidance of occupational hazards. The U.S. Bureau of Labor Statistics (2006) reports that health care and social assistance workers rank second highest in percentage of nonfatal workplace injuries reported in 2004, the latest year for which statistics are available. (www.bls.gov/iif/oshsum. htm#04Summary%20Tables).

The survey reports the number of new work-related illness cases that are recognized, diagnosed, and reported during the year. Some conditions, for example, long-term latent illnesses caused by exposure to carcinogens, often are difficult to relate to the workplace and are not adequately recognized and reported. The overwhelming majority of the reported new illnesses are easier to directly relate to workplace activity, for example, contact dermatitis, carpal tunnel syndrome, or back injuries.

The cumulative weight lifted by a nurse providing direct patient care in a typical 8-hour workday is estimated to be 1.8 tons. Unfortunately, nurses accept back pain as part of their job, with 52% to 63% of nurses reporting musculoskeletal pain that lasts for more than 14 days; in 67% of cases, pain was a problem for at least 6 months (Nelson et al., 2007).

The newest approach to this serious occupational problem has been the use of safe patient handling policies—at the facility level, state level, or national level. More information about developing a safe patient handling policy can be found at: Patient Care Ergonomics Resource Guide: Safe Patient Handling and Movement, VA Hospital, Tampa, FL, and Department of Defense, 2001. Revised August 31, 2005. Available at: www.visn8.med.va.gov/patientsafetycenter/. The Occupational Safety & Health Administration also

TABLE 18-6	THOUGHT DISTORTIONS

Thought distortion	Example
All-or-nothing thinking: seeing things only in absolutes	If I leave this job, no one will respect me.
Overgeneralization: interpreting every small setback as a never-ending pattern of defeat	Everyone here is so smart; I'm a real loser.
Dwelling on negatives: ignoring multiple positive experiences	I made a mistake. I'm not good enough to be a nurse.
Jumping to conclusions: assuming that others are reacting negatively without definite evidence	I don't know why I study. Everyone thinks I'm going to fail the NCLEX anyway.
Pessimism: automatically predicting that things will turn out badly	It's only a matter of time before everything falls apart for me.
Reasoning from feeling: thinking that if one feels bad, one must be bad	My head hurts because I'm a bad person.
Obligations: living life around a succession of too many "shoulds," "shouldn'ts," "musts," "oughts," and "have-tos."	I should marry Joe. Everyone likes him.

Source: Compiled from Frisch, N., & Frisch, L. (2002). *Psychiatric Mental Health Nursing* (3rd ed). Clifton Park: Delmar Cengage Learning.

has Guidelines for Nursing Homes: Ergonomics for the Prevention of Musculoskeletal Disorders, OSHA 3182, 2003. Available at: www.osha.gov/ergonomics.

There are numerous suggestions for safeguarding against various hazards in the workplace. Occupational hazards can be divided into four major categories: (1) infectious agents, (2) environmental agents, (3) physical agents, and (4) chemical agents. See "Exploring the Web" at the end of this chapter and Table 18-7.

INFECTIOUS AGENTS Infectious agents can be transferred through direct contact with an infected patient or through exposure to infected body fluids. The major infectious agents for health care workers are HIV, herpes, tuberculosis, and hepatitis. A recent survey of fifty-eight hospitals found that 44% of the needle stick injuries were sustained by nurses compared to 15% by medical practitioners (IHCWSC, 2006). Nurses have the largest amount of direct patient contact and are at the greatest risk for exposure to blood-borne pathogens. The chance of a seroconversion, which occurs when a serological test for antibodies changes from a negative reading to a positive reading, varies according to the disease exposure. The estimated risk for infection for HIV after needle exposure is from 0.29% to 0.56%. The risk for hepatitis B ranges between 6% and 30% for nonimmunized personnel, whereas hepatitis C carries an estimated risk of 6% (Lee, Botteman, Xanthakos, & Nicklasson, 2005).

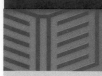

EVIDENCE FROM THE LITERATURE

Citation: Waters, T. R. (2007, Aug.). When Is It Safe to Manually Lift a Patient? *American Journal of Nursing, 107*(8), 53–59.

Discussion: According to the U.S. Bureau of Labor Statistics, in 2005, nursing ranked eighth among occupations reporting work-related musculoskeletal disorders involving days away from work, with more than 9,000 cases of such disorders and a median of seven missed days of work per injury. Nurses' aides, orderlies, and attendants ranked second, behind laborers and freight, stock, and material movers.

Musculoskeletal disorders are often caused by the cumulative effect of repeated patient-handling tasks and high-risk tasks such as lifting, transferring, and repositioning patients. Extensive laboratory-based research has documented high levels of biomechanical stress on caregivers' spines, shoulders, hands, and wrists from patient lifting and repositioning.

Many of these injuries are preventable. A strong body of research has demonstrated that mechanical lifting equipment, as part of a program promoting safe patient handling and movement, can significantly reduce musculoskeletal injuries among health care workers.

Note that for most patient-lifting tasks, the maximum recommended weight limit is 35 pounds—but even less when the task is performed under less than ideal circumstances, such as lifting with extended arms, lifting when near the floor, lifting when sitting or kneeling, lifting with the trunk twisted or the load off to the side of the body, lifting with one hand or in a restricted space, or lifting during a shift lasting longer than eight hours.

In 2003, the American Nurses Association launched its Handle with Care campaign, "a profession-wide effort to prevent back and other musculoskeletal injuries." See www.nursingworld.org/handlewithcare. The ANA also released a position statement, Elimination of Manual Patient Handling to Prevent Work-Related Musculoskeletal Disorders. See www.nursingworld.org. Search for "manual patient handling."

Implications for Nursing: Nurses should work to avoid back injuries by following these guidelines. Check the Web sites for patient-handling information.

TABLE 18-7	SAFEGUARDS FOR OCCUPATIONAL HAZARDS

Infectious Agents

- Do not recap needles.
- Use needle-free intravascular access devices.
- Place needle disposal containers near point of use of needles.
- Use personal protective equipment.
- Report all needle-stick injuries immediately.
- Wash hands before and after each patient contact.

(continues)

TABLE 18-7	SAFEGUARDS FOR OCCUPATIONAL HAZARDS (CONTINUED)

Physical Agents

- Follow standards of care for dealing with radiation/laser equipment.
- Assess work area for amount of noise.
- Eliminate excessive noise in the workplace.
- Implement good body mechanics. Get equipment and help to lift heavy patients.
- Follow ergonomic safety guidelines from OSHA (Department of Government Affairs, 2006b).

Environmental Agents

- Develop a zero tolerance, no abuse policy to protect nurses and all staff.
- Develop a violence reduction plan to protect staff.
- Rotate shifts clockwise—day to evening to night (Rogers, 1997).
- Assess for dangerous chemicals, mold, and fungus in your workplace.
- Review Occupational Safety and Health Administration (OSHA) standards at your facility for environmental agents.
- Develop an agency/facility plan to work with victims of terrorism.
- Maintain air quality, avoid fumes from glutaraldehyde, ethylene oxide, and laser plume smoke.

Chemical Agents

- Utilize effective ventilation systems.
- Develop standards of care for handling gaseous waste, chemotherapy, disinfectants, and anesthetics.
- Protect pregnant nurses from handling chemotherapy during the first trimester.
- Use appropriate nonlatex barrier protections.
- Develop policies and procedures to ensure safety from latex allergies.

Although the majority of infectious agents are transmitted through blood, the herpes simplex virus can be transmitted by direct contact with an infected lesion. Hepatitis A is transmitted primarily via diarrhea as a result of poor hygienic practices among health care workers. The overall incidence of tuberculosis (TB) is gradually increasing, and there are certain regional differences. For example, in 2004, the rate of cases per 100,000 population differed by states: 1.0 in Wyoming, 7.1 in New York, 8.3 in California, and 14.6 in the District of Columbia. The overall rate for TB in the United States in 2004 was 4.9 per 100,000 people, and in 2000, the rate was only 3.5 per 100,000 people (CDC, 2006).

ENVIRONMENTAL AGENTS Another group of occupational hazards is environmental agents. These include all the agents within the hospital that may lead to injury. The most prevalent include violence, shift work, air quality, mold and fungus, and bioterrorism. Nurses are at risk for workplace violence. Employment in a health care facility is considered one of the most dangerous jobs in the United States. In a recent study, nearly half a million nurses per year reported being victims of some type of violence in the workplace (Department of Government Affairs, 2006a).

Poor air quality in the workplace is yet another environmental risk that may lead to symptoms such as shortness of breath, eye and nose irritation, headaches, contact dermatitis, joint pain, memory problems, and reproductive difficulties. Glutaraldehyde, a chemical used to disinfect many commonly used instruments, can emit a hazardous gas. Ethylene oxide, a chemical commonly used to sterilize surgical equipment, has been reported to have carcinogenic effects. Lasers used in operating rooms can emit hazardous gaseous material in the form of either laser plume or chemical byproducts of laser smoke. Laser treatment carries the risk of eye and skin injury if the instruments are not handled properly. It is essential that nurses be protected from the byproducts of lasers by high-efficiency smoke evacuators. (Andersen, 2004). Air quality can also be influenced by mold and fungus, which are often found in carpeting and in ceiling tiles. The presence of mold and fungus can lead to asthma and other respiratory problems. Most hospitals have some type of bioterrorist alert plan. Nurses play an active role in dealing with any type of bioterrorist disaster.

PHYSICAL AGENTS   Physical agents are another occupational hazard and include radiation, noise, and lifting patients. Radiation exposure is common among health care workers. Radiation is used for both diagnostic and treatment interventions. Persons exposed to excessive amounts of radiation are at risk for cancer. Nurses can protect themselves from the effects of radiation by following agency guidelines and wearing a dosimeter that measures the amount of radiation exposure. Pregnant nurses working with radiation should declare their pregnancy to their employer as soon as possible (Duke University, 2006). Noise is another physical hazard that can lead to hearing loss. Excessive noise that occurs over a long period of time can also lead to irritability and inability to concentrate. High levels of noise are deleterious for both nurses and patients. Special care units are especially noisy with alarms, ventilators, suction equipment, monitors, call lights, and so on.

CHEMICAL AGENTS   Another occupational hazard is chemical agents such as anesthetic agents, antineoplastic drugs, disinfectants, latex gloves, hazardous drugs, and drug and alcohol abuse. Questions still remain as to the negative effects of anesthesia on health care workers. Nurses working in the operating room should continue to protect themselves by ensuring proper ventilation and appropriate disposition of waste products (Allen, 2004).

Latex glove exposure is another type of chemical concern for nurses. It has been reported that approximately 8% to 13% of health care workers

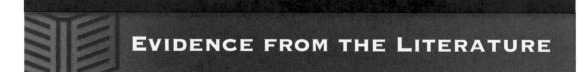

EVIDENCE FROM THE LITERATURE

Citation: Nelson, A., Fragala, G., & Menzel, N. (2003, Feb.). Myths and facts about back injuries in nursing. *American Journal of Nursing, 103*(2), 32–36.

Discussion: Manual lifting and other patient-handling tasks are high-risk activities for both nurses and patients. The prevalence of work-related back injuries in nursing is among the highest of any profession internationally. Annual prevalence rates of nursing-related back pain range from 33.9% in New Zealand to 47% in the United States to 66.8% in the Netherlands. The year 2000 incidence rate for back injuries involving days away from work was 181.6 per 10,000

(continues)

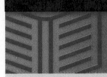

EVIDENCE FROM THE LITERATURE
(CONTINUED)

full-time workers in nursing homes and 90.1 for hospitals, compared with incidence rates of 98.4 for truck drivers, 70 for construction workers, 56.3 for miners, 47.1 for agricultural workers, and 43.2 for workers in manufacturing. The rising rate of obesity also increases the risk of injury to nurses and other health care workers who handle patients. Patients studied in a Veterans Administration hospital who required lifting ranged from 91 lbs. to 387 lbs. and averaged 169 lbs. The need to protect nurses from injury must direct efforts to the following in the future:

- Ergonomic assessment of patient care environments
- Engineering controls, such as new ceiling-mounted mechanical lifting devices designed to reduce manual patient handling
- Standardized protocol for assessing the handling and moving of patients
- Algorithms for deciding about the number of personnel and type of equipment needed to handle and move patients safely
- A new education model that includes hospital-unit peer leaders who would ensure that workers use equipment competently and who could help change nursing practice

Several misconceptions about how best to prevent musculoskeletal injuries when handling and moving patients are discussed in this article, which is the first of a two-part series.

Several emerging technologies and strategies that can improve nursing safety for both patients and nurses, based on engineering and administrative controls, are also discussed.

Implications for Practice: Attention to the facts should help nurses prevent back injuries. These back injuries have the potential to disrupt or end a nurse's career.

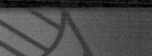

CASE STUDY 18-1

Y ou are a nurse admitting Mrs. Zakima, an 84-year-old female. You received the following report from the emergency room. Her vital signs are BP 140/70, RR 30, HR 80. The patient has bilateral rales, 2+ pitting pedal edema, weighs 350 pounds, and is 5′ 5″ tall. Mrs. Zakima is a transfer from a nursing home. She is being admitted for symptoms related to congestive heart failure. She has a past history of hypertension, diabetes, rheumatoid arthritis, dementia, and MRSA. Mrs. Zakima is being admitted to your unit. In preparing the room that she will be admitted to, what do you need to keep in mind with regards to noise, safety, and universal precautions?

What safety precautions would you put in place to protect yourself, that is, ergonomics, universal precautions, and so forth?

After reviewing her chart, you find she is taking the following medications: methotrexate, zestril, toprol, and lasix. What other precautions should you take with this patient?

are allergic to latex (AANA, 2006). Reactions to latex range from simple contact dermatitis to a more systemic reaction to an anaphylactic crisis. Yet another concern for nurses is the potential for personal misuse of drugs and/or alcohol. The ANA estimates 6% to 8% of nurses may have a substance-abuse problem. This is similar to the national average for drug abuse. Nurses should be aware of the potential for addiction and abuse.

SOCIAL HEALTH

Social health is another significant element of health. The essence of social health is interacting with other people. Having the ability to relate to others is essential for life. Few can survive completely alone. It is human nature to seek out others and grow in relationships (Dossey et al., 2005).

IMPACT OF SOCIAL RELATIONSHIPS

The positive effects of social support on health outcomes have been documented in the literature (Breedlove, 2005). If these interactions are frequent, that only adds to good health. In other words, the more you see your friends, the healthier you become. The variety of those relationships may also keep you healthy. The greater the diversity of the relationships, such as professional, family, neighborhood, or church relationships, the more likely you are to remain healthy.

SPIRITUAL HEALTH

Spiritual health is the last area of health. Spirituality is an elusive term that is difficult to define. It can be viewed as the essence of being, that which gives meaning and direction in life, and the principles of good living. It may also be your relationship with a higher being, other individuals, or your environment (Dossey et al., 2005). Koenig (1999) has extensively researched religion and health. His findings lend some scientific support to the positive effects of prayer and religious involvement.

Little has been said about the spiritual needs of nurses (McEwan, 2004). Nurses function in a fast-paced and stressful environment, which often leads to job dissatisfaction, burnout, and potentially suboptimal patient care. Some hospitals are addressing the spiritual well-being of nurses as a way to cope with these current demands by offering the RISEN (Re-Investing Spirituality and Ethics in our Network) program. The RISEN program helps nurses become more conscious and committed to their own spiritual growth in order to facilitate the healing process in others (Ollier, 2004).

KEY CONCEPTS

- Clinical ladders can guide nursing development.

- There are numerous types of advance practice nurses (APNs) within both the hospital and community settings. Some examples of these roles include the CNS, NP, and CRNA.

- To provide quality patient care, nurses need to first take care of themselves and maintain a healthy lifestyle.

- Health is not just the absence of disease; it is the state of complete balance of six elements of health, i.e., physical, intellectual, emotional, professional, social, and spiritual health.

- Nurses' physical health encompasses good nutrition, proper exercise, and adequate sleep.

- An important piece of intellectual health is adequate financial planning. Now is the time to begin saving.

- To stay healthy, you must make a conscious decision to maintain each of the six elements of health.

- Establishing short-term, intermediate, and long-term goals will shape your career.

KEY TERMS

anger

certification

clinical ladders

competency

401K

emotional health

health

intellectual health

money market account

physical health

professional health

Roth IRA

social health

spiritual health

REVIEW QUESTIONS

1. You have $1,000 that you would like to deposit into an account. Which of the following would offer the highest interest rate with the greatest flexibility in accessing the money?
   A. money market account
   B. passbook savings account
   C. traditional bank checking account
   D. traditional IRA

2. The optimal method to decrease fatigue when rotating shifts is to
   A. rotate clockwise.
   B. rotate counterclockwise.
   C. rotate nights to days only.
   D. rotate evenings to days only.

3. The process of certification allows the registered nurse to
   A. demonstrate clinical expertise.
   B. demonstrate educational expertise.
   C. demonstrate clinical and/or educational expertise.
   D. demonstrate advanced nursing degrees.

REVIEW ACTIVITIES

1. Your best friend is getting married next month, and you are the maid of honor. You have already purchased a nonrefundable airline ticket to attend the bridal shower. You work in a very small intensive care unit. You have been working 10- and 12-hour shifts and are near exhaustion. Your head nurse calls you two days before you are to leave for the shower and asks you to work the weekend. One of the staff has been involved in a serious car accident, and there is no one else to work. What would you do?

2. You were recently hired on a nursing unit. What equipment and supplies do you need to protect yourself from occupational hazards?

3. Finally, you have graduated and moved to the city of your choice and are working at the health care facility of your choice. You are starting to apply all the knowledge and skills that you gained at school. You are around all types of nursing mentors and role models and are witnessing firsthand the activities of new and experienced staff nurses, as well as those of advance practice nurses. Develop some SMART goals regarding where you will be 1, 3, 5, or 10 years from now.

EXPLORING THE WEB

- Calculate your BMI and determine your life expectancy and health risks at:
  www.healthstatus.com

- Try one of the following sites to retrieve information on dietary supplements, nutrition, and alternative medicine:
  www.mypyramid.gov
  www.nutritionsite.com

- Retirement Information Sites:

  Charles Schwab:
  www.schwab.com
  Click on *Retirement Planning*

  Social Security:
  www.ssa.gov

  Fidelity Investments:
  www.fidelity.com
  Click on *Retirement Center*; then follow the different retirement options.

  Vanguard:
  www.vanguard.com
  Click on *Personal Investors*; then click on the *Planning & Advice* tab.

  Valueline:
  www.valueline.com
  Click on *What's New? Retirement Planners.*

  Morningstar:
  www.morningstar.com
  Click on *Retirement.*

- Resources for Violence Prevention:

  The ANA's Workplace Violence: Can You Close the Door? Call (800) 274–4ANA:
  www.nursingworld.org

  Guidelines for Preventing Workplace Violence for Healthcare and Social Service Workers. U.S. Department of Labor, OSHA 3148–1996, available online:
  www.osha-slc.gov

- Resources for Needle-Sticks:

  Safer Needle Devices: Protecting Health Care Workers:
  www.osha-slc.gov

- American Nurses Association:
  www.nursingworld.org

  Centers for Disease Control and Prevention:
  www.cdc.gov

- Resources for Latex Allergy:

  ANA's position paper on Latex Allergy:
  www.nursingworld.org
  or call (800) 274–4ANA

  OSHA:
  www.osha-slc.gov

- Resource for Back Strain:

  Occupational Safety and Health Administration's ergonomics information:
  www.osha-slc.gov
  or call (202) 693–1999

- General Interest and Nursing Issues:

  Centers for Disease Control:
  www.cdc.gov

  National Institutes of Health:
  www.nih.gov

  National League for Nursing:
  www.nln.org

  ANA certification listing:
  www.nursingworld.org

  Center for Nursing:
  www.nursingcenter.com

  National Council of State Boards of Nursing:
  www.ncsbn.org

  General nursing interest site:
  www.allnurses.com

  Health care information:
  www.medscape.com
  www.docguide.com

- Specialty Issues:

  American Association of Nurse Anesthetists:
  www.aana.com

  Flight nursing:
  www.flightweb.com

Small Business Administration:
www.sbaonline.sba.gov

Service Corps of Retired Executives:
www.score.org

Traveling nurses:
www.springnet.com
www.healthcareers-online.com

REFERENCES

Allen, G. (2004). Evidence for practice: Surgical team members' exposure to inhalational anesthetics. *Association of Operating Room Nurses Journal, 79*(1), 235.

American Association of Nurse Anesthetists. (AANA). (2006). *AANA latex glove protocol.* Retrieved January 30, 2006, from www.aana.com/crna/prof/latex.asp.

American Nurses Association. (ANA). (2000). Press release. Retrieved February 25, 2000, from www.ana.org

American Nurses Credentialing Center Certification. (2009). Available at www.nursecredentialing.org/certification.aspx.

Andersen, K. (2004). Safe use of lasers in the operating room: What perioperative nurses should know. *AORN Journal, 79*(1), 171.

Battaglia, C. (1996) Murmurs. Long Branch, NJ: Vista Publishing.

Benner, P. (1984). *From novice to expert.* Menlo Park, CA: Addison-Wesley.

Breedlove, G. (2005). Perceptions of social support from pregnant and parenting teens using community-based doulas. *Journal of Perinatal Education, 14*(3),15–22.

Centers for Disease Control and Prevention. (CDC). (2006). *Guidelines for preventing the transmission of Mycobacterium tuberculosis in health-care settings.* Retrieved January 20, 2006, from www.cdc.gov.

Dawson, D., & Reid, K. (1997). Fatigue, alcohol and performance impairment. *Nature, 338*(6639), 235.

Department of Government Affairs. (2006a). *Health care worker safety.* Retrieved January 30, 2006, from www.anapoliticalpower.org

Department of Government Affairs. (2006b). *Safe patient handling and the OSHA ergonomics standard.* Retrieved January 30, 2006, from www.anapolitical-power.org

Dossey, B. M., Keegan, L., & Guzzetta, C. E. (2005). Holistic nursing: A handbook for practice. Sudbury, MA: Jones and Bartlett Publishers.

Duke University Medical Center. (2006). *Radiation safety considerations for nurses at Duke.* Retrieved January 30, 2006, from www.safety.duke.edu/RadSafety/nurses/default.asp.

Ellis, A. (1997). *Anger: How to live with it and without it.* New York: Citadel Press, Kensington.

Erickson, J., Holm, L., Chelminiak, L., & Ditomassi, M. (2005). Why not nursing. *Nursing 2005, 35*(7), 46–49.

Frank, M. B. (2005). Practicing under the influence of fatigue (PUIF): A wake-up call for patients and providers. *The National Association of Neonatal Nurses, 5*(2), 55–61.

Frisch, N. C., & Frisch, L. E. (2006). *Psychiatric Mental Health Nursing* (3rd ed.). Clifton Park, NY: Delmar Cengage Learning.

Guidelines for Nursing Homes: Ergonomics for the Prevention of Musculoskeletal Disorders. (2003). OSHA. Available at: www.osha.gov/ergonomics.

Healthy People 2010 document, available at www.healthypeople.gov/LHI/lhiwhat.htm.

Holistic Online. (2006). *Therapeutic benefits of laughter.* Retrieved January 28, 2006, from www.holistic-online.com/Humor_Therapy/humor_therapy_benefits.htm.

Hughes, R. G., & Rogers, A. E. (2004). First do no harm: Are you tired. *American Journal of Nursing, 104*(3), 36–38.

Institute of Medicine. (IOM). (2004). Keeping patients safe: Transforming the work environment of nurses. Washington, DC: National Academies Press.

International Health Care Worker Safety Center. (IHCWSC). (2006). Uniform needlestick and sharp injury report 58 hospitals, 2001. University of Virginia. Retrieved January 28, 2006, from www.healthsystem.virginia.edu/internet/epinet/soi01.cfm.

Johns, M. W. (1991). A new method for measuring daytime sleepiness: the Epworth Sleepiness Scale. *Sleep. 14*(6), 540–545.

Koenig, H. G. (1999).The healing power of faith. *Annals of Long-Term Care, 7*(10), 381–384.

Lee, J. M., Botteman, M. F., Xanthakos, N., & Nicklasson, L. (2005). Needlestick injuries in the United States: Epidemiologic, economic and quality of life issues. *American Association of Occupational Health Nurses Journal, 53*(3), 117–134.

McEwan, W. (2004). Spirituality in nursing? What are the issues? *Orthopaedic Nursing, 23*(5), 321–326.

Mee, C. (2005). Nursing 2005 salary survey. *Nursing 2005, 35*(10), 321–326.

Merriam-Webster. (2005). Merriam-Webster's online dictionary. Retrieved March 26, 2006, from www.m-w.com.

Nelson, A., Fragala, G., & Menzel, N. (2003, Feb.). Myths and facts about back injuries in nursing. *American Journal of Nursing, 103*(2), 32–36.

Nelson, A. L., Collins, J., Knibbe, H., Cookson, K., de Castro, A. B., Whipple, K. L. (2007, Mar.). Safer patient handling. *Nursing Management,* 26–31.

Nightingale, F. (1969). Notes on Nursing. New York: Dover. (Original work published 1860.)

Ollier, C. (2004). Body and spirit: Nurturing strategies help nurses cope with on the job stress. *COR Health, LLC, 4*(12), 5–8.

Orman, S. (2008). *The Road to Wealth.* New York: Penguin Group.

Patient Care Ergonomics Resource Guide: Safe Patient Handling and Movement, VA Hospital, Tampa, FL, and Department of Defense, 2001. Revised August 31, 2005. Available at: www.visn8.med.va.gov/patientsafetycenter/.

Rogers, B. (1997). Health hazards in nursing and health care: An overview. *American Journal of Infection Control, 25*(3), 248–261.

Silbiger, S. (2005). *The 10-day MBA.* New York: Harper Collins.

Stromberg, M. F., Niebuhn, B., Prevost, S., Fabrey, L., Muenzen, P., Spence, C., et al. (2005, May). More than a title. *Nursing Management, 36*(5), 36–46.

Thomas, S. P. (2003). Anger: The mismanaged emotion. *Medsurg Nursing, 12*(2), 351–357.

U.S. Department of Health and Human Services. (2001). *Healthy People 2010: Goals.* Retrieved January 2, 2002, from www.healthypeople.gov.

U.S. Bureau of Labor Statistics. (2006). *Injuries and illnesses.* Retrieved January 12, 2006, from www.bls.gov/iif/oshsum.htm#04Summary%News%20Release.

Waters, T. R. (2007, Aug.). When Is It Safe to Manually Lift a Patient? *American Journal of Nursing, 107*(8), 53–59.

World Health Organization. (WHO). (2006). *Benefits of physical activity.* Retrieved December 30, 2005, from www.who.int/ moveforhealth/advocacy/information_sheets/benefits.en.index.html.

SUGGESTED READINGS

American Journal of Nursing. (2006, Jan. supp.). Your guide to certification. 106, 50–63.

Blocks, M. (2005). Practical solutions for safe handling. *Nursing 2005, 35*(10), 44–45.

Hader, R. (2005). Salary survey 2005. *Nursing Management, 36*(7), 18–27.

Hunt, L. (2005). Sit-down comedy. Meet Ivy Push, nursing's funny girl. *American Journal of Nursing, 105*(7), 110–111.

Institute of Medicine. (IOM). (2006). *Keeping patients safe: Transforming the work environment of nurses.* Retrieved August 21, 2006, from www.iom.edu/Default.aspx?id=16173.

National Institutes of Health. (NIH). *Body mass index calculator.* Retrieved February 2, 2002, from www.nhlbi.nih.gov/guidelines/obesity/bmi_tbl.htm.

Nelson, R. (2005). AJN reports: Is there a doctor in the house? A new vision for advanced practice nursing. *American Journal of Nursing, 105*(5), 28–29.

Steefel, L. (2005). New doctoral degree aims to advance nursing practice. *Nursing Spectrum: New York & New Jersey edition, 17*(5), 14–15.

Tracey, C., & Nicholl, H. (2006). Mentoring and networking. *Nursing Management—UK, 12*(10), 28–32.

Wesorick, B. (2006). *Clinical practice model resource center.* Retrieved August 22, 2006, from www.cpmrc.com.

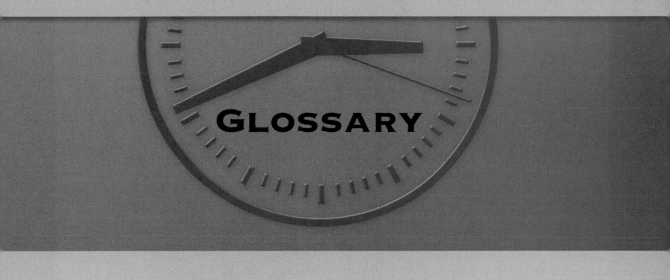

GLOSSARY

360-degree feedback Performance evaluation system in which an individual is assessed by a variety of people in order to provide a broader perspective about his or her performance.

401K Retirement savings account that both employee and for-profit employer contribute to.

403b Retirement savings account that both employee and not-for-profit employer contribute to.

accounting Activity that nurse managers engage in to record and report financial transactions and data.

activity log Time management technique to assist in determining how both personal and professional time is used by periodically recording activities.

administrative law Body of law created by administrative agencies in the form of rules, regulations, orders, and decisions that protect the rights of citizens.

assault Offer to touch or threat of touching another in an offensive manner without that person's permission.

autocratic leadership Centralized decision-making style in which the leader makes decisions and uses power to command and control others.

autonomy An individual's right to self-determination and individual liberty.

battery Touching of another person without that person's consent.

benchmarking Continuous process of measuring products, services, and practices against the toughest competitors or those customers recognized as industry leaders.

beneficence The duty to do good to others and to maintain a balance between benefits and harms.

budget A plan that provides formal quantitative expression for acquiring and distributing funds over the ensuing time period.

capital budget Accounts for the purchase of major new or replacement equipment.

capitation Health care payment of a fixed amount of money established to cover the cost of health care services delivered to a patient during a specified length of time, e.g., one year.

care delivery model Method to organize the work of caring for patients.

case management Strategy to improve patient care and reduce hospital costs through coordination of care.

certification   Process by which a non-governmental agency or association asserts that an individual licensed to practice a profession has met certain predetermined standards specified by that profession for practice.

certified registered nurse anesthetist   Advanced clinical nursing specialist who manages the patient's anesthesia needs before, during, and after surgery or other procedures.

change   Making something different from what it was.

change agent   One who is responsible for implementation of a change project.

civil law   That body of law that governs how individuals relate to each other in everyday matters.

clinical ladder   A promotional model that acknowledges that staff members have varying skill sets based on their education and experience. As such, depending on skills and experience, staff members may be rewarded differently and carry differing responsibilities for patient care and the governance and professional practice of the work unit.

clinical pathway   Care management tool that outlines the expected clinical course and outcomes for a specific patient type.

co-insurance   Form of cost-sharing in which the patient pays a percentage of the fee for approved health care services after the deductible amount has been paid.

co-payment   Fixed health care fee paid by the patient to the health care provider at the time of service; this amount is paid in addition to the money the health care provider will receive from the insurance company.

common law   Body of law that develops from precedents set by judicial decisions that, over time, have the force of law, as distinguished from legislative enactments.

competence   Ability of the nurse to act with and integrate the knowledge, skills, values, attitudes, abilities, and professional judgment that underpin effective, quality nursing, and are required to practice safely and ethically in a designated role and setting.

compromising   Finding a middle-ground solution where neither party meets all their goals.

conflict   Disagreement about something of importance to each person involved.

connection power   Strength that comes from the extent to which nurses are connected with others having power.

consensus   Situation in which all group members agree to live with and support a decision, regardless of whether they totally agree.

constitution   A set of basic laws that specifies the powers of the various segments of a government and how these segments relate to each other.

construction budget   Budget that is developed when renovation or new structures are planned.

contingency theory   Leadership theory that acknowledges that other factors in the environment influence outcomes as much as leadership style and that leader effectiveness is contingent upon or depends upon something in addition to the leader's behavior.

contract law   Rules that regulate certain transactions between individuals and/or legal entities such as businesses.

customers   Everyone internal or external to the organization who receives the product or service of the workers, e.g., patients, nurses, physicians, community, etc.

dashboard   Documentation tool providing a snapshot image of pertinent information and activity reflecting a point in time.

deductible   Predetermined out-of-pocket fee paid by a patient for health care services before reimbursement through health insurance begins to be paid.

defamation Intentionally false communication either published or publicly spoken.

delegation Transfer of responsibility for the performance of a task from one individual to another while retaining accountability for the outcome.

democratic leadership Style in which participation is encouraged and authority is delegated to others.

direct care Time spent providing hands-on care to patients.

disease management Systematic way to coordinate health care interventions for populations of people with conditions in which their self-care efforts are significant.

employee-centered leadership Style with a focus on the human needs of subordinates.

ethical dilemma A conflict between two or more ethical principles for which there is no obviously correct decision.

ethics The branch of philosophy that concerns the distinction between right from wrong on the basis of a body of knowledge, not just on the basis of opinions.

evidence-based care Clinically competent care based on the best scientific evidence available.

evidence-based practice Conscientious, explicit, and judicious use of current best evidence in making decisions about the care of individual patients.

expert power Power derived from the knowledge and skills nurses possess.

false imprisonment Imprisonment that occurs when people are incorrectly led to believe they cannot leave a place.

fee for service Payment of a fee for delivery of a health care service, e.g., payment of a fee to a nursing or medical practitioner for a Pap test.

fidelity The principle of promise keeping; the duty to keep one's promise or word.

formal leadership Leadership in which a person is in a position of authority or in a sanctioned role within an organization that connotes influence.

full-time equivalent Measure of the work-time commitment of a full-time employee.

functional nursing Care delivery model that divides nursing work into functional roles that are then assigned to individual team members.

goal Specific aim or target that a unit wishes to attain within the time span of one year.

good samaritan laws Laws that have been enacted to protect the health care professional from legal liability for actions rendered in an emergency when the professional is giving service without pay.

Gross Domestic Product (GDP) Economic measure of a country's national income and output within a year that reflects the market value of goods and services produced within the country.

group process Stages that a group progresses through as it matures, consisting of the following: forming, storming, norming, performing, and adjourning.

health disparities Persistent inequalities between the health outcomes of people in minority groups versus non-minority groups, due to such variables as gender, sexuality, age, ethnicity, socioeconomic group, lifestyle, and/or health care access.

Health Maintenance Organization (HMO) Prepaid managed care health plan providing comprehensive health care coverage for designated services through an approved group of health care providers.

indirect care Activities that support patient care but are not done directly to the patient.

informal leader Individual or member of a group who demonstrates leadership outside the scope of a formal leadership role rather than as the head or leader of the group.

information power Nurses who influence others with the knowledge they provide to the group are using information power.

innovation Process of creating new services or products.

inpatient unit Hospital unit that provides care to patients 24 hours a day, 7 days a week.

job-centered leadership Leadership style that focuses on work schedules, cost, and efficiency, with less attention given to developing work groups and high-performance goals.

justice The principle of fairness that is served when an individual is given that which he or she is due, owed, deserves, or can legitimately claim.

knowledge workers Workers who are involved in serving others through their special knowledge.

laissez-faire leadership Passive and permissive leadership style in which the leader defers decision making.

leadership Process of influence whereby the leader influences others toward goal achievement.

learning organizations Organizations that are based on five learning disciplines and that demonstrate responsiveness and flexibility.

legitimate power Power derived from the position a nurse holds in a group; it indicates the nurse's degree of authority.

living will Document voluntarily signed by patients that specifies the type of care they desire if and when they are in a terminal state and cannot sign a consent form or convey this information verbally.

malpractice Professional's wrongful conduct in discharge of professional duties or failure to meet standards of care for the profession, which results in harm to an individual entrusted to the professional's care.

managed care program Provides comprehensive health care to participating policyholders of a health care organization through the use of a network of providers and facilities.

management Process of planning, organizing, coordinating, and controlling resources and staff to achieve organizational goals.

margin Profit.

medicaid Joint federal and state program providing health insurance coverage for medically indigent and disabled persons who qualify on the basis of low income and resources.

medicare U.S. government federally funded single-payer program providing health insurance coverage for persons over age 65 and some disabled persons.

mission statement A formal expression of the purpose or reason for existence of an organization.

modular nursing Care delivery model that is a kind of team nursing that divides a geographical space into modules of patients with each module having a team of staff led by an RN to care for its patients.

money market account Similar to a bank checking account, though it often requires a larger minimum amount of money to open and often has a higher interest rate.

morality Behavior in accordance with custom or tradition; usually reflects personal or religious beliefs.

motivation Whatever influences our choices and creates direction, intensity, and persistence in our behavior.

negligence Failure to provide the care a reasonable person would ordinarily provide in a similar situation.

nonmaleficence The principle of doing no harm.

nonproductive hours Paid time not devoted to patient care; includes benefit time such as vacation, sick time, and education time.

operational budget Accounts for the income and expenses associated with day-to-day activity within a department or organization.

outcome elements of quality The end products of quality care. Outcomes review the status of patients that may result from health care; outcome elements ask the question, "How is the patient better as a result of health care?"

Pareto principle   Principle developed by Pareto, a 19th century economist, which states that 20% of focused effort results in 80% of results, or conversely, that 80% of unfocused effort results in 20% of results.

patient acuity   Measure of nursing workload that is generated for each patient based on his or her needs.

patient-centered care   Care delivery model in which care and services are brought to the patient.

patient classification system (PCS)   System for identifying different patients based on their acuity, functional ability, or resource needs.

patient-focused care   A model of differentiated nursing practice that emphasizes quality, cost, and value.

philosophy   Statement of beliefs based on core values; rational investigations of the truths and principles of knowledge, reality, and human conduct.

physical health   Encompasses nutrition and exercise coupled with a balanced amount of rest; health preventive behaviors such as avoiding smoking; and health screening behaviors that detect health problems early, such as an annual Pap smear.

Point of Service plan (POS)   Managed care option that offers enrollees the right to obtain health care services from an approved, participating, or network provider.

power   Ability to create, get, and use resources to achieve one's goals.

Preferred Provider Organization (PPO)   Health care delivery system that is similar to an HMO and provides services contracted with medical health care providers (e.g., hospitals and physicians) who have agreed to provide designated services as they are needed to a group of people at a discounted fee.

Primary Health Care (PHC)   "The first level of contact of individuals, the family, and community with the national health system, bringing health care as close as possible to where people live and work, and constituting the first element of a continuing health care process".

primary nursing   Care delivery model that clearly delineates the responsibility and accountability of the RN and reinforces the RN as the primary provider of nursing care to patients.

process elements of quality   Elements that identify what nursing and health care interventions must be in place to deliver quality care. Process elements include such things as managing the health care process, utilizing clinical practice guidelines and standards for nursing and medical interventions, passing medications, and so on.

productive hours   Hours worked and available for patient care.

profit   Determined by the relationship of income to expenses.

public law   General classification of law, consisting generally of constitutional, administrative, and criminal law. Public law defines a citizen's relationship with his or her government.

quality assurance   Quality inspection approach to ensure that minimum standards of care exist in health care institutions, primarily hospitals.

quality improvement   Management philosophy to improve the organizational structure and the level of performance of key processes in the organization to achieve high quality outcomes.

referent power   Power derived from how much others respect and like any individual, group, or organization.

relative value unit (RVU)   Index number assigned to various health care services based on the relative amount of resources (labor and capital) used to produce the service.

respect for others   Acknowledgment of the right of people to make their own decisions.

resume   Brief summary of a person's background, training, and experience, as well as his or her qualifications for a position.

reward power   Power to reward others.

Roth IRA   Individual retirement account that is much less restrictive than an IRA; first introduced in 1998.

sentinel event   Unexpected occurrence involving death or serious physical or psychological injury to a patient.

shared governance   Situation in which nurses and managers work together to define their roles and expected outcomes, holding everyone accountable for their role and expected outcomes.

skill mix   Percentage of RN staff to other direct care staff, LPNs, and NAP.

social health   Ability to relate to and interact with others.

sources of power   Combination of conscious and unconscious factors that allow an individual to influence others to do as the individual wants.

spiritual health   Human capacity to find strength from within; results from a connection with a higher being or power.

stakeholder   Provider, employer, customer, patient, or payer who may have an interest in, and seek to influence, the decisions and actions of an organization.

stakeholder assessment   A systematic consideration of all potential stakeholders to ensure that the needs of each of these stakeholders are incorporated in the planning.

structure elements of quality   Elements that identify what structures must be in place in a health care system/unit to deliver quality care. Structure elements consist of such things as a well constructed hospital, quality patient care standards, quality staffing policies, environmental standards, and the like.

supervision   Provision of guidance or direction, oversight, evaluation, and follow-up by the licensed nurse for the accomplishment of a delegated nursing task by assistive personnel.

SWOT analysis   A tool that is frequently used to conduct environmental assessments. SWOT stands for Strengths, Weaknesses, Opportunities, and Threats.

team   Small number of people with complementary skills who are committed to a common purpose, performance goals, and approach for which they hold themselves accountable.

team nursing   Care delivery model that assigns staff to teams that are then responsible for a group of patients.

time management   Set of related common-sense skills that helps a person use his or her time in the most effective and productive way possible.

tort   A civil wrong for which a remedy may be obtained.

total patient care   Care delivery model in which nurses are responsible for the total nursing care for their patient assignment for the shift they are working.

transformational leader   Leader who is committed to a vision that empowers others.

uncompensated care   Health care that goes unpaid and for which health care providers fail to be reimbursed for their services by either the patient or an insurance program.

Universal Health Care (UHC)   Government-sponsored system that ensures health care coverage for all eligible residents of a nation regardless of income level or employment status.

variance   Difference between what was budgeted and the actual cost.

veracity   The obligation to tell the truth.

workplace advocacy   Activities nurses undertake to address problems in their everyday workplace setting.

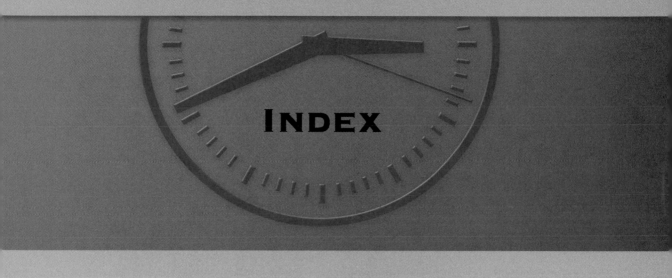

INDEX